Introduction to Veterinary Bacteriology

Charles M.
SCANLAN

D.V.M., Ph.D.

Introduction to Veterinary Bacteriology

Iowa State
University
Press / Ames

To Glenda and Matthew

Charles M. Scanlan, D.V.M., Ph.D., is associate professor, Department of Veterinary Microbiology and Parasitology, Texas Veterinary Medical Center, Texas A&M University, College Station, Texas.

© 1988 Iowa State University Press, Ames, Iowa 50010
All rights reserved

Composed by Iowa State University Press from author-provided disks

Printed in the United States of America

First edition, 1988

Library of Congress Cataloging-in-Publication Data

Scanlan, Charles M. (Charles Mack)
   Introduction to veterinary bacteriology.

   Bibliography: p.
   Includes indexes.
   1. Veterinary bacteriology. I. Title.
SF780.3.S32   1988   636.089′6014   88–618
ISBN 0–8138–0159–1

Contents

SECTION V.   BACTERIAL DISEASES OF DOMESTIC ANIMALS

Part 1.   Bovine Diseases

Part 2.   Ovine Diseases

Part 3.   Porcine Diseases

Part 4.   Equine Diseases

Part 5.   Canine Diseases

Part 6.   Feline Diseases

SECTION VI.   DETERMINATIVE BACTERIOLOGY

Part 1.   Aerobic Extracellular Bacteria

Part 2.   Anaerobic Extracellular Bacteria

Part 3.   Obligate Intracellular Bacteria

SECTION VII.   ZOONOTIC BACTERIAL DISEASES

Preface

This text on the principles of veterinary bacteriology and selected bacterial diseases of domestic animals is presented in outline format. It is primarily a treatise on the fundamentals of pathogenic bacteriology and the bacterial diseases of cattle, sheep, swine, horses, dogs, and cats. The scope and arrangement of subjects treated in this book are the direct outcome of my experiences in the instruction of students in veterinary medicine and in veterinary practice. The factual information, principles, and concepts presented in the text are designed to fulfill three clearly defined goals. First, it is intended for use by veterinary students experiencing their first exposure to veterinary pathogenic bacteriology. To that end, emphasis is placed on correlating and interfacing the fundamentals of bacteriology, immunology, and pathology with the clinical aspects of various bacterial agents, so that the student acquires not only the basic required information on bacterial pathogens of domestic animals but also an appreciation of the complexity of bacterial pathogenesis. Second, the text serves as a reference base for the infectious disease and medicine courses that have traditionally been presented during the clinical years of the professional curriculum. Third, the text provides a concise update and review of veterinary bacteriology for the veterinary practitioner, for whom it also has been written. The text is intended to supplement and complement the numerous veterinary books on various aspects of immunology, pathology, medicine, and therapy that are currently available to the profession.

I am grateful to Susan H. Poythress and Sophia T. Alexshonis for their assistance in preparation of the manuscript and to Annie S. Miley and the Biomedical Learning Resources Center for the illustrations.

Overview of Organization and Content

The text is made up of seven sections. The content, objectives, and format of each section are briefly described below so that readers can use the text efficiently.

SECTION I. GENERAL BACTERIOLOGY

The 2 chapters in this section emphasize the current classification schema and nomenclature of procaryotic organisms and their bacterial structural components and functions. In Chapter 2, the general characteristics of the 54 genera of extracellular and facultative intracellular bacteria and the 9 genera of obligate intracellular and cell-associated bacteria, which are described in Sections III and IV, respectively, are summarized.

SECTION II. BACTERIAL PATHOGENESIS

The 3 chapters in this section initiate the interfacing of the bacterial virulence factors, host immune mechanisms, and associated pathology to help explain the host bacterial interaction and therefore the pathogenicity of bacterial diseases.

SECTION III. EXTRACELLULAR AND FACULTATIVE INTRACELLULAR BACTERIA

Of the 57 chapters in this section, 54 describe genera that contain bacterial pathogens of domestic animals or man. One chapter describes the family Enterobacteriaceae, one summarizes the culture requirements of bacteria that are commonly isolated from domestic animals, and one summarizes the host range of selected bacteria.

Each genus description has the following format:

I. GENUS NAME

This section contains a list of pathogens and nonpathogens, under the headings Species, Hosts, Specific Diseases, and Nonspecific Diseases. The pathogenic species of domestic animals and man are listed in alphabetical order. The hosts, which include domestic animals and man, are listed by animal species in alphabetical order. The disease name is printed in capital letters if the disease is also discussed in a separate chapter in Section V. An opportunistic infection or infection in which the disease is poorly defined begins with a lowercase letter. Specific human disease agents are included in some genera, but they generally are not discussed in the disease overview.

Some nonpathogenic species are listed, particularly if they must be distinguished from similar pathogenic species.

Selected characteristics of the genus or selected species are sometimes described.

II. HABITAT AND ECOLOGY

The natural habitat and ecology of the genus or selected species are described.

III. CELLULAR, CULTURAL, AND BIOCHEMICAL CHARACTERISTICS

A. Cellular characteristics

The gram reaction, cellular morphology, and motility of the genus and selected species are described.

B. Cultural characteristics

The oxygen requirements of the genus and selected species are described as obligate aerobic, facultative anaerobic, or obligate anaerobic.

Bacteria that form colonies on blood agar and/or MacConkey agar when incubated aerobically at 37°C are classified as having nonfastidious growth requirements, whereas bacteria that do not form colonies on these media or under these incubation conditions are considered to have fastidious growth requirements. The culture and identification procedures for aerobic nonfastidious bacteria and the anaerobic bacteria are presented in Section VI. Culture procedures for the aerobic fastidious bacteria are briefly described under each appropriate genus.

C. Biochemical characteristics

The catalase and oxidase reactions are determined for the gram-positive and gram-negative bacteria, respectively. The metabolism of bacteria are classified as fermentative, respiratory, or both.

IV. DISEASE OVERVIEW

The diseases caused by each pathogenic species in domestic animals are outlined. The 55 chapters that include the 54 genera and the family Enterobacteriaceae are placed in 11 parts based on their similarities and common properties. This format allows the utilization of traditional systematic bacteriologic classification schema.

SECTION IV. OBLIGATE INTRACELLULAR
AND CELL-ASSOCIATED BACTERIA

The 10 chapters in this section are arranged in 4 parts with a format similar to that in Section III. The 9 genera are grouped within their respective families.

SECTION V. BACTERIAL DISEASES OF DOMESTIC ANIMALS

These 45 chapters are arranged in 6 parts: bovine, ovine, porcine, equine, canine, and feline bacterial diseases. Each chapter has a common format that includes etiology, transmission, clinical features, pathogenesis, pathology, diagnosis, and immunization (except 1 chapter on feline extracellular bacterial diseases, which is presented as an overview of these infections in cats). The topics were selected because of their unique mechanisms of pathogenesis, prevalence, or economic significance.

SECTION VI. DETERMINATIVE BACTERIOLOGY

These 6 chapters, which describe the diagnostic procedures for bacteria, are organized into 3 parts. The aerobic extracellular bacteria that will grow on blood agar and/or MacConkey agar when incubated aerobically at 37°C are discussed in Part 1, the anaerobic extracellular bacteria in Part 2, and the obligate intracellular bacteria in Part 3.

SECTION VII. ZOONOTIC BACTERIAL DISEASES

The important zoonotic bacterial diseases that are acquired by veterinarians are presented in the only chapter in this section.

SECTION I

General Bacteriology

1 | Classification and Nomenclature of Procaryotic Organisms

I. TAXONOMIC GROUPS
  A. Classification is the arrangement of bacteria into taxonomic groups on the basis of their similarities or relationships.
  B. Bacterial taxonomic ranks from kingdom to subspecies
    1. Kingdom
       a. All procaryotic organisms are placed in the kingdom Procaryotae. The procaryotes include the bacterial pathogens of domestic animals and man, while eucaryotes include yeasts, fungi, and protozoa, as well as higher plants, domestic animals, and man.
         (1) Bacteria possess a primitive genetic structure known as a procaryotic nucleus, which has no nuclear membrane, no nucleolus, and very little, if any, nucleoprotein.
         (2) Eucaryotic cells have a true nucleus, where the nuclear membrane surrounds the chromosomes.
    2. Divisions
       a. Bacterial pathogens of domestic animals and man are classified in three divisions based on cell wall type (Table 1.1).

Table 1.1. Divisions of procaryotes

Division	Type of Cell Wall
Firmicutes	Gram-positive
Gracilicutes	Gram-negative
Tenericutes	No rigid cell wall

    3. Classes
       a. Class designations are seldom used in the determinative bacteriology of veterinary bacterial pathogens.
    4. Orders
       a. Like classes, orders of bacteria are seldom used in systematic classification schema. Exceptions are the orders Chlamydiales and Rickettsiales, which contain the obligate intracellular pathogens.
    5. Families
       a. Some families represent groups of related genera such

as the family Enterobacteriaceae; other families are groups of genera that are based on practical convenience and have limited applicability in understanding their characteristics.

6. Genera
   a. The bacterial genus is usually a well-defined group that is clearly separated from other genera.
   b. The genus names of bacteria often indicate the morphology of the species (e.g., *Streptococcus*, chains of spherical cells; *Bacillus*, rod-shaped cells; and *Spirochaeta*, spiral-shaped cells), the organism's discoverer or scientist (e.g., *Coxiella*, Cox; *Escherichia*, Escherich; *Pasteurella*, Pasteur; and *Salmonella*, Salmon), as well as various other characteristics.

7. Species
   a. The species is the basic taxon of bacteria. It is used in all genera except for *Leptospira* and *Salmonella*, in which the serovar is the basic taxon.
   b. A species is a collection of strains that share many properties.

8. Subspecies
   a. Subspecies is the lowest taxonomic rank in nomenclature. A species may be divided into two or more subspecies. It is often used to facilitate the description of organisms within a species with notable differences in host range or other important characteristics (e.g., *Campylobacter fetus* ss *venerealis* and *C. fetus* ss *fetus*).

C. Taxonomic classification and terminology within the species
   1. Strains
      a. A strain is made up of descendants derived from an initial single colony isolated from an exogenous source, such as a pathologic lesion (e.g., *Fusobacterium necrophorum* strain 2101 isolated from a case of bovine foot rot).
      b. A type strain serves as the permanent example of the species.
      c. A reference strain is often used for comparative infectious disease studies (e.g., *Brucella abortus* strain 2308, which was isolated from a Wisconsin cow with brucellosis, is frequently used in bovine brucellosis experiments).
   2. Biovars
      a. Biovars have special biochemical or physiological properties (e.g., *F. necrophorum* biovars A, B, and C differ in their biological properties).

3. Serovars
    a. Serovars (serotypes) have distinctive antigenic properties.
    b. Bacterial serology is based on the many antigenic differences found in structures on the surface of bacteria. Capsular, somatic, and flagellar antigens are used in serotyping bacteria (Fig. 1.1).

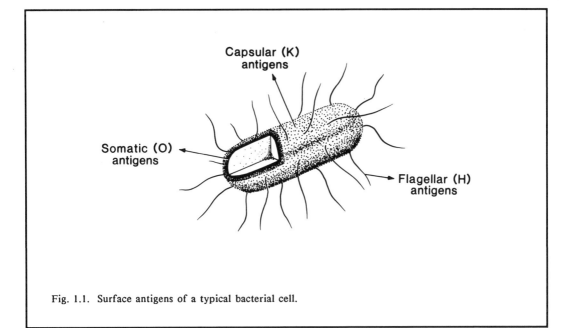

Fig. 1.1. Surface antigens of a typical bacterial cell.

II. NOMENCLATURE

A. Nomenclature is the scientific naming of organisms. In this text, the bacterial classification is based on two reference sources.
    1. Bacteria in the divisions Firmicutes, Gracilicutes, and Tenericutes are described in *Bergey's Manual of Systematic Bacteriology*, first edition, 1984.
    2. Genera described since the publication of *Bergey's Manual of Systematic Bacteriology* are documented in the *International Journal of Systematic Bacteriology*.
B. Binomial nomenclature is based on the genus and species of bacteria (e.g., *Streptococcus equi*).

III. BACTERIAL PATHOGENS OF DOMESTIC ANIMALS AND MAN

A. Only bacteria associated with diseases of domestic animals or man or of medical importance are listed (Table 1.2).

Table 1.2. Classification of medically important bacteria

	Kingdom Procaryotae	
Division Firmicutes	Division Gracilicutes	Division Tenericutes

Division Firmicutes	Division Gracilicutes	Division Tenericutes

Cocci
  Family Microccocaceae
    Genus *Micrococcus*
    Genus *Staphylococcus*
  Other genera
    Genus *Peptococcus*
    Genus *Peptostreptococcus*
    Genus *Streptococcus*
 	
Endospore-forming rods
  Genus *Bacillus*
  Genus *Clostridium*
 	
Regular nonsporing rods
  Genus *Erysipelothrix*
  Genus *Lactobacillus*
  Genus *Listeria*
 	
Irregular, nonsporing rods
  Genus *Actinomyces*
  Genus *Bifidobacterium*
  Genus *Corynebacterium*
  Genus *Eubacterium*
  Genus *Propionibacterium*
 	
The mycobacteria
  Family Mycobacteriaceae
    Genus *Mycobacterium*
 	
Nocardioforms
  Genus *Nocardia*
  Genus *Rhodococcus*
 	
Uncertain affiliation
  Genus *Dermatophilus*
	The spirochetes
	Order Spirochaetales
	  Family Spirochaetaceae
	    Genus *Borrelia*
	    Genus *Treponema*
	  Family Leptospiraceae
	    Genus *Leptospira*
	
	Aerobic helical/vibrioid bacteria
	  Genus *Campylobacter*
	
	Aerobic rods and cocci
	  Family Pseudomonadaceae
	    Genus *Pseudomonas*
	  Family Legionellaceae
	    Genus *Legionella*
	  Family Neisseriaceae
	    Genus *Acinetobacter*
	    Genus *Moraxella*
	    Genus *Neisseria*
	  Other genera
	    Genus *Alcaligenes*
	    Genus *Bordetella*
	    Genus *Brucella*
	    Genus *Francisella*
	
	Facultative anaerobic rods
	  Family Enterobacteriaceae
	    Genus *Citrobacter*
	    Genus *Edwardsiella*
	    Genus *Enterobacter*
	    Genus *Escherichia*
	    Genus *Klebsiella*
	    Genus *Morganella*
	    Genus *Proteus*
	    Genus *Providencia*
	    Genus *Salmonella*
	    Genus *Serratia*
	    Genus *Shigella*
	    Genus *Yersinia*
	  Family Vibrionaceae
	    Genus *Aeromonas*
	    Genus *Vibrio*
	  Family Pasteurellaceae
	    Genus *Actinobacillus*
	    Genus *Haemophilus*
	    Genus *Pasteurella*
	
	Anaerobic rods
	  Family Bacteroidaceae
	    Genus *Bacteroides*
	    Genus *Fusobacterium*
	Anaerobic cocci
	  Family Veillonellaceae
	    Genus *Veillonella*
	
	The rickettsias and chlamydias
	Order Rickettsiales
	  Family Rickettsiaceae
	    Genus *Cowdria*
	    Genus *Coxiella*
	    Genus *Ehrlichia*
	    Genus *Neorickettsia*
	    Genus *Rickettsia*
	  Family Anaplasmataceae
	    Genus *Anaplasma*
	    Genus *Eperythrozoon*
	    Genus *Haemobartonella*
	Order Chlamydiales
	  Family Chlamydiaceae
	    Genus *Chlamydia*
		Class Mollicutes
		Order Mycoplasmatales
		  Family Mycoplasmataceae
		    Genus *Mycoplasma*
		    Genus *Ureaplasma*

2	Bacterial Structure and Function

I. BACTERIAL STRUCTURAL COMPONENTS AND THEIR FUNCTIONS (Fig. 2.1)

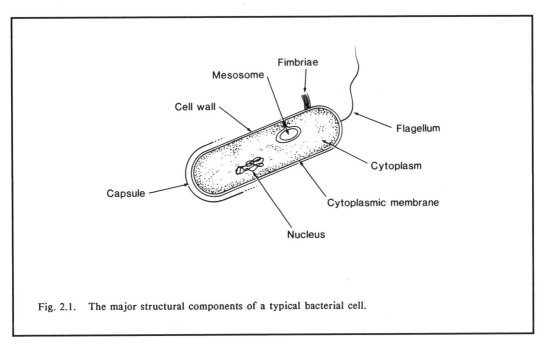

Fig. 2.1.   The major structural components of a typical bacterial cell.

A.   Cell wall
1.   All bacterial pathogens of domestic animals and man possess a complex rigid cell wall except the mycoplasmas and ureaplasmas, which lack a cell wall and are surrounded only by a cytoplasmic membrane.
   a.   Peptidoglycan (murein) gives rigidity to the cell wall and is located adjacent to the cytoplasmic membrane. It is composed of a disaccharide polymer with alternating monomers of N-acetylglucosamine and N-acetylmuramic acid that are linked by beta 1-4 glycoside bonds and peptides. The peptides consist of four or five amino acids, including D-alanine, L-alanine, D-glutamic acid, L-lysine, and diaminopimelic acid.

      b.   The peptidoglycan layer is thick in gram-positive bacteria, thin in gram-negative bacteria, and absent in the genera *Mycoplasma* and *Ureaplasma.*

         (1) Peptidoglycan often makes up 80 to 90 percent of the gram-positive cell wall but only about 10 percent of the gram-negative cell wall.

2. Traditionally bacteria have been described and often classified based on their staining reaction with the Gram stain, cellular morphology, and cellular arrangement.

      a.   The Gram stain, developed by the Danish bacteriologist Hans Christian Gram in the nineteenth century, will stain most aerobic and anaerobic bacteria. The gram-positive bacteria stain purple, and the gram-negative stain pink.

         (1) There are differences in the cell wall structure of gram-positive and gram-negative bacteria. The cell wall makes up approximately 20 percent of the total dry weight of the bacterium.

         (2) Cell wall components of gram-positive and gram-negative bacteria are listed (Table 2.1).

Table 2.1. Cell wall components of gram-positive and gram-negative bacteria

Component	Gram-positive	Gram-negative
Lipid and/or lipoprotein	+ or −	+
Lipopolysaccharide	−	+
Peptidoglycan	+	+
Polysaccharide	+	+
Protein	+	+
Teichoic acid	+	−

      b.   The cellular morphology of most bacteria are described as either a coccus (spherical-shaped cell), or bacillus (rod-shaped cell). The spirochetes are bacilli with a helical shape, and the mycoplasmas and ureaplasmas are pleomorphic due to the absence of a cell wall.

         (1) Extracellular and obligate intracellular bacteria are measured in micrometers (um), but mycoplasmas and ureaplasmas are often measured in nanometers (nm).

           (a) Cocci are approximately 1 um in diameter.

           (b) Most bacilli range from 0.5 to 1.0 um in width by 1 to 5 um in length. For convenience, bacilli are commonly grouped according to size as large (e.g., *Bacillus* and *Clostridium*), medium (e.g., Enterobacteriaceae and *Pseudomonas*), and small (e.g., *Bordetella*, *Brucella*, and *Pasteurella*).

           (c) The spirochetes in the genera *Leptospira* and *Treponema* range from 0.1 to 0.4 um in width by 5 to 30 um in length.

    (d) The mycoplasmas and ureaplasmas range in size from 50 to 250 nm.

    (e) The chlamydiae are spherical and range from 0.2 to 1.0 um in diameter. Most rickettsiae are coccobacilli and are approximately 0.3 um in width by 0.5 um in length.

   (2) The weight of a medium-sized bacilli is approximately 10^{-9} g.

  c. Cellular arrangement is used to describe some bacteria that form chains or clusters of cells.

   (1) The streptococci generally form chains of cells and the staphylococci grapelike clusters.

 3. Structural types

  a. Gram-positive bacteria (Fig. 2.2)

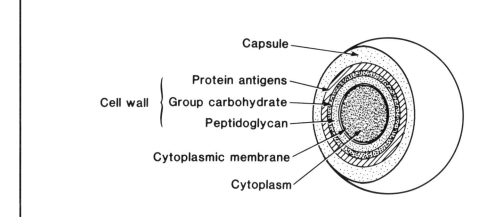

Fig. 2.2. Cross section of an encapsulated streptococcal cell.

   (1) The cell wall has a single thick layer (20 to 80 nm) of peptidoglycan, which may make up 50 to 90 percent of the cell wall. Teichoic acids, polysaccharides, proteins, and sometimes lipids are other cell wall components.

    (a) Teichoic acids make up 20 to 40 percent of the cell wall of gram-positive bacteria. Teichoic acids are polymeric chains of glycerol or ribitol molecules linked to each other by phosphodiester bridges.

    (b) Acid-fast bacteria contain high levels of lipid in their cell walls. These lipids make the bacteria difficult to stain, but once stained the cells resist decoloration with acidified aqueous or organic solvents, whereas non-acid-fast bacteria decolorize easily in a few seconds.

  (2) The acid-fast bacterial pathogens of domestic animals are in the genera *Mycobacterium* and *Nocardia*. These genera have two levels of acid-fastness. True acid-fast bacteria are in the genus *Mycobacterium* and partially acid-fast bacteria in the genus *Nocardia*. Acidified organic solvents are used to decolorize the mycobacteria and acidified aqueous solvents to decolorize the nocardiae.

b.   Gram-negative bacteria (Fig. 2.3.)

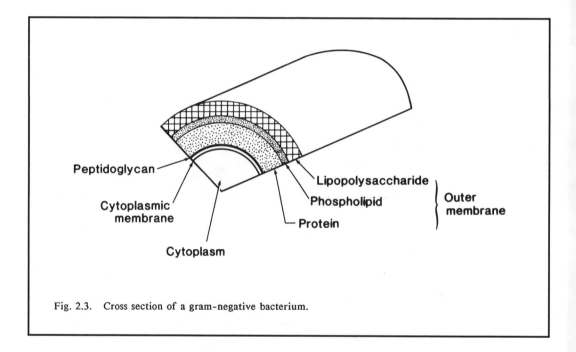

Fig. 2.3.   Cross section of a gram-negative bacterium.

  (1) The cell wall has a very thin layer (2 to 3 nm) of peptidoglycan, which is often present as a monolayer or bilayer and is separated from the cytoplasmic membrane by the periplasmic space. The outer membrane is external to the peptidoglycan layer and is composed of phospholipids, lipopolysaccharides, and proteins.

    (a) Lipopolysaccharides (LPSs) are a class of macromolecules unique to gram-negative bacteria that have great compositional and structural diversity but are constructed according to a common architectural principle. LPSs are composed of the core polysaccharide, Lipid A, and O antigens. Lipid A is the principal toxic component of the LPS; however, the endotoxicity of Lipid A moieties extracted from various species and strains of gram-negative bacteria vary considerably in potency. Chemical components of Lipid A include glucosamine-4-phosphate, ethanolamine, and a variety of long chain fatty acids. The endotoxic potency of Lipid A has been correlated with beta-OH fatty acids, especially beta-OH myristic acid. A trisaccharide of 2-keto-3-deoxyoctonic acid (KDO) links the Lipid A to the core polysaccharide via a ketoacetic linkage in most pathogenic bacteria. The inner portion of the core oligosaccharide is frequently composed of ethanolamine, heptoses, and phosphate, whereas the outer portion contains hexoses such as glucose, galactose, and N-acetylglucosamine. The O antigens are extensions of the outer portion of the core oligosaccharide and are made up of repeating oligosaccharide units each composed of 3 or 4 different hexoses. These O antigens are responsible for the serologic specificity of the smooth gram-negative bacteria. The O antigens are synthesized on the inner surface of the cytoplasmic membrane. Rough gram-negative bacteria either lack the enzymes to synthesize O antigens or lack the enzymes to attach the O antigens to the core polysaccharide.

(b) Porin proteins form pores or channels in the outer membrane of the bacterium, which allows nutrients to diffuse through the cell wall. The diameter of the channel in porin proteins imposes a size limitation on the nutrients that a cell can employ. The cutoff point in enteric bacteria is approximately 600 daltons, allowing entry of molecules about the size of trisaccharides and tetrapeptides.

(c) Other proteins in the outer membrane provide specific transport systems for nutrients whose passage through the pores might be too slow (e.g., the beta-galactosidase permease for lactose in the lactose-positive enteric bacteria).

(2) All the obligate intracellular pathogens of domestic animals in the orders Chlamydiales and Rickettsiales are gram-negative.

    c. Spirochetes
       (1) The spirochetes are slender, helically coiled bacteria. They have a three-layered outer envelope called the peptidoglycan-cytoplasmic membrane complex.
       (2) The periplasmic flagella provide a means of motility for the spirochetes. Each flagellum extends the length of the bacterium and is located between the cytoplasmic membrane and the peptidoglycan layer.
       (3) The spirochetes are classified as gram-negative but stain poorly with the Gram stain.
       (4) Pathogens are in the aerobic genera *Borrelia* and *Leptospira* and the anaerobic genus *Treponema*.
    d. Cell wall-free bacteria
       (1) Bacterial pathogens in the genera *Mycoplasma* and *Ureaplasma* do not have a cell wall and are enclosed only by the cytoplasmic membrane. The cells are pleomorphic and are often classified as gram-negative.
    e. Cell wall-defective bacteria
       (1) Protoplasts are derived from gram-positive bacteria and are bound only by a cytoplasmic membrane.
       (2) Spheroplasts are derived from gram-negative bacteria and retain some residual cell wall material.
       (3) L-forms are morphologically equivalent to protoplasts and spheroplasts and can be derived from either gram-positive or gram-negative bacteria.
          (a) Stable L-forms are unable to revert to their vegetative cell forms, whereas transitional L-forms can synthesize their cell wall components and revert to normal vegetative cells.
          (b) L-forms may achieve a state of latency and persist for long periods in the tissues of infected animals. They may serve as sources for relapse.

B. Capsule
    1. The capsule or slime layers of bacteria are often amorphous structures that are loosely attached to the cell wall. Some capsules are extensions of the cell wall. Their function is antiphagocytic.
    2. The chemical composition of the capsule depends on the species of bacteria.
      a. The capsules of most bacteria are polysaccharides. Polysaccharide capsules are generally simple polymers composed of one or a few different sugars.
       (1) The streptococci in Lancefield groups A and C have hyaluronic acid capsules. Hyaluronic acid is a disaccharide polymer with alternating monomers of D-glucuronic acid and *N*-acetylglucosamine.
      b. *Bacillus anthracis* has a polypeptide capsule.

C. Endospores
1. Endospores are resistant stages in the life cycle of the gram-positive genera *Bacillus* and *Clostridium*. Endospores are extremely resistant to environmental influences and will survive in the environment for extremely long periods of time. Spores are formed inside the vegetative cell (sporangium) in response to adverse environmental and nutritional conditions.
   a. In a culture of sporeforming bacteria, physiological and environmental factors lead at some point to an arrest in vegetative growth. Then after a number of hours a single endospore is formed in each cell in the population.
   b. Sporogenesis is all events (genetic, morphological, biochemical, and physiological) leading to the conversion of a vegetative cell into a spore. Sporulation comprises those stages of sporogenesis that concern only the synthesis and assembly of spore components.
2. Endospore formation proceeds through well-defined, morphologically identifiable stages. First, genome condensation occurs in a structure called the forespore. Second, the forespore develops inside the vegetative cell. This is initiated by invagination of the cytoplasmic membrane in the subpolar region, thus separating the cytoplasm into the forespore and sporangial cytoplasm. Third, the spore cortex is laid down between the two layers formed by the invaginating membrane. The spore cortex is responsible for the resistance of the spore and occupies approximately half the volume of the spore. The formation of spores during sporulation occurs over a period of 4 to 8 hours after the cell stops growing.
   a. Spores have a chemical composition similar to parent vegetative cells, but no free water is present. Calcium dipicolinate makes up 5 to 15 percent of the dry weight of the spore but is absent from vegetative cells. It is largely responsible for the environmental resistance of the spores.
   b. The basic organization of the endospores of the aerobic bacteria in the genus *Bacillus* is comparable to that of the endospores of the anaerobic bacteria in the genus *Clostridium* (Fig. 2.4).

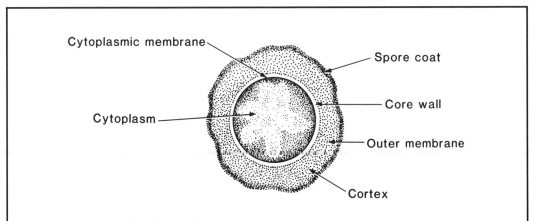

Fig. 2.4.   Cross section of a bacterial spore.

     c. Pathogenic bacteria in the genus *Bacillus* produce spores in aerobic conditions, and bacteria in the genus *Clostridium* produce spores in anaerobic conditions. If spores can be demonstrated in anaerobic culture, the bacteria should be considered as belonging to the genus *Clostridium*.

   3. Endospore germination proceeds through several well defined stages.

     a. Germination and outgrowth are two stages in the transformation of the spore to a vegetative cell.

       (1) In germination, the dormant state is lost in a series of degradative reactions lasting only a few minutes, followed by outgrowth lasting a few hours in which the spore gradually develops into a vegetative cell.

       (2) Outgrowth comprises the period up to the time of cell division and the return to vegetative growth.

     b. Endospores of *Bacillus* are released from the sporangium before germination, but the endospores of *Clostridium* germinate within the sporangium.

   4. The location of the spore in the cell may be central, terminal, or subterminal. The shape of the spore may be oval or round.

     a. The location and shape of the endospore is a useful aid in the identification of the species in the genera *Bacillus* and *Clostridium* (Fig. 2.5).

D. Flagella

   1. Flagella are found on the surface of many gram-positive and gram-negative bacteria and occur most commonly although not exclusively among the rod-shaped bacteria. They are responsible for the motility of bacterium.

     a. Spirochetes in the genera *Borrelia*, *Leptospira*, and *Treponema* are motile by means of periplasmic flagella, also called axial filaments.

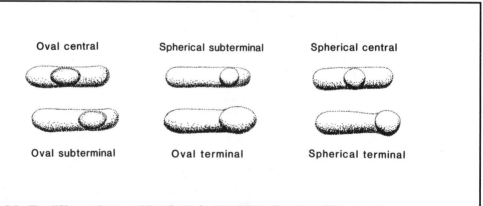

Fig. 2.5. The different shapes and locations of endospores in bacterial cells.

2. Flagella have three morphologically distinct parts: filament, hook, and basal component (Fig. 2.6).
   a. The filament is a long helical structure composed of subunits of a single protein called flagellin. The proteins are helically arranged into a cylindrical structure. The filaments are 12 to 20 nm in diameter and are often several times the length of the bacterial cell.
   b. The hook is composed of subunits of a single protein that is immunologically distinct from the filament protein.
   c. The basal component is anchored to the bacterial cell wall.
3. Flagella are classified by their arrangement on bacteria (Fig. 2.7).

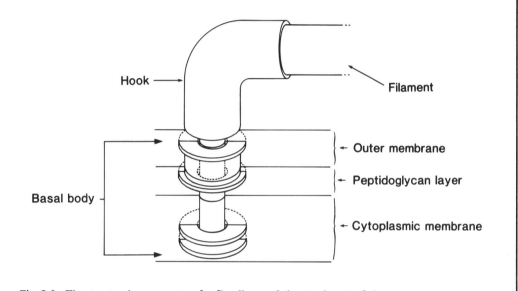

Fig. 2.6. The structural components of a flagellum and the attachment of the basal body to the bacterial cell wall. The two lower rings are embedded in the cytoplasmic membrane and the two upper rings in the peptidoglycan layer and the outer membrane.

   a. Peritrichously flagellated
      (1) The flagella are distributed over the whole cell.
         (a) Motile bacteria in the family Enterobacteriaceae have this arrangement. The number of flagella per cell can range from as low as 5 to over 100.
   b. Polar flagellated
      (1) A single flagellum or a bundle of flagella are found at one or both poles of the bacterium. When there is only one polar flagellum present it is called monotrichous, but if two or more are present it is called multitrichous.

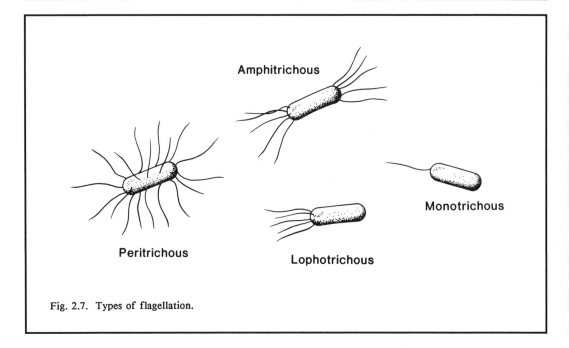

Fig. 2.7. Types of flagellation.

       (a) Amphitrichous bacteria have flagella at both poles.

       (b) Lophotrichous bacteria have several flagella at one pole.

       (c) Monotrichous bacteria have a single polar flagellum.

   4. Motile gram-positive bacteria have only peritrichous flagella, whereas motile gram-negative bacteria have either peritrichous or polar flagella.

E. Fimbriae

   1. Fimbriae (pili) are shorter and thinner than flagella and are found on the surface of many gram-negative bacteria and a few gram-positive bacteria. They are thin, hairlike, straight, rigid structures that penetrate through the cell wall and are attached to the cytoplasmic membrane. Fimbriae are composed of a protein called pilin. They are often classified as F antigens.

      a. Fimbriae may have either a peritrichous or polar arrangement.

      b. Fimbriated strains of bacteria may revert to a nonfimbriated phase, depending on the culture conditions.

   2. Fimbriae have two basic functions.

      a. Bacterial conjugation is achieved by a conjugation bridge composed of fimbriae that connect two cells. These fimbriae are found in many species in the Enterobacteriaceae and a few other bacteria.

      b.   Fimbriae can serve as adherence antigens, such as the K88 (F4) and K99 (F5) fimbriae of enterotoxigenic *Escherichia coli* (ETEC).

F.   Periplasm

   1.   The periplasm is the space located between the cell wall and the cytoplasmic membrane. It serves as a buffer component between the internal environment of bacterial cells and the external environment.

      a.   The physiological role of the periplasmic space in gram-positive bacteria is largely unknown.

      b.   In gram-negative bacteria, the periplasm contains a variety of hydrolytic enzymes and proteins that aid the transport of various compounds, including sugars, amino acids, and inorganic ions, into and out of the bacterial cytoplasm.

G.   Cytoplasmic membrane

   1.   The cytoplasmic membrane separates the cell wall and periplasm from the cytoplasm. It is about 10 nm across and is composed of a lipid bilayer in which proteins are embedded. The lipids maintain the structural integrity of the membrane, and the proteins are responsible for the specialized functions of the membrane.

      a.   The lipid bilayer is primarily composed of phospholipids. The polar head groups are exposed to the aqueous phase on the surfaces of the membrane, and the hydrocarbon tails are buried in the interior. The relative amounts and types of lipids vary from species to species.

         (1) The cytoplasmic membranes of *Mycoplasma* and *Ureaplasma*, like eucaryotic cells, contain sterols. All other bacterial pathogens of domestic animals lack sterols.

      b.   There are at least three kinds of proteins associated with the cytoplasmic membranes of bacteria. One group of proteins comprises biosynthetic enzymes responsible for the synthesis of the cell wall, in particular the cytoplasmic membrane, peptidoglycan, outer membrane, and capsule. A second group comprises transport enzymes responsible for the transport of nutrients and electrolytes from the external milieu into the cell. A third class of proteins located in the cell membrane comprise the cytochrome enzymes of the electron transport system.

         (1) The membrane proteins are distributed across the bilayer asymmetrically and vary in heterogeneity.

         (2) There is a rough correlation between the metabolic activity of a membrane and its protein content.

         (3) The relative amounts of proteins and lipids vary from species to species.

            (a) The cytoplasmic membranes of gram-positive bacteria are composed of about 75 percent protein and 25 percent lipid.

    2.   A mesosome is a specialized convoluted invagination of the cytoplasmic membrane. Mesosomes occur in both gram-positive and gram-negative bacteria but are more prominent in gram-negative bacteria. The genome of some bacterial species are attached to the mesosome, which is involved in DNA segregation during cell division.

H.   Cytoplasm

    1.   Nuclear body

        a.   Bacteria have a single circular chromosome. The double-stranded DNA is not bound by a nuclear membrane as is the genome of eucaryotic cells.

           (1)   The chromosomal DNA of *E. coli* is about 1 mm long, has a molecular weight of 2.6×10^9, and has approximately four million base pairs. The chromosomal DNA encodes for about 4,000 proteins.

        b.   The bacterial chromosome replicates semiconservatively and bidirectionally from the origin. The replicated genome segregates between the daughter cells; then cross walls form as the parent cell divides into two daughter cells. This process is called binary fission.

    2.   Ribosomes

        a.   Ribosomes are distributed throughout the cytoplasm and are the sites of protein synthesis.

        b.   Ribosomes are complexes of ribosomal RNA (rRNA) and proteins. The bacterial ribosome has a sedimentation coefficient of 70S and consists of two subunits whose sedimentation coefficients are 50S and 30S. The 50S subunit contains one 23S rRNA molecule, one 5S rRNA molecule, and 32 different proteins. The 30S subunit contains one 16S rRNA molecule and 21 different proteins.

           (1)   The ribosomes of eucaryotic organisms have sedimentation coefficients of 80S and consist of two subunits whose sedimentation coefficients are 60S and 40S.

    3.   Plasmids and episomes

        a.   Extrachromosomal DNA may be present in the bacterium as either plasmids or episomes.

           (1)   Plasmids are small, extrachromosomal, self replicating, circular strands of DNA that replicate autonomously from the bacterial chromosome. Plasmids are usually less than one-twentieth the size of the bacterial chromosome. There are usually multiple copies of each plasmid in the bacterial cell.

               (a)   The plasmids contain genes that code for as few as 2 or 3 proteins or as much as 20 to 25 percent of the total cellular protein.

           (2)   Episomes are plasmids that are capable of integrating into the bacterial chromosome.

   b. Different plasmids provide a variety of functions
       (1) R (resistance) factors are plasmids that contain genes
            that code for antibiotic resistance. These factors are
            capable of transferring resistance between strains of
            the same bacterial species and between closely related
            bacterial species. Plasmids are responsible for 60 to
            90 percent of the resistance genes in gram-negative
            pathogens. They also occur in many gram-positive
            pathogens. R factors usually carry resistance to
            several antibiotics and frequently combine with each
            other to produce new combinations of resistance
            determinants. Drug resistance can spread through a
            population of gram-negative bacteria in epidemic
            fashion. An example of an R factor is beta-lactamase,
            an extracellular enzyme that specifically hydrolyzes
            the amide bond in the beta-lactam ring of penicillin,
            rendering the antibiotic inactive.
       (2) F (fertility) factors are plasmids that promote the
            transfer of the donor bacterial chromosome at a high
            frequency of recombination (Hfr) into the recipient
            bacterial chromosome during conjugation.
       (3) Colicinogenic (Col) factors are found in many species
            of enterobacteria and code for bacteriocins, which are
            extracellular toxins that inhibit the growth of strains
            of the same or different species of bacteria. The
            presence of a Col factor in a bacterial strain confers
            immunity on that strain to the particular bacteriocin
            produced.
            (a) Colicines are the subset of bacteriocins produced
                 by the coliform bacteria.
            (b) Bacteriocin typing is used to differentiate
                 strains within a bacterial species by observing
                 the pattern of growth inhibition of a series of
                 test strains.
       (4) Virulence factors may be encoded in the genetic
            material of plasmids and episomes. These factors
            include hemolysins, fimbrial adherence antigens, and
            exotoxins. For example, plasmids in hemolytic strains
            of ETEC may encode for the hemolysin, fimbrial
            antigens, and enterotoxins. Both the fimbrial antigens
            and enterotoxins are necessary to produce intestinal
            disease.
 4. Cytoplasmic granules
   a. The presence and amount of these storage particles vary with
       the type of bacterium and its level of metabolic activity.
   b. There are three common types of cytoplasmic granules.
       (1) Glycogen is a polymer of D-glucose. It serves as a
            carbohydrate reserve.

(2) Volutin granules are composed of a poly-hexa-meta phosphate. These granules serve as a reserve for high-energy phosphate.

(3) Poly-beta-hydroxybutyric acid is a lipid reserve.

II. TRANSFORMATION, TRANSDUCTION, AND CONJUGATION

A. There are three types of gene transfer that can alter the DNA content of bacteria.

1. Transformation occurs when plasmids or exogenous bacterial chromosomal DNA is taken up by competent recipient bacteria and undergoes recombination with the bacterial chromosome to transform the bacterium, which then expresses the new genes.

   a. Competency is usually a transitory state in bacterial cultures when the cells are capable of transferring the naked DNA across the bacterial cell wall.

   b. Transformation is primarily a laboratory manipulation and probably does not occur in nature. The frequency of transformation is low even under optimal conditions.

2. Transduction occurs when fragments of bacterial chromosomal DNA are transferred into a recipient bacterium by a bacteriophage. Most bacteriophages are highly adapted to specific bacterial species, strains, or serovars.

   a. During the bacteriophage infection, a piece of bacterial DNA becomes enclosed within the bacteriophage. When the phage infects the recipient bacterium, the DNA from the donor bacterium is released and undergoes recombination with the chromosome of the recipient bacterium.

   b. Lysogenization by certain converting phages may produce changes in the serotype of the bacterium (e.g., *Salmonella*) or transfer a toxin to a nontoxigenic bacterium converting it to a toxigenic strain (e.g., *Clostridium botulinum*).

3. Conjugation occurs when DNA is transferred from one bacterium to another through fimbriae in a form of sexual recombination. Conjugation is very common in gram-negative bacteria. Conjugative chromosomal transfer may occur between strains or species within a genus, or between species of different genera.

   a. Genetic material can be transferred from one bacterial cell to another through fimbriae, which serve as a conjugation bridge between cells. Generally only a portion of the chromosome is transferred, since the conjugation bridge may rupture spontaneously before chromosome transfer is completed. The F^+ cell is the genetic donor and the F^- cell the recipient. The integration of genes from the exogenetic chromosome segment donated by the F^+ cell into the chromosome of the F^- endogenote is achieved by recombination.

III. CLASSIFICATION OF BACTERIA BY OXYGEN REQUIREMENTS

A. Obligate aerobes, obligate anaerobes, and facultative anaerobes
1. Obligate aerobic bacteria require oxygen for growth and have a respiratory metabolism.
    a. The terminal electron acceptor is molecular oxygen.
    b. Respiration yields 38 adenosine 5'-triphosphate (ATP) from one molecule of glucose.
    c. The end products of respiration are carbon dioxide and water.
2. Obligate anaerobic bacteria require oxygen-free conditions for growth and have a fermentative metabolism.
    a. The terminal electron acceptors are organic compounds.
    b. Fermentation yields two ATP from one molecule of glucose. Almost all clinically significant bacteria use the Embden-Meyerhof-Parnas pathway.
    c. Fermentation is metabolism in which organic compounds serve as both electron donors and electron acceptors. The number of moles of carbon, hydrogen, and oxygen must be the same in the products as in the substrates.
3. Facultative anaerobic bacteria will grow in the presence or absence of oxygen. These bacteria grow fermentatively under anaerobic conditions but switch preferentially to respiration under aerobic conditions.
    a. Under aerobic conditions, facultative anaerobes, like *E. coli*, will catabolize part of the carbohydrate substrate, such as a glucose, via fermentative pathways not involving oxygen.
B. Microaerophilic and capnophilic bacteria
1. Microaerophilic bacteria require oxygen for growth but prefer a reduced oxygen concentratiion of 3 to 15 percent.
2. Capnophilic bacteria prefer a carbon dioxide concentration between 3 and 10 percent.
    a. Carbon dioxide is required by most bacteria and usually is available as a product of metabolism.
        (1) Slow-growing or fastidious organisms may not generate enough carbon dioxide so it must be supplied exogenously.
        (2) Many pathogenic bacteria require the addition of 5 to 10 percent carbon dioxide to the incubator atmosphere for primary isolation in vitro from clinical materials.
3. Some bacteria prefer both a reduced oxygen concentration and an increased carbon dioxide concentration.
    a. A candlejar, a closed container in which a candle is allowed to burn until the available oxygen will no longer support combustion, has both a reduced oxygen and an increased carbon dioxide concentration.

IV. BACTERIAL METABOLISM AND GROWTH REQUIREMENTS
  A. Bacteria differ markedly with regard to the optimal temperature range for their growth.
    1. Psychophilic bacteria grow best at temperatures below 20°C.
    2. Mesophilic bacteria grow best between 25°C and 40°C. Most medically important bacterial species are mesophiles.
    3. Thermophilic bacteria grow best between 55°C and 80°C.
  B. Hydrogen ion concentration
    1. The optimal pH for most pathogenic bacteria of domestic animals and man is 7.2 to 7.4.
  C. Chemorganotropes and chemolithotropes
    1. Bacteria that derive their energy from organic compounds are known as chemorganotropes, and bacteria that derive their energy from inorganic compounds are known as chemolithotropes.
      a. The bacterial pathogens of domestic animals are chemorganotropes. Most facultative anaerobes and obligate anaerobes have the ability to ferment various carbohydrates, and some can utilize amino acids as a source of energy. The products of these fermentations vary with the bacterial species. Fermentations are usually classified according to the main fermentation end products.
    2. Most bacterial pathogens in veterinary medicine can utilize carbohydrates as a source of carbon and energy. These bacteria, which are referred to as saccharolytic, can utilize carbohydrates via the fermentative and/or oxidative metabolic pathways. Glucose can be degraded by three major metabolic pathways. Bacteria utilize one or more of these pathways for glucose metabolism, depending on their enzymatic composition and the presence or absence of oxygen.
      a. The Embden-Meyerhof-Parnas pathway is an anaerobic pathway that utilizes glucose in the absence of oxygen. This fermentative pathway is utilized exclusively by the obligate anaerobic bacteria and by the facultative anaerobic bacteria in the absence of oxygen. In this pathway, glucose is degraded to pyruvic acid, which is then oxidized to form lactic acid or a variety of organic acids. Bacteria that possess the appropriate enzyme systems can further degrade these acids into carbon dioxide, alcohols, and other organic compounds.
      b. The Entner-Douderoff pathway is an aerobic pathway that utilizes glucose in the presence of oxygen. This oxidative pathway is utilized by some obligate aerobic bacteria and by some facultative anaerobic bacteria in the presence of oxygen. In this pathway, glucose is degraded to pyruvic acid, which enters the tricarboxylic acid (TCA) cycle where molecular oxygen is the terminal electron acceptor. The final products are water and carbon dioxide.
      c. The hexose monophosphate pathway is utilized by many

facultative anaerobic bacteria, which are capable of growing in the presence of oxygen but are nonoxidative. This pathway allows these bacteria, which are incapable of utilizing the TCA cycle and passing hydrogen on to molecular oxygen, to degrade glucose to pyruvic acid.

3. Asaccharolytic bacteria are incapable of utilizing carbohydrates as a source of energy. These bacteria derive their energy from other types of organic compounds such as amino acids, organic acids, an alcohols. They are frequently referred to as nonfermentors.

V. LABORATORY IDENTIFICATION CRITERIA FOR BACTERIA
A. Presumptive identification criteria
1. The majority of the medically important bacteria can be identified to the genus level, or placed into a group of genera, based on the following criteria.
   a. Cellular properties
      (1) Gram reaction
      (2) Cellular morphology
      (3) Cellular arrangement
         (a) The plane of cell division in staphylococci is random, resulting in the formation of cells that resemble clusters of grapes, whereas the streptococci divide in a single plane, resulting in pairs or chains of cells.
         (b) All gram-positive and gram-negative bacilli divide in only one plane forming pairs of cells and chains of varying length.
   b. Culture requirement and colony morphology
      (1) Nutritional requirement and ability to grow on different kinds of media
      (2) Atmospheric requirements
         (a) Obligate aerobic
         (b) Facultative anaerobic
         (c) Obligate anaerobic
   c. Biochemical characteristics
      (1) Mode of carbohydrate utilization, particulary glucose
      (2) Catalase reactions of gram-positive bacteria
      (3) Oxidase reactions of gram-negative bacteria
2. The definition and identification of the various bacterial species is based on a set of physiological and biochemical characteristics including the degradation of carbohydrates, amino acids, and a variety of other substrates.
   a. There is often considerable variation among the different strains within a species.
   b. Many bacterial species have been subdivided further by a variety of techniques, including biological characteristics, biochemical reactions, antigen analysis, and susceptibility

to bacteriophages that infect and lyse bacteria. The resulting biovars, serovars, and phagovars often have considerable pathogenic and epidemiologic significance.

3. Bacterial pathogens of domestic animals are frequently classified into two groups: extracellular and facultative intracellular bacteria and the obligate intracellular and cell-associated bacteria.

B. Extracellular and facultative intracellular bacteria

1. Fifty-four genera of extracellular and facultative intracellular bacteria and their staining reactions, cellular characteristics, and oxygen requirements are listed in Table 2.2.

2. The majority of the aerobic gram-positive and gram-negative bacterial pathogens of domestic animals and man will grow on blood agar and/or MacConkey agar when incubated in air at 37°C.

   a. Blood agar will support their growth and will determine their hemolytic patterns. The hemolytic patterns adjacent to bacterial colonies are classified as nonhemolytic (gamma hemolysis), complete (beta hemolysis), and partial (alpha hemolysis). One aerobic species, *Staphylococcus aureus*, and one anaerobic species, *Clostridium perfringens*, will produce a double zone of hemolysis, which is a complete zone of hemolysis adjacent to the colony surrounded by a partial zone of hemolysis.

   b. MacConkey agar, which contains bile salts, is a selective media for some gram-negative pathogens. Most enteric gram-negative bacteria will grow, but the media inhibits most gram-positive bacteria and some gram-negative bacteria. Lactose-positive bacteria form red colonies and lactose-negative bacteria colorless colonies.

3. Bacteria that will not grow on blood agar and/or MacConkey agar when incubated aerobically at 37°C are considered to have fastidious growth requirements. These microorganisms require either supplemental growth factors or different incubation conditions.

   a. These fastidious bacteria include the obligate anaerobic bacteria and most species in the aerobic genera *Borrelia*, *Brucella*, *Campylobacter*, *Francisella*, *Haemophilus*, *Legionella*, *Leptospira*, *Mycobacterium*, *Mycoplasma*, *Taylorella*, and *Ureaplasma*.

4. Bacterial growth in culture has four phases (Fig. 2.8).

   a. In the lag phase, the bacterial cells increase in size and metabolic activity, but there is no detectable multiplication.

   b. In the logarithmic phase, the cells divide by binary fission so that there is a linear relationship between the logarithmic number of cells and time. The generation time (between cell divisions) varies greatly between bacterial species. *E. coli* has an approximate generation time of 20

Table 2.2. Characteristics of genera of extracellular and facultative intracellular bacteria

Genus	Staining Reaction		Cellular Characteristic				Oxygen Requirement	
	Gram	Acid-fast	Cocci	Rods	Motility[a]	Endospores	Aerobic[b]	Anaerobic
Acinetobacter	−			+	−		+	
Actinobacillus	−			+	−		+	
Actinomyces	+			+	−		+	
Aeromonas	−			+	+		+	
Alcaligenes	−			+	+		+	
Bacillus	+			+	−	+	+	
Bacteroides	−			+	−			+
Bifidobacterium	+			+	−			+
Bordetella	−			+	+		+	
Borrelia	−			+	+		+	
Brucella	−			+	−		+	
Campylobacter	−			+	+		+	
Citrobacter	−			+	+		+	
Clostridium	+			+	+	+		+
Corynebacterium	+			+	−		+	
Dermatophilus	+			+	+		+	
Edwardsiella	−			+	+		+	
Enterobacter	−			+	+		+	
Erysipelothrix	+			+	−		+	
Escherichia	−			+	+		+	
Eubacterium	+			+	−			+
Francisella	−			+	−		+	
Fusobacterium	−			+	−			+
Haemophilus	−			+	−		+	
Klebsiella	−			+	−		+	
Legionella	−			+	+		+	
Leptospira	−			+	+		+	
Listeria	+			+	+		+	
Micrococcus	+		+		−		+	
Moraxella	−			+	−		+	
Morganella	−			+	+		+	
Mycobacterium	+	+		+	−		+	
Mycoplasma[c]	−				−		+	
Neisseria	−		+		−		+	
Nocardia	+	+		+	−		+	
Pasteurella	−			+	−		+	
Peptococcus	+		+		−			+
Peptostreptococcus	+		+		−			+
Propionibacterium	+			+	−		+	
Proteus	−			+	+		+	
Providencia	−			+	+		+	
Pseudomonas	−			+	+		+	
Rhodococcus	+			+	−		+	
Salmonella	−			+	+		+	
Serratia	−			+	+		+	
Shigella	−			+	−		+	
Staphylococcus	+		+		−		+	
Streptococcus	+		+		−		+	
Taylorella	−			+	−		+	
Treponema	−			+	+			+
Ureaplasma[c]	−				−		+	
Veillonella	−		+		−			+
Vibrio	−			+	+		+	
Yersinia	−			+	+		+	

[a] Some or all species in the genus are motile.
[b] Includes both obligate aerobes and facultative anaerobes.
[c] Lacks a cell wall.

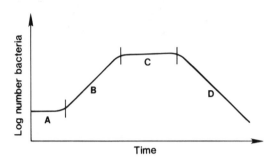

Fig. 2.8. A typical bacterial growth curve in culture media illustrating the
lag phase (*A*), logarithmic growth phase (*B*), stationary phase (*C*), and decline
or death phase (*D*).

minutes, but a *Mycobacterium* species may require 20 to 24
hours. A strain of *E. coli* with a 20-minute generation time
will have a 64-fold increase in 6 hours, whereas a
Mycobacterium species with a 24-hour generation time will
require 6 days to attain a 64-fold increase. Most bacterial
pathogens have generation times in the range of 20 minutes
to 2 hours.

  c. In the stationary phase, cell division decreases and finally
stops, usually because of an exhaustion of an essential
nutrient in the medium.

  d. In the decline phase, the bacterial cells begin to die, and
both viable and total cell counts decline as autolysis of
the cells occur.

5. Several biochemical tests are used in presumptive identification
of bacteria.

  a. The catalase test is used primarily with gram-positive
bacteria to determine the presence of the enzyme catalase.
Reactions are either positive or negative.

    (1) Most aerobic bacteria are catalase-positive, whereas
most obligate anaerobic bacteria are catalase-negative.

  b. The oxidase test is used primarily with gram-negative
bacteria to determine the presence of cytochrome oxidase,
which is used in the electron transport systems of some
aerobic bacteria. Reactions are either positive or negative.

    (1) Although all aerobic bacteria possess a respiratory
chain, the cytochrome components of respiratory chains
of various bacteria vary markedly. Oxidase-positive
bacteria possess cytochrome oxidase, while members of
the family Enterobacteriaceae and genus *Acinetobacter*
lack cytochrome oxidase and are oxidase-negative.

  c. Glucose and lactose fermentation media are used to determine
if bacteria can utilize these carbohydrates.

(1) Glucose is a six-carbon monosaccharide. Lactose is a disaccharide composed of glucose and galactose.
  d. Oxidation-fermentation media are used to determine whether a bacterium can utilize glucose by oxidative and/or fermentative metabolic pathways.
   (1) Saccharolytic bacteria, which utilize glucose, produce acid; however, asaccharolytic bacteria grown in this medium produce a neutral or slightly alkaline reaction.
  e. Motility media are used to determine the motility of bacteria.
   (1) Generally all species and strains of bacteria in a genus are all either motile or nonmotile.
  f. Coagulase tests evaluate the ability of a bacterium to produce enzymes capable of clotting plasma. The coagulation reactions are either positive or negative.
   (1) Traditionally rabbit plasma has been used as a substrate for the *Staphylococcus* species.
C. Obligate intracellular and cell-associated bacteria
 1. The nine genera of the obligate intracellular and cell-associated bacteria that have species that are pathogens of domestic animals (*Anaplasma*, *Chlamydia*, *Cowdria*, *Coxiella*, *Ehrlichia*, *Eperythrozoon*, *Haemobartonella*, *Neorickettsia*, and *Rickettsia*) are aerobic, gram-negative, and nonmotile. These organisms will not grow on cell-free media.

VI. COMPARISON OF PROCARYOTIC AND EUCARYOTIC CELLS
 A. Bacterial cells differ markedly from the eucaryotic cells of domestic animals and man in nuclear organization, cytoplasmic organelles, and chemical composition (Table 2.3).

Table 2.3. Differential properties of procaryotic and eucaryotic cells

Characteristic	Procaryotic Cells	Eucaryotic Cells
Nuclear body		
Nuclear membrane	–	+
Chromosome	Single, circular	Multiple, linear
DNA	+	+
Histones	–[a]	+
Ribosomes		
Cytoplasmic	70S	80S
Mitochondria	–	70S
Endoplasmic reticulum	–	+
Cell wall components		
Peptidoglycan	+	–
Sterols	–[b]	+

[a]Histonelike proteins are associated with the bacterial chromosome.

[b]Sterols are present in the cytoplasmic membranes of the genera *Mycoplasma* and *Ureaplasma*.

SECTION II

Bacterial Pathogenesis

| 3 | Bacterial Virulence Factors |

Pathogenic bacteria are able to overcome the host's body defense mechanisms and invade and proliferate in the tissues. They produce toxins and enzymes that cause destruction and death of tissue cells, resulting in clinical symptoms of disease and occasionally death of the infected animal.

I. ROLE OF CAPSULE, CELL WALL, FLAGELLA, AND FIMBRIAE IN DISEASE
  A. Antiphagocytic factors
    1. Capsules
      a. The capsules and slime layers on the surface of bacteria contribute to the disease-producing potential of extracellular bacteria by preventing phagocytosis by neutrophils and macrophages. These antiphagocytic substances prevent phagocytic cells from forming sufficient contact with the encapsulated bacteria to allow phagocytosis to take place.
      b. Encapsulated pathogenic bacteria are invariably more virulent than nonencapsulated strains of the same bacterial species. Encapsulated bacteria tend to resist phagocytosis in the nonimmmune host, proliferate, and establish a focus of infection, whereas nonencapsulated bacteria are usually phagocytized and killed.
        (1) Virulent strains of *Francisella tularensis* have a capsule, but avirulent strains do not.
        (2) Encapsulated strains of *Bacillus anthracis* are virulent and nonencapsulated mutants avirulent.
    2. Cell wall antigens
      a. Gram-negative bacteria
        (1) Smooth strains of gram-negative bacteria have a hydrophobic surface and tend to resist phagocytosis, whereas rough strains have a hydrophilic surface and are readily phagocytized.
          (a) Members of the family Enterobacteriaceae, which are recovered from extraintestinal infections, are invariably smooth. If polysaccharide slime layers are present on their surface, these antigens are often considered to be extensions of the O antigens of their lipopolysaccharides.
      b. Gram-positive bacteria
        (1) The outer membrane proteins of gram-positive bacteria frequently exhibit antiphagocytic activity.

(a) The M protein antigen of *Streptococcus equi* has strong antiphagocytic activity and is a primary virulence factor of the bacterium.

(b) The M protein antigens of *Streptococcus pyogenes* have antiphagocytic activity and play a significant role in the pathogenesis of the infection. Specific types of M protein antigens have been associated with both rheumatic fever and glomerulonephritis, which are postinfection complications.

(c) Protein A of *Staphylococcus aureus*, which can bind to the Fc portion of immunoglobulins, imparts antiphagocytic activity by competing with the Fc receptors on the surfaces of neutrophils and macrophages.

(2) Teichoic acids exhibit some antiphagocytic activity.

B. Adherence and colonization factors

1. Fimbriae

a. Some fimbriae act as adhesins, allowing bacteria to adhere and colonize various epithelial surfaces of the host.

(1) The specificity of these fimbrial antigens often determines the host and tissue specificity of various pathogenic bacteria.

(2) The adhesive properties of fimbriae, which act as lectins by binding to select monosaccharides, can be detected by measurement of the adherence of bacteria to epithelial cells or by their ability to promote hemagglutination.

b. Gram-negative bacteria

(1) Numerous fimbrial (F) antigens have been demonstrated to adhere to the enterocytes of the small intestine. These colonization factor antigens on human and animal strains of enterotoxigenic *Escherichia coli* (ETEC) are usually serotype- and species-specific.

(a) The K88, K99, and 987P fimbrial antigens on porcine ETEC strains adhere to specific glycoproteins present on the mucosal surface of the small intestine. The K99 antigen will also adhere to the intestinal mucosa of calves and lambs. K88 and K99 are now classified as F4 and F5, respectively.

(2) Fimbriae of *Moraxella bovis* will adhere to the cornea of cattle.

c. Gram-positive bacteria

(1) Pathogenic strains of *Corynebacterium renale* have fimbriae, which endow the bacteria with the ability to adhere and colonize the epithelial surface of the renal

pelvis of cattle. Nonfimbriated strains of *C. renale* are avirulent.

2. Cell wall structures
   a. Gram-negative bacteria
      (1) Some gram-negative enterics can colonize the mucosal surface of the intestines. The mechanisms of adherence are poorly understood.
      (2) *Campylobacter fetus* ss *venerealis* can colonize the epithelial surfaces of the bovine female genital tract.
   b. Gram-positive bacteria
      (1) Virulent strains of *S. equi* adhere to the equine pharyngeal epithelium. The M protein extends through the the hyaluronic acid capsule and mediates attachment to the epithelial cells.

3. Cytoplasmic membrane
   a. Mycoplasmataceae
      (1) These organisms colonize and firmly adhere to the mucosal epithelium.

C. Invasive factors
   1. Some pathogenic bacteria have invasive properties that endow them with the ability to penetrate intact skin and mucous membranes.
      a. Skin
         (1) *F. tularensis* and the pathogenic leptospires can invade intact skin.
      b. Mucous membranes
         (1) Brucellae, salmonellae, shigellae, *Listeria monocytogenes*, and *Treponema pallidum* can invade mucous membranes.
         (2) Virulent shigellae penetrate the epithelial cells of the intestinal mucosa. This depends on the presence of smooth lipopolysaccharide antigen on the bacterial cell surface, particularly the chemical composition of the O side chain polysaccharide.
             (a) *Shigella* species penetrate the lining of epithelial cells of the human large bowel but do not invade beyond the submucosa. Although shigellae can produce exotoxins capable of killing the epithelial cells, invasiveness is a more important determinant of virulence than is exotoxin production, since noninvasive toxigenic strains do not cause disease as do invasive nontoxigenic strains.
      c. Meninges
         (1) *Haemophilus influenzae* type b often causes an acute bacterial meningitis in infants and young children from 3 months to 6 years of age. The organisms initially

colonize the nasal pharynx and then invade into the bloodstream, with subsequent localization in the brain. The other encapsulated types (a, c, d, e, and f) also are invasive and cause systemic manifestations of the disease but not meningitis.

    (a) The capsular polysaccharide is the major antigenic determinant and confers type specificity on the organism. Type b has pentoses (ribose and ribitol) as the sugar components, whereas types a, c, d, e, and f have either hexose or hexosamine moieties.

D.   Genotypic variation of cell surface antigens

    1.   Immune modulation

        a.   The cell surface and flagellar antigens of some bacteria are able to undergo phase variation, in which the bacterium is able to switch from the production of one antigenic type to another. This periodic alteration of a surface structure helps the bacterium to avoid elimination by the host's immune system.

        b.   Gram-negative bacteria

           (1) *C. fetus* ss *venerealis* possesses both O and W cell wall antigens. Antigenic variation of the W antigens, which are the most important in eliciting protective immunity, occurs only in vivo under the selective pressure of the immune response, while the O antigens are stable. Alteration in the antigenic structure of the W antigens can occur when specific immunoglobulins are present. Therefore the successful destruction of a major portion of the bacterial population in the bovine female reproductive tract leaves a residual portion of bacteria that possess antigenic determinants differing from those of the original population. The residual bacterial population may multiply and be largely eliminated in turn by a second immune response, leaving a residual population of a third antigenic type. This process may be repeated indefinitely. Because *C. fetus* ss *venerealis* is an infection of the mucous membranes of the female genital tract and because the sIgA-producing system has a poor immunologic memory, the bacteria may reutilize antigens without stimulating a secondary immune response.

E.   Phenotypic variation of cell surface antigens

    1.   Comparison of bacteria in vivo and in vitro

        a.   Gram-negative bacteria

           (1) Members of the family Enterobacteriaceae isolated from disease processes are invariably smooth, but when

cultured on bacteriologic media, they often revert to rough forms.

(a) Most rough gram-negative bacteria, when inoculated into an animal, will revert to the smooth form.

b. Gram-positive bacteria

(1) *Streptococcus pneumoniae*, the cause of human pneumococcal pneumonia, has a polysaccharide capsule that plays a major role in antiphagocytic defense. The smooth strains are virulent, and the rough strains avirulent. Smooth strains with a capsule are not phagocytized, but rough strains without a capsule are phagocytized and killed.

(a) Capsular size varies at different stages of in vivo growth and can be roughly correlated with virulence. During the logarithmic growth phase when capsular polysaccharide synthesis is maximal, the bacteria are maximally virulent. Later in the growth cycle, when polysaccharide synthesis is reduced, the capsules are smaller and the bacteria less virulent.

(b) When cultured on artificial media, the smooth encapsulated bacteria often revert to rough, nonencapsulated forms.

2. Effects of temperature

a. Gram-negative bacteria

(1) *Yersinia enterocolitica* is motile by means of peritrichous flagella when cultured at $20^{\circ}C$ but is nonmotile at $37^{\circ}C$.

(2) *Yersinia pestis*, the etiologic agent of plague, produces both fraction 1 and V/W antigens at $37^{\circ}C$, but these antigens are not expressed at $25^{\circ}C$. The enzymes necessary for the synthesis of these virulence factors are inactive at $25^{\circ}C$.

(a) Fraction 1 (F1) is a protein capsular antigen. It is antiphagocytic and is associated with the resistance of the bacterium to phagocytosis.

(b) The V antigen is protein and the W antigen a lipoprotein. The V/W antigens are antiphagocytic and are associated with the capacity for intracellular survival and multiplication following phagocytosis.

(c) Fleas are primary vectors in the transmission of the disease to rodents and man. The flea infected with *Y. pestis* ($25^{\circ}C$) lacks both F1 and V/W antigens, but in rodents and man ($37^{\circ}C$) the bacteria express both F1 and V/W antigens.

b. Gram-positive bacteria
(1) *L. monocytogenes* is motile by means of peritrichous flagella when cultured at 20°C but nonmotile at 37°C.
F. Intracellular parasitism
1. Facultative intracellular bacteria
a. Facultative intracellular bacteria can grow and proliferate both extracellularly and intracellularly within eucaryotic cells.
(1) Traditionally the *Brucella* species, *L. monocytogenes*, *Salmonella* serovars, and *Mycobacterium* species have been the primary facultative intracellular pathogens of domestic animals and man.
(2) The in vivo growth of the *Brucella* species and *Mycobacterium* species is primarily in macrophages. These bacteria often prevent the fusion of the phagosomes and lysosomes within the macrophages.
2. Obligate intracellular bacteria
a. The obligate intracellular bacteria can only grow and proliferate within nucleated cells or erythrocytes of the host.
(1) Anaplasmataceae
(a) Members of the genera *Anaplasma*, *Eperythrozoon*, and *Haemobartonella* grow in or on erythrocytes.
(2) Chlamydiaceae
(a) The two *Chlamydia* species can parasitize a variety of nucleated cell types, where they grow in the cytoplasm.
(3) Rickettsiaceae
(a) *Cowdria ruminantium*, *Coxiella burnetii*, and *Rickettsia rickettsii* parasitize vascular endothelial cells.
(b) *Ehrlichia* species parasitize leukocytes.
(c) *Neorickettsia helminthoeca* parasitize reticular cells of lymphoid tissue.
G. Toxins associated with cell surface structures
1. Endotoxin
a. The lipopolysaccharide (LPS) in the cell wall of gram-negative bacteria can cause hypotension, shock, fever, intravascular coagulation, and death.
b. The endotoxicity of the LPS resides in the Lipid A.
c. The clinical manifestations of endotoxicity are only manifested when the gram-negative cells are lysed, releasing large amounts of free LPS.
(1) Under normal physiologic conditions, live, intact gram-negative bacteria continuously shed small amounts of the outer membrane; however, insufficient amounts of LPS are shed to manifest an endotoxin response.
(2) In broth medium, it has been estimated that

approximately 5 percent of a gram-negative bacterium's
outer membrane is shed into the medium per generation.
d.   The toxicity of the LPS can be manifested in numerous ways.
(1) Endotoxin stimulates leukocytes, perhaps through
prostaglandin production, to release endogenous
pyrogens, which act on the hypothalmus to trigger
fever.
(2) Endotoxin can cause a leukopenia and a hyperglycemia.
(3) Endotoxin can activate both the alternate complement
pathway, leading to local tissue damage, and the
clotting system, leading to disseminated intravascular
coagulation.
(4) Endotoxin may induce circulatory abnormalities that
result in increased vascular permeability and shock,
impaired blood circulation, organ damage, and death.

II. ROLE OF EXOTOXINS AND EXTRACELLULAR ENZYMES
A.   Exotoxins
1.   General properties and characteristics
a.   Bacterial exotoxins vary greatly in their mode of action and
potency.
b.   Most toxins are proteins liberated from either intact or
lysed bacterial cells.
2.   Hemolysins
a.   Hemolysins lyse erythrocytes. Some hemolysins also will
lyse other types of cells, including phagocytic cells.
b.   The hemolytic reactions and modes of action of the various
hemolysins vary markedly.
(1) *S. aureus* hemolytic toxins
(a) The alpha, delta, and epsilon toxins produce zones
of complete hemolysis on sheep blood agar, while
beta toxin produces a zone of incomplete
hemolysis.
(b) Alpha toxin is secreted as an inactive protease,
which after activation by a membrane-bound
proteolytic enzyme, hydrolyzes structural membrane
proteins of erythrocytes. The alpha toxin is the
most potent of the four hemolytic membrane toxins
produced by *S. aureus*.
(c) Beta toxin degrades the sphingomyelin of the
erythrocyte membrane by hydrolysis. A red cell's
susceptibility to this sphingomyelinase is
directly related to the amount of sphingomyelin
accessible to the toxin.
(d) Delta toxin lyses erythrocytes by a detergentlike
activity.
c.   Some hemolysins are closely related.
(1) Streptolysin O is an oxygen-labile hemolysin. It is

produced by numerous pathogenic streptococci and is immunologically related to numerous other hemolysins, including pneumolysin of *S. pneumoniae*, botulinolysin of *Clostridium botulinum*, tetanolysin of *C. tetani*, chauveolysin of *C. chauvoei*, and theta toxin of *C. perfringens*.

3. Leukotoxins
    a. Leukotoxins kill and often lyse phagocytic cells.
    b. The mode of action of various leukotoxins varies markedly.
        (1) *S. aureus* leukocidin
            (a) The Panton-Valentine leukocidin is composed of two polypeptides, a fast (F) component with MW 32,000 and a slow (S) component with MW 38,000. The two polypeptides are distinguished by their electrophoretic mobility. The components interact synergistically and interrupt the phospholipids of the phagocytic cell membrane. This exotoxin is active against the neutrophils and macrophages of rabbits and man.
        (2) *Fusobacterium necrophorum* leukotoxin
            (a) This leukotoxin has a MW of less than 500 daltons and is highly active against the neutrophils and macrophages of cattle and sheep. It is considered to be the primary virulence factor of the bacterium.

4. Inhibitors of protein synthesis
    a. Diphtheria toxin of *Corynebacterium diphtheriae*
        (1) Diphtheria toxin inhibits protein synthesis via enzymatic depletion of an enzyme required for the assembly of peptides on the mRNA template. Diphtheria toxin inhibits polypeptide chain elongation by catalyzing the inactivation of eucaryotic elongation factor 2 (EF-2), which is required for translocating polypeptide tRNA from the acceptor site to the donor site on the eucaryotic ribosome. EF-2 is inactivated by being coupled with the adenosine diphosphate ribose resulting from the cleaves of nicotinamide adenine diphosphate (NAD).
            (a) The protein holotoxin is a single polypeptide chain with MW 62,000 that is activated by proteolytic cleavage into fragment A (MW 24,000) and fragment B (MW 38,000). Fragment B binds to the ganglioside Gm_1 on the cell membrane of susceptible cells and facilitates the entry of fragment A into the cytoplasm of the cell. Fragment A has the enzymatic activity.
            (b) Man is the only animal species with receptors for fragment B, thus allowing fragment A to gain

access to the cell cytoplasm. All human cells are
sensitive to the holotoxin (Table 3.1).

Table 3.1. Biological activities of diphtheria
holotoxin fragments A and B

Fragments	In Vitro	In Vivo	
	Tissue culture	Man	Other animals
A	+	−	−
B	−	−	−
A + B	+	+	−

Note: + = cells sensitive; − = cells resistant.

   b.   Exotoxin A of *Pseudomonas aeruginosa*
      (1) The mode of action of exotoxin A is similar to that of
          diphtheria toxin.
   c.   Cytotoxins of *Salmonella* and *Shigella*
      (1) The cytotoxins produced by some strains of *Salmonella*
          and *Shigella* will inhibit protein synthesis in
          eucaryotic cells.
         (a) Shiga toxin, produced by *S. dysenteriae*, is a
             multicomponent protein complex that inhibits
             eucaryotic cytoplasmic protein biosynthesis by
             inactivating the 60S ribosomal subunits in a
             catalytic manner.
 5.   Enterotoxins
   a.   Choleragen of *Vibrio cholerae*
      (1) This heat-labile enterotoxin (choleragen) causes the
          loss of water and electrolytes into the intestinal
          lumen with a subsequent watery diarrhea, the
          predominant characteristic of cholera. The
          pathogenesis of *V. cholerae* depends on the ability of
          the bacteria to adhere and colonize the mucosal surface
          of the small intestine, multiply at the site of
          infection, and secrete choleragen. Cholera is a
          prototype toxigenic disease in which the clinical signs
          are solely attributable to the action of the
          enterotoxin.
         (a) The holotoxin is composed of one A_1 subunit, one
             A_2 subunit, and five B subunits. The B subunits
             are responsible for binding to the ganglioside Gm_1
             on the cell membranes of the small intestinal
             enterocytes. The A_1 subunit enters the cell and
             activates adenylate cyclase, which enzymatically
             degrades adenosine 5'-triphosphate (ATP), leading
             to increased intracellular levels of cyclic
             adenosine-3',5'-monophosphate (cAMP), which
             stimulates the hypersecretion of electrolytes and

water. The A_2 subunit may serve as a stabilizer
of the A complex before its action on the cell.

   (b) Neither fragment A nor B alone has toxic activity.
Both are required for the full manifestation of
toxicity.

  b. Heat-labile enterotoxin of *E. coli*

    (1) The ETEC produces a heat-labile enterotoxin (LT) very
similar to choleragen of *V. cholerae*.

      (a) LT is a holotoxin composed of fragments A and B.
The B subunit of LT binds to the gangliosides on
the small intestinal enterocytes, while the A
subunit possesses the biological activity.

      (b) The B fragment of LT differs by a limited number
of amino acid residues from choleragen, while the
A fragment shares some regions of homology with
the analogous subunit of choleragen.

      (c) The LT is plasmid-mediated. The LT gene consists
of a promoter, followed by a ribosome-binding
sequence, the information for the A polypeptide, a
second ribosome-binding sequence, and the
information for the B polypeptide. Both the A and
B peptide reading regions have information coding
for an amino terminal peptide.

    (2) Heat-labile enterotoxins similar to the LT of *E. coli*
have been demonstrated in some strains of *Salmonella*,
Shigella, and *Y. enterocolitica*.

  c. Heat-stable enterotoxins of *E. coli*

    (1) Some ETEC produce heat-stable enterotoxins (ST), which
are composed of 18 or 19 amino acid residues. The ST
activates guanylate cyclase, which enzymatically
degrades guanosine 5'-triphosphate (GTP), with a
subsequent increase in cyclic guanosine-3',5'-
monophosphate (cGMP).

      (a) The two types of ST, ST_A and ST_B, are controlled
by different plasmids.

      (b) Some plasmids will code for both LT and ST.

    (2) Heat-stable enterotoxins similar to the ST of *E. coli*
have been demonstrated in some strains of *Salmonella*
and *V. cholerae*.

6. Neural toxins

  a. Botulism toxins of *C. botulinum*

    (1) Seven immunologically distinct toxin types are
produced; however, each toxin has an identical mode of
action. Botulinum toxins depress the formation and/or
release of acetylcholine from cholinergic motor nerve
endings, resulting in a flaccid paralysis.

      (a) On a gram for gram basis, botulism toxin is the

most potent toxin known to produce intoxication in man.

 (2) The different toxin types vary in their host specificity. Man is susceptible to toxin types A, B, E, and F but cattle only to types C and D. The differences in host range and susceptibility to toxin types have been postulated to be due to differences in intestinal absorption (i.e., the antigenically different toxins are absorbed differently from the intestinal tracts by man and various domestic animals) or by differences in toxin receptor sites (i.e., the molecular configuration of the toxins may differ to the extent that attachment to receptor sites may be possible in one species but not another).

 b. Tetanus toxin of *C. tetani*

 (1) Tetanospasmin is responsible for the neurological signs of tetanus. This protein is released from lysed bacterial cells as a single polypeptide chain with MW 150,000. This inactive prototoxin is nicked by a proteolytic enzyme into two polypeptide chains: the H-chain (MW 100,000) and the L-chain (MW 50,000). The H-chain and L-chain remain held together by one or more disulfide bonds. The activated toxin affects the motor cells within the cerebrospinal axis by blocking presynaptic and postsynaptic inhibition in the central nervous system, resulting in hyperflexia and spasms of skeletal muscle.

 (a) On a gram for gram basis, tetanus toxin is the second most potent toxin known to produce intoxication in man.

 (2) Tetanus has been reported in all domestic animals; however, their susceptibility varies markedly.

 c. Lethal toxins of *C. perfringens*

 (1) *C. perfringens* produces a variety of exotoxins and extracellular enzymes in the alimentary tract. The lethal toxins are absorbed by the intestinal tract and transported hematogenously to the central nervous system where they manifest their toxicity.

 (a) Alpha toxin is an oxygen-stable hemolysin with phospholipase C enzymatic activity. It degrades phospholipids on eucaryotic cells, resulting in tissue necrosis, and exhibits several toxic effects, being hemolytic, dermonecrotic, and lethal.

B. Extracellular enzymes

 1. Coagulases

  a. Several types of coagulase enzymes can cause the clotting of plasma by reacting with prothrombin to form thrombin, which in turn acts on fibrinogen to form fibrin.

(1) Coagulases are significant virulent factors of *Staphylococcus intermedius.*

2. Collagenases and elastases
   a. These enzymes degrade collagen and elastin, which are major components of connective tissue.
      (1) *Bacteroides melaninogenicus* produces collagenase, which plays a significant role in the pathogenesis of infections caused by this obligate anaerobic gram-negative bacterium.
      (2) Kappa toxin of *C. perfringens* is a collagenase.
3. Fibrinolysins
   a. They activate the plasma system, leading to the breakdown of fibrin.
      (1) *S. pyogenes* produces streptokinase, which has fibrinolytic activity. Streptokinase converts plasminogens to plasmin, which in turn promotes the lysis of fibrin blood clots, thus allowing the rapid spread of streptococcal infections by preventing the formation of a fibrin barrier around the infection.
4. Hyaluronidase
   a. This enzyme hydrolyzes hyaluronic acid, which is a major constituent of the ground substance in connective tissue.
      (1) *S. pyogenes* produces hyaluronidase. The bacterium also has a hyaluronic acid capsule.
5. Lipases and esterases
   a. These enzymes hydrolyze lipids.
6. Lysozyme
   a. This enzyme hydrolyzes the peptidoglycan found in the cell walls of gram-negative and gram-positive bacteria.
7. NADase
   a. Nicotinamide adenine dinucleotidase (NADase) cleaves the nicotinamide portion from the coenzyme nicotinamide adenine dinucleotide (NAD).
      (1) *S. pyogenes* produces NADase.
8. Neuraminidases
   a. *V. cholerae* produces a neuraminidase that is unable to remove N-acetylneuraminic acid from the Gm_1 gangliosides on human intestinal enterocytes but is able to convert other gangliosides to Gm_1, thus synthesizing even more receptor sites to which choleragen can bind.
   b. *H. influenzae* produces a neuraminidase.
   c. *S. pneumoniae* releases a toxic neuraminidase during autolysis of the cell. It is called purpura-producing principle.
9. Nucleases
   a. Deoxyribonucleases (DNAse) hydrolyze deoxyribonuclic acid (DNA).

      b.   Ribonucleases (RNAse) hydrolyze ribonucleic acid (RNA).
10. Proteases
      a.   A variety of bacteria proteases degrade proteins to peptides
         and amino acids.
11. Ureases
      a.   Bacterial ureases hydrolyze urea to form ammonia and carbon
         dioxide.
12. Pigments
      a.   *P. aeruginosa* produces pyocyanin, which inhibits
         mitochondrial respiratory activity in eucaryotic cells.
13. Immunosuppressive factors
      a.   *P. aeruginosa* produces an extracellular immunosuppressive
         factor, which inhibits cell-mediated immunity.

III. ROLE OF IRON IN BACTERIAL INFECTIONS
    A.   Effects of iron on bacterial levels of catalase and cytochromes
       1.   The catalase and cytochrome contents are markedly reduced in many
           bacteria when grown on iron-poor media.
           a.   The iron requirements of the cytochromes are met first, but
              the levels of catalase and peroxidases are reduced.
              (1) The virulence of *Y. pestis* is correlated with catalase
                    activity.
    B.   Effects of iron on toxin production
       1.   Diphtheria toxin of *C. diphtheriae*
           a.   Diphtheria toxin is produced maximally when iron
              concentrations are suboptimal for bacterial growth. The
              amount of inorganic iron in the external and internal milieu
              is a critical factor regulating toxin production, which is
              depressed until the level of iron is critically reduced.
              (1) The capacity of *C. diphtheriae* to elaborate toxin comes
                    from the tox gene, which is carried by the beta-
                    bacteriophage. The tox gene is a prophage that
                    programs the structure of the toxin. The lysogenized
                    bacterial cells are responsible for toxin biosynthesis.
                    For maximum toxin production, phage multiplication must
                    be initiated and lysis delayed, since phage liberation
                    results in lysis of the bacteria with cessation of
                    toxin synthesis.
       2.   Tetanospasmin of *C. tetani*
       3.   Alpha toxin of *C. perfringens*
    C.   Effects of serum and iron on bacterial growth in vitro
       1.   Nonimmune serum may have a bacteriostatic effect, a bactericidal
           effect, or no effect on bacterial growth. Both the
           bacteriostatic and bacteriocidal effects can be abolished by
           saturation of the iron-binding capacity of serum transferrin with
           iron.
    D.   Bacterial mechanisms for acquiring iron from serum
       1.   Bacteria that can grow in serum must possess a specific mechanism
           for acquiring iron from partially saturated transferrin.

      a.   A direct interaction must take place between receptors on the bacterial cell and the iron transferrin complex.

      b.   Iron-chelating compounds of low molecular weight are secreted by the bacteria, which are capable of removing iron from the transferrin molecule. The resulting iron chelate is then taken up by the bacterial cells. These bacterial iron-binding compounds are called siderochromes. Their formation is sometimes induced by media with a low iron content.

           (1) Examples of siderochromes include aerobactin and enterobactin of *E. coli*, mycobactin of *M. tuberculosis*, and determinate P of *Y. pestis*.

           (2) Strains of *Y. pestis* with determinant P have the ability to acquire extracellular iron. This ability to acquire iron from the host is an essential virulence factor.

E.   Host iron and its availability to bacteria

   1.   A distinction must be made between various iron-containing compounds present in the host and their availability to bacteria.

      a.   The iron contained in ferratin, hemosiderin, hemoglobin, and myoglobin is not freely available to bacteria.

           (1) Bacterial hemolysins lyse red blood cells, releasing the iron-containing hemoglobin molecules and thus providing a potential source of iron for the bacterium.

      b.   The iron associated with transferrin and lactoferrin may become available to bacteria.

           (1) These two iron-binding proteins often play a critical role in host resistance to bacterial infections by making iron unavailable to bacteria.

           (2) Transferrin is present in serum and is a critical component in maintaining the homostasis of iron.

               (a) The antibacterial effects of serum appear to be due in part at least to the high affinity of transferrin for iron, which makes it almost completely unavailable as free iron.

               (b) Transferrin either alone or more usually in concert with specific antibody can have a powerful inhibitory effect on bacterial growth. When enough iron is added to saturate the iron-binding capacity of transferrin, the antibacterial activity of serum is greatly reduced. Antibody and complement cannot function effectively against most bacterial infections in the absence of unsaturated transferrin.

           (3) Lactoferrin is present in milk and some other body secretions.

F. Bacterial infection and iron
   1. The availability of iron to bacteria in injured or dead tissue is often significantly different from normal healthy tissue.
      a. The lysis of erythrocytes can provide large amounts of iron.
         (1) Bacterial hemolysins are often critical virulence factors.
      b. In conditions in which serum iron levels are elevated, such as hemolytic anemias, animals may become extremely susceptible to bacterial infection.
   2. Iron metabolism often undergoes change during the inflammatory processes induced by bacterial infections.
      a. The level of serum iron is decreased in most inflammatory processes.
         (1) Small amounts of endotoxin can cause a decrease of serum iron. Endotoxin appears to liberate iron-chelating compounds from the leukocytes.
         (2) Iron-free lactoferrin is released from areas of inflammation and possibly from the liver.

4	Pathology of Bacterial Diseases

The different types of inflammation, exudates, and lesions produced by pathogenic bacteria vary with the virulence and pathogenicity of the infective bacterium, resistance of the host, and the tissues affected. Most infections are caused by the normal bacterial flora.

I. NORMAL BACTERIAL FLORA
   A. Composition and clinical significance
      1. It is important for the veterinarian and clinical microbiologist to be aware of the normal bacterial flora of domestic animals. This knowledge aids in anticipating what organisms are most commonly associated with infections involving a given portal or anatomic source and is also useful in determining the potential clinical significance of isolates.
      2. The bacterial flora of healthy domestic animals is composed of both aerobic and anaerobic commensal and pathogenic bacteria that

exist in a symbiotic equilibrium. The presence of the commensals helps prevent the pathogenic bacteria from invading the host's tissues and producing disease.

    a.   The majority of bacterial infections of domestic animals are caused by bacterial species that are part of the permanent or transient normal flora.

        (1) Some bacterial species are regular members of the normal flora, and others seem to be associated almost exclusively with a state of disease.

        (2) Some of the bacterial species are almost ubiquitous on the skin, the various mucous membranes, or gastrointestinal tract of their specific domestic animal host or hosts. Other bacterial species have very specific ecologic preferences.

    b.   Treatment with broad spectrum antimicrobial drugs often disrupts the composition of the normal bacterial flora, causing changes that occasionally result in serious infection.

    c.   Aerobic and anaerobic bacteria reside as normal flora on the skin and mucous membrane surfaces of the nasal pharynx, oral pharynx, mouth, gastrointestinal tract, orifices of the external genitalia, urethra, and vagina.

        (1) Anaerobic bacteria are widely distributed in tissues that have a low oxygen tension and redox potential. With few exceptions, all the pathogenic anaerobic bacteria are part of the normal flora, and they are all opportunistic pathogens.

  B.   Distribution

    1.   Skin

        a.   Various anaerobic bacterial species constitute the majority of the skin flora, while the micrococci, staphylococci, and streptococci are the predominant aerobic bacteria.

           (1) The majority of the resident skin microflora are commensals and lack pathogenic potential.

           (2) The bacterial flora of the skin tends to exist in microcolonies of 10^2 to 10^3 organisms and is not evenly distributed.

        b.   The skin is an efficient barrier to bacterial invasion by either the resident microflora or exogenous bacteria from the environment, provided that the integrity of the skin is not breached.

    2.   Internal body organs

        a.   The internal body organs in healthy animals are sterile, except for the gastrointestinal tract.

           (1) The local and systemic host defense mechanisms effectively maintain the sterility of the internal body organs.

        b.   The mucous membranes of organ systems with a portal of exit to the external surfaces of the body often have a normal microbial flora.

3. Mucous membranes
    a. Alimentary tract
        (1) The tissues of the alimentary tract provide an enormous range of colonizable surfaces, extending from the keratinized epithelial cells of the stratified squamous tissues of the upper tract to the mucus-covered tissues of the intestine.
        (2) The upper alimentary tract, including the mouth, pharynx, and esophagus, has both a resident and transient bacterial flora.
            (a) The oral cavity is heavily colonized with bacteria, including specific pathogens that cause tooth decay and gingivitis.
            (b) The pharynx and esophagus have a similar microbial flora.
        (3) The gastrointestinal system has a very complex ecosystem of microorganisms (discussed in the gastrointestinal tract section).
    b. Respiratory system
        (1) The upper respiratory tract, particularly the nasal pharynx, is heavily colonized with bacteria, while the lower respiratory tract, including the trachea, bronchi, and bronchioles, is normally sterile or only transiently colonized by inhaled bacteria.
    c. Urinary tract
        (1) The urinary tract, except for the urethra, is normally sterile.
    d. Female genital system
        (1) The mucous membranes of the vagina and external cervix are heavily colonized with bacteria, but the remainder of the female genital tract is usually sterile.
        (2) The vaginal microbial flora includes aerobic and anaerobic bacteria, as well as mycoplasmas, ureaplasmas, and yeasts. The vaginal secretions may contain up to 10^8 bacteria/ml.
4. Gastrointestinal tract
    a. Establishment of the gastrointestinal flora
        (1) In the newborn domestic animal, bacteria can be found in the gastrointestinal tract within the first few hours of life. The first bacteria to colonize the intestines are *Escherichia coli*, other coliforms, streptococci, and some of the clostridia, including *C. perfringens*, followed by the lactobacilli. During the first few weeks of life, the many species of anaerobic bacteria that eventually form the major population of the lower small intestine, cecum, and large intestine

slowly become established. Anaerobic bacteria include the bacteroides, bifidobacteria, clostridia, eubacteria, fusobacteria, spirochetes, and anaerobic gram-positive and gram-negative cocci. These bacteria play an essential role in the health and well-being of an animal by preventing the establishment of pathogens, and once established, they remain throughout life, under normal condition.

(2) The young animal in which the intestinal anaerobes are not yet established is very susceptible to enteric infection.

b. Gastrointestinal flora of young and adult animals

(1) In monogastric animals, the empty stomach is sterile due to the gastric acidity, which precludes bacterial growth. The abomasum of the neonatal ruminant is similar to the stomach of monogastric animals.

(2) In ruminants, the microbial flora of the rumen, reticulum, and omasum is primarily composed of protozoa and a very complex bacterial flora, which varies markedly with the composition and energy content of the ration.

(3) The duodenum, jejunem, and upper ileum have a scanty bacterial flora compared with the lower ileum, cecum, and large intestine, which are heavily colonized with bacteria.

(4) There are two distinct bacteria populations within the digestive tracts of both monogastric and ruminant animals. The first occurs in the fluid phase as single cells or as floating colonies. These bacteria are often associated with or adhered to the ingesta. The second is adhered to the lining cells of the intestine and is often physiologically integrated into the overall chemical functions of the tissues.

(5) Obligate anaerobes make up approximately 99.9 percent of the intestinal flora; the majority of the remaining flora are facultative anaerobic, gram-negative enterics. The facultative anaerobes help maintain the anaerobic environment of the lower small intestine and large intestine by utilizing any free oxygen, thus lowering the redox potential and enabling the anaerobes to survive and proliferate.

(6) The types of microorganisms multiplying in the intestines depend on both dietary substances that are not digested and absorbed by the host and nutrients supplied directly by the host, including desquamated mucosal cells and protein and other substances secreted into the intestinal lumen.

5. Fecal flora
   a. Animals of the same species tend to have a similar type of fecal flora but show some differences from those of other species.

II. BACTERIA-INDUCED INFLAMMATORY PROCESSES
   A. Types of inflammation
   1. Serous inflammation
      a. Serous inflammation is often the initial response in an acute bacterial infection. The exudate is characterized by excessive fluid with a low content of protein and phagocytic cells and often precedes other types of exudate.
   2. Serofibrinous inflammation
      a. When strands of fibrin are found within the serous exudate, it is frequently referred to as serofibrinous inflammation.
   3. Fibrinous inflammation
      a. The exudate contains an excessive amount of fibrin.
         (1) Pasteurellae pneumonias are characterized by a fibrinous exudate.
   4. Catarrhal inflammation
      a. This a relatively mild inflammation involving a mucous membrane. The exudate is characterized by a profuse secretion of mucus with some destruction and desquamation of epithelial cells.
         (1) Mild gastrointestinal infections are often characterized by a catarrhal inflammation.
   5. Suppurative inflammation
      a. The infection causes an intense concentration of infiltrated neutrophils at the inflammatory focus and necrosis of host tissues. Pyogenic bacteria chemotactically attract phagocytic cells, which attempt to phagocytize and kill the bacteria. During this process, many neutrophils as well as some macrophages are lysed, liberating numerous enzymes and toxic compounds that damage host tissues.

III. BACTERIAL INFECTIONS OF BODY SYSTEMS AND TISSUES
   A. Integument
   1. Bacterial dermatitides include folliculitis, impetigo, and pyoderma.
      a. Folliculitis is an infection of the hair follicles.
      b. Impetigo is a superficial pustular dermatitis.
      c. Pyoderma is a skin disease characterized by a pustular exudate, which may be either superficial or deep.
   2. Bacterial dermatitides are often secondary to predisposing conditions that permit the normal bacterial flora to initiate an infection of the epidermis.
      a. The staphylococci and streptococci are the most common

etiologic agents of these nonspecific bacterial infections.
   3. Dermatophilosis
      a. *Dermatophilus congolensis* is the only bacterial pathogen of
         domestic animals that is restricted to the epidermis.
B. Subcutis and connective tissue
   1. Bacteria-induced abscesses can occur in any body organ or tissue
      but are most commonly found in the subcutaneous tissues.
      a. Abscesses frequently result from the spread of contiguous
         infections.
      b. Abscesses may become encapsulated by fibrous connective
         tissues or form fistular draining tracts.
   2. Cellulitis is characterized as a diffuse bacterial infection of
      connective tissue with a rapid spread in subcutaneous tissues and
      fascial planes.
      a. The clostridia are commonly incriminated as agents of
         cellulitis.
C. Circulatory system
   1. Blood
      a. Extracellular and facultative intracellular bacteria
         (1) Bacteremia is a disease condition in which
             extracellular bacteria are present in the blood. The
             affected animal may or may not be symptomatic.
         (2) Septicemia is a disease condition in which
             extracellular bacteria are present in the blood and the
             affected animal is symptomatic.
         (3) Toxemia is the presence of toxins in the blood. The
             toxins may be either endotoxins or exotoxins.
             (a) Endotoxemia is the presence of bacterial
                 endotoxins in the blood. Lipid A is responsible
                 for the nonspecific endotoxic activity of the
                 lipopolysaccharide found in gram-negative
                 bacterial cell walls.
             (b) Most bacterial exotoxins are protein and have a
                 specific toxic effect on the host.
      b. Obligate intracelluar and cell-associated bacteria
         (1) Erythrocytes are parasitized by bacteria in the genera
             Anaplasma, *Eperythrozoon*, and *Haemobartonella*.
         (2) Leukocytes are parasitized by bacteria in the genera
             Ehrlichia and *Neorickettsia*.
   2. Blood vessels
      a. Vascular endothelial cells are parasitized by *Cowdria*
         ruminantium, *Coxiella burnetii*, and *Rickettsia rickettsii*.
         These obligate intracellular gram-negative bacteria
         proliferate in the vascular endothelial cells, causing a
         vasculitis.
   3. Heart and pericardium
      a. Endocardium

(1) Mural and valvular endocarditis result from the bacterial localization on and colonization of the endocardium and heart valves. The mechanisms by which bacteria localize on the endocardium and heart valves of domestic animals have not been clearly delineated, but it has been postulated that damaged endothelium and recurrent bacteremia are required to initiate the lesions.

(2) Common etiologic agents are *Erysipelothrix rhusiopathiae* and the group D streptococci.

b. Myocardium

(1) Bacterial myocarditis occurs in a variety of systemic diseases, due to the hematogenous dissemination of the organisms, or is initiated by direct extension from bacterial lesions of the endocardium and pericardium. Primary bacterial myocarditis is rare, but traumatic pericarditis and myocarditis resulting from the penetration of foreign bodies from the reticulum occurs frequently in the bovine.

c. Pericardium

(1) Bacterial pericarditis is often the result of hematogenous infection, but it also may be initiated by traumatic permeation from an infectious process in adjacent tissue. The pericardial exudate is either purulent or fibrinous in character.

D. Musculoskeletal system

1. Skeletal muscle

a. Bacterial infections of skeletal muscle (myositis) are most often acquired when exogenous bacteria implanted in muscle from penetrating wounds but also may result from the extension of an infectious process in contiguous tissues.

(1) Primary infection of skeletal muscle is exemplified by blackleg, which is caused by *Clostridium chauvoei*.

(2) Secondary myositis can be caused by a variety of bacterial species, including pathogens in the genera *Staphylococcus* and *Streptococcus*.

2. Bones

a. Osteomyelitis is a bacterial infection of the bone marrow. Most infections are acquired via the hematogenous route.

b. Bacterial infections of bone (osteitis) can result either from systemic infections that localize in bone or from trauma, such as fractures infected with either the endogenous bacterial flora or exogenous bacteria. Osteomyelitis often occurs concurrently with osteitis.

(1) Systemic infections that localize in bone and result in an osteitis include brucellosis and tuberculosis. Spondylitis due to *Brucella suis* is common in swine.

(2) Traumatic implantation of *Actinomyces bovis* in the jawbones of cattle results in a proliferative osteomyelitis.

3. Joints
   a. Bacteria-induced arthritis primarily affects the articular cartilages, synovial membranes, and joint capsule.
   b. Bacteria may enter a joint from the blood, from a focus of infection in adjacent soft tissues and bone, or through a puncture wound. Most arthritides are hematogenous in origin, and the direct spread of infection from adjacent tissue to joints is uncommon.
   c. Hematogenous polyarthritis is a common sequela to navel ill in calves, foals, and piglets.
      (1) Hematogenous bacteria localize in the synovial layer of the articular capsule with subsequent penetration into the joint. Most infections result from an intermittent or sustained bacteremia. The arthritis is intially polyarticular, but many joints clear the infection and only the larger joints of the limbs tend to have progressive infections. The arthritis is usually characterized by either a purulent or fibrinous inflammation, depending on the bacterial agent. Bacteria in the genus *Staphylococcus* and *Actinomyces pyogenes* produce a purulent reaction, and bacteria in the genus *Streptococcus* produce a fibrinous exudate.

E. Respiratory system
   1. Upper respiratory infections
      a. Nasal mucosa
         (1) Inflammation of the nasal mucosa is termed rhinitis.
         (2) Porcine atrophic rhinitis is caused by *Bordetella bronchiseptica*. The infection causes inflammation of the nasal mucous membranes and hypoplasia of the nasal turbinates.
      b. Trachea and bronchi
         (1) Bacterial infections of the trachea, bronchi, or both the trachea and bronchi, are called tracheitis, bronchitis, and tracheobronchitis, respectively.
         (2) *B. bronchiseptica* can cause a primary tracheobronchitis in dogs. The bacteria colonize the epithelial lining of the trachea and primary bronchi but do not invade beyond the basement membrane.
   2. Lower respiratory infections
      a. Lungs
         (1) Pneumonia is a term used to describe inflammatory processes and lesions of the lung.
         (2) The distribution of bacteria-induced pneumonic lesions is largely dependent on the route of infection.

Pathogenic bacteria can enter the lungs either via the bronchogenous or the hematogenous route.

(3) Most infections are acquired by inhalation.

    (a) The lower respiratory tract is constantly exposed to bacteria inhaled on dust particles or aerosolized from the nasal, oral, and pharyngeal mucosa in droplet nuclei. Most of these bacteria, however, impact on the respiratory membranes that line the nasal passages, trachea, bronchi, and bronchioles and are rapidly removed or inactivated by the pulmonary clearance mechanisms. Some bacteria may reach the alveoli, where most are phagocytized and killed by pulmonary alveolar macrophages. When these host defense mechanisms fail, bronchopneumonia may result.

    (b) Bronchopneumonias, in which the anterior and ventral portions of the lungs are the first and most extensively affected, are acquired via the bronchi. The inhaled bacteria initiate a focus of infection around the infected bronchiole. The pneumonic area may eventually involve the entire lobule supplied by the bronchiole. The pneumonic processes in the apical and cardiac lobes may progress and eventually involve the anterior part of the diaphragmatic lobes.

(4) Pneumonic lesions, which are initiated via the hematogenous route, are distributed through the pulmonary parenchyma.

(5) Types of pneumonic lesions

    (a) Suppurative pneumonias are generally caused by pyogenic bacteria. The cellular exudate is primarily composed of neutrophils.

    (b) Fibrinous pneumonias are often caused by *Pasteurella* species and *Staphylococcus* species. Fibrin and neutrophils predominate in the exudate. Most extracellular bacteria cause fibrinous pneumonias.

    (c) Interstitial pneumonic lesions are often caused by *Chlamydia psittaci* and *Mycoplasma* species.

    (d) Lung abscesses can form in hepatized tissues as sequelae to pneumonia or from hematogenous bacterial emboli. The emboli are scattered throughout both lungs, but the largest number of foci establish infections near the pleural surface.

(6) Bacteria-induced pneumonic lesions tend to be similar regardless of the causative bacterium and progress through four successive stages.

(a) The congestive stage, which develops within hours
     after the pathogenic bacteria establish an
     infectious focus, is characterized by hyperemia,
     and the alveoli are filled with a serous exudate.
     After about 2 days, the red hepatization stage
     develops in the consolidated areas of the lungs.
     Red hepatization results from the hemorrhage by
     diapedesis into the alveoli. The cellular exudate
     is composed of erythrocytes, lymphocytes,
     macrophages, and neutrophils. Gray hepatization
     represents the stage between the initial
     consolidation of the affected lung tissue and
     resolution of the lesions. The alveoli are filled
     with leukocytes and fibrin. Under normal
     conditions, the resolution of the pneumonic
     lesions begin about 1 week after the onset of the
     pneumonias. The bacterial pathogens are cleared,
     and the fibrin and leukocytes that filled the
     alveoli are gradually removed.

b. Pleura
    (1) Bacterial pleuritis may result from direct extension
         from the lung infections or by the hematogenous route
         without involvement of the pulmonary parenchyma.
         (a) The pleural exudate may be serous, purulent,
              fibrinous, or fibrinopurulent.
    (2) Pyothorax results from the accumulation of a pleural
         exudate in the pleural cavity.
         (a) Canine pyothorax is commonly caused by *Actinomyces
              viscosus* and *Nocardia asteroides*. These bacteria
              produce a pyogranulomatous exudate.

F. Alimentary infections
    1. Upper alimentary infections
        a. Oral cavity
            (1) Inflammatory processes of the oral mucosa, gums,
                 pharynx, tongue, and tonsils are called stomatitis,
                 gingivitis, pharyngitis, glossitis, and tonsilitis,
                 respectively. In bacterial infections, the lymphoid
                 tissues of the palate, pharyngeal mucosa, and tonsils
                 are often edematous and hyperplastic.
            (2) The inflammatory reactions may be catarrhal,
                 diphtheretic, purulent, or ulcerative.
                 (a) Catarrhal stomatitis is a mild superficial
                      inflammation that may progress to a purulent or
                      ulcerative stomatitis.
                 (b) A diphtheritic membrane forms on the pharyngeal
                      mucosa in calf diphtheria.
        b. Esophagus
            (1) Bacteria-induced esophagitis is rare in domestic
                 animals.

2. Lower alimentary infections
   a. Forestomachs of ruminants
      (1) Inflammatory processes of the reticulum and rumen are called reticulitis and rumenitis, respectively.
      (2) Rumenitis with ulceration of the epithelium allows the colonization of these lesions by the normal rumen microflora.
         (a) Ruminal lesions are the primary foci of infection in the bovine rumenitis-liver abscess complex. The ruminal acidosis is caused by overeating of high-carbohydrate rations.
      (3) Traumatic reticuloperitonitis, in which the reticulum is perforated by foreign bodies, is almost always followed by a local or diffuse bacterial peritonitis and occasionally by a pericarditis.
         (a) *A. pyogenes* and *Fusobacterium necrophorum* are commonly isolated from the purulent exudate.
   b. Stomach and intestines
      (1) Gastritis refers to an inflammatory process of the stomach of monogastric animals or the abomasum of ruminants, while enteritis applies generally to an inflammation of any portion of the intestine but common usage frequently refers only to the small intestine.
         (a) Bacteria-induced conditions involving both the stomach and intestines are referred to as gastroenteritis and of both the small and large intestines as enterocolitis.
         (b) Inflammatory processes of the colon and rectum are called colitis and proctitis, respectively.
      (2) Enteric infections are induced either by ingestion of pathogens or by proliferation of indigenous microflora to an infective dose level.
         (a) Bacterial pathogens commonly ingested include *E. coli, Salmonella* serovars, and *Treponema hyodysenteriae*.
         (b) Endogenous bacterial flora, which can proliferate and produce enteric disease, includes *E. coli, Salmonella* serovars, and *C. perfringens*.
      (3) Most bacterial enteric infections are characterized by one of the following: diarrhea, dysentery, enterotoxicosis, or enterotoxemia.
G. Liver, gall bladder, and bile ducts
   1. Liver
      a. Inflammation of the hepatic parenchyma is termed hepatitis.
      b. Bacteria can gain entrance into the hepatic parenchyma by several routes.
         (1) Hematogenous bacteria are transported to the liver via the hepatic artery, portal veins, or umbilical veins.
            (a) Bovine liver abscesses are initiated by bacterial

emboli containing *F. necrophorum* via the hepatic portal system from the primary infectious foci in the ruminal wall.

 (b) Neonatal bacterial hepatitis is a common sequela of umbilical infections when bacteria are transported by umbilical vessels from an infected umbilicus.

 (2) Ascending bacteria via the bile ducts can initiate a bacterial hepatitis.

 (3) Bacteria are implanted into the hepatic parenchyma by foreign bodies.

  (a) Foreign body penetration of the liver from the reticulum of cattle and sheep is common.

 (4) Contiguous infections in the peritoneal cavity can invade the capsule of the liver.

 2. Gall bladder and bile ducts

  a. Inflammation of the gall bladder and bile ducts is termed cholecystitis and chalangitis, respectively. These conditions can be initiated either by hematogenous bacteria or by bacteria that ascend the ducts from the intestine.

H. Urinary system

 1. Kidneys

  a. Nephritis is a general term referring to any inflammatory process that may involve one or both kidneys, whereas inflammation primarily of the glomerular tufts, interstitial tissue, and renal pelvis is termed glomerulitis, interstitial nephritis, and pyelonephritis, respectively. Diffuse glomerulitis affecting the glomeruli in both kidneys is commonly termed glomerulonephritis.

  b. Most infections are acquired via the hematogenous route, but some may result via ascending infections from the ureters.

  c. Diseases

   (1) Glomerulonephritis occurs in a variety of infectious diseases, especially porcine erysipelas, salmonellosis, and streptococcal infections.

   (2) Interstitial nephritis is commonly associated with *Leptospira canicola* infections in dogs.

   (3) Pyelonephritis is commonly caused by *Corynebacterium renale* in cattle, in which the bacteria adhere to the epithelium of the renal pelvis by fimbriae.

 2. Urinary bladder

  a. The majority of bacteria-induced urinary bladder infections (cystitis) are acquired via ascending infections through the ureters, but cystitis of hematogenous origin can occur.

  b. Cystitis occurs in all domestic animal species by a variety of bacteria. The most common agents include *E. coli*, *Proteus* species, other coliforms, staphylococci, and streptococci.

I. Female genital system
    1. Vagina and cervix
        a. Bacterial infection of the vagina and cervix are termed
            vaginitis and cervicitis, respectively. Most infections
            result in a cervicovaginitis and are acquired from an
            extension of an endometritis or from exogenous bacteria
            entering through the orifice of the vulva. A few infections
            are acquired hematogenously.
            (1) Cervicitis is not considered to be a separate entity
                 and generally results from an extension of a metritis
                 or vaginitis.
        b. Bacteria-induced exudates of cervicovaginitis are usually
            catarrhal in nature but may be serous or fibrinopurulent.
    2. Uterus
        a. Endometritis is a term used to describe bacterial infections
            of the endometrium. Most uterine infections are initiated
            as an endometritis, in which the uterine mucosa is mainly
            involved, but many infections progress to involve other
            tissues of the uterus.
            (1) *Campylobacter fetus* ss *venerealis* infections of the cow
                 are manifested as a mild endometritis with very little
                 involvement of uterine tissues other than the uterine
                 mucosa.
        b. Metritis infers involvement of the entire wall of the uterus
            and often is characterized by a purulent exudate. Common
            complications and sequelae of metritis are uterine abscess,
            pyometra, and salpingitis.
            (1) Pyometra is an accumulation of pus in the uterine lumen
                 and is characterized as an acute or chronic suppurative
                 infection. Pyometra occasionally occurs in the bitch,
                 cow, and queen but is rare in the ewe, mare, and sow.
    3. Oviducts
        a. Bacterial salpingitis, an inflammation of the oviducts, is
            usually bilateral and secondary to an infection in the
            uterus. Bacterial infections of the Fallopian tubes are
            more common in the cow and sow than in other domestic
            animals.
J. Mammary glands
    1. Bacteria-induced inflammation and infection of the mammary glands
        (mastitis) occurs in all species of domestic animals, but the
        primary economic impact is in dairy cows.
    2. Bovine mastitis
        a. Mastitis in dairy cows can be caused by more than 50 species
            of bacteria. The majority of the infections are caused by
            Streptococcus agalactiae, other streptococci, and
            Staphylococcus aureus. Other common agents include *E. coli*,
            Klebsiella pneumoniae, other coliforms, *Pasteurella* species,
            and *Pseudomonas aeruginosa.*

(1) The portal of entry for most infections is the teat orifice and canal. Brucellosis and tuberculosis are generally acquired by the hematogenous route, as are infections produced by the enterobacteria that occur secondarily to a puerperal infection of the uterus.

3. Canine and feline mastitis

   a. Most of the cases of bacteria-induced mastitis of bitches and queens are caused by the staphylococci and streptococci, and most infections gain entrance via tissues in the nipples and adjacent skin. The primary infections frequently spread by the lymphatics to involve adjacent glands.

4. Equine mastitis

   a. Clinical mastitis in the mare occasionally occurs, and most infections are acquired by the teat orifice and canal. The staphylococci, streptococci, and enterobacteria are commonly incriminated.

5. Ovine mastitis

   a. Commonly isolated bacteria from ewes include *Mycoplasma agalactiae*, *Pasteurella haemolytica*, and *S. aureus*.

6. Porcine mastitis

   a. Acute mastitis in sows commonly occurs shortly after parturition, and coliforms are frequently incriminated. *S. aureus* may produce a chronic granulomatous mastitis, particularly in older sows.

K. Male genital system

   1. Inflammation of the epididymis, prostate, seminal vesicles, spermatic cord, and testes is termed epididymitis, prostatitis, seminal vesiculitis, funiculitis, and orchitis, respectively. Inflammation involving both the penis and prepuce is called balanoposthitis.

   2. Bacterial infections of the various tissues and organs of the male genital system can develop either hematogenously or by ascending infection through various ducts and accessory glands.

      a. In ascending infections, an epididymitis precedes the orchitis. An epididymitis and orchitis frequently coexist.

L. Central nervous system

   1. Inflammatory processes involving the brain, spinal cord, both the brain and spinal cord, and meninges are called encephalitis, myelitis, encephalomyelitis, and meningitis, respectively.

   2. Bacteria can invade the central nervous system by various routes.

      a. Bacteria can reach the central nervous system via the peripheral nerves.

         (1) *Listeria monocytogenes* can invade the brain stem along the cranial nerves in the perineural lymphatics of the trigeminal and facial nerves. These infections produce characteristic microabscesses in the brain stem.

      b. Bacteria can be implanted directly in penetrating injuries or during surgical procedures.

        c.   Some bacterial infections of the central nervous system result from the direct extension of infections in adjacent tissues either by extension along the peripheral nerves or by erosion of the bone encasing the brain and spinal cord.

        d.   Bacteria can reach the central nervous system via the hematogenous route.

           (1) Although many bacteria are found in bacteremias and septicemias, only a few bacterial species and strains are highly invasive for the central nervous system.

M. Eyes

    1. Inflammation of the conjunctiva and cornea are called conjunctivitis and keratitis, respectively. When both the conjunctiva and cornea are involved, the condition is termed keratoconjunctivitis.

    2. Conjunctivitis frequently occurs in domestic animals without concurrent involvement of the cornea; however, in severe cases of conjunctivitis a keratitis commonly occurs.

        a.   Most bacterial infections are acquired from either endogenous ocular flora or exogenous bacteria.

N. Ear

    1. Otitis externa, an inflammation of the outer ear, commonly occurs in dogs and cats.

        a.   Common bacterial pathogens include *P. aeruginosa*, *Proteus* species, and staphylococci.

    2. Otitis media is an inflammation of the middle ear (tympanic cavity), which is separated from the external ear by the tympanic membrane and connects to the pharynx by the Eustachian tube.

        a.   Most bacterial infections occur via penetration of the tympanic membrane or ascend the Eustachian tube from the pharynx. Hematogenously acquired infections are considered to be rare in domestic animals.

5	Bacterial Infection and Immunity

Bacterial infectious diseases are complex interactions between bacteria and host, each seeking survival within one ecosystem. The effect of bacterial infectious disease is the sum of microbial activity plus the associated host response. Interfacing the bacterial virulence factors and the host's immune mechanisms help to explain the host bacterial interaction and therefore the pathogenicity of bacterial disease.

I. ROLE OF LEUKOCYTES IN BACTERIAL INFECTIONS
  A. Granulocytic cells
    1. Neutrophils are the most important population of granulocytic phagocytes involved in host defense against invading bacteria and are most effective in extravascular tissues. Neutrophils are the primary cells responsible for the containment and elimination of acute bacterial infections that invade the body, especially infections caused by extracellular pyogenic bacteria.
    2. Eosinophils possess an innate capacity to phagocytize particulate matter but are seldom able to phagocytize and kill most common bacterial pathogens.
    3. Basophils like eosinophils do not play a significant role in the host's antibacterial defense.
  B. Monocytes and macrophages
    1. Monocytes and macrophages are effective phagocytic cells and are generally regarded as the first line of defense against facultative intracellular and obligate intracellular bacteria, such as *Brucella abortus*, *Chlamydia psittaci*, *Listeria monocytogenes*, *Mycobacaterium bovis*, and *Salmonella typhimurium*.
    2. Monocytes are found in the peripheral blood but are more effective against invading bacteria once they have migrated into the tissues and have become macrophages.
      a. Monocytes and macrophages are aided in phagocytosis by surface receptors for some immunoglobulin classes and complement components that bind to bacteria opsonized with immunoglobulin or complement.
    3. Macrophages occur in the tissues both as free cells, which can migrate throughout the body, or as fixed cells in specialized tissues and organs.
      a. Fixed macrophages are called histocytes in connective tissue, Kupffer cells in the liver, and alveolar macrophages in the lungs.
      b. Bone marrow, lymph nodes, spleen, and the central nervous system contain both fixed and free macrophages.

4. Macrophages are the predominant phagocytic cell found in most chronic infections and in those infections caused by facultative intracellular pathogens.
   a. Macrophages can serve as effector cells in both nonspecific and specifically acquired cell-mediated immunity. These macrophages have acquired an increased bactericidal ability.

C. Lymphocytes
   1. Lymphocytes cannot phagocytize bacteria.
   2. B-lymphocytes (B-cells) can differentiate into plasma cells, which produce immunoglobulins.
      a. Humoral immunity plays a significant role in defense against extracellular bacterial infections, and to a lesser extent in facultative intracellular and obligate intracellular bacterial infections.
   3. T-lymphocytes (T-cells) can serve a variety of functions in cell-mediated immune responses.
      a. Cell-mediated immunity often is important in defense against facultative intracellular and obligate intracellular bacterial infections.

II. NEUTROPHILS AND PHAGOCYTOSIS

A. Three factors are necessary for neutrophils to be effective in host defenses.
   1. The neutrophils must migrate to the area of infection.
      a. Neutrophils diapedese from the peripheral blood into tissues and are attracted along chemotactic gradients to the proximity of the invading bacteria. The rapid accumulation of neutrophils at the infected site follows the release of a variety of chemotactic factors during acute bacterial infections.
      b. Cytotaxins are substances that directly stimulate the directional migration of phagocytic cells. Cytotaxins include various components of complement and numerous products from bacteria and damaged tissue cells.
      c. Cytotaxigens are substances that cause a chemical change in a noncytotaxin, thus converting it to a cytotaxin. Enzymes, which serve as cytotaxigens, include trypsin, collagenases, plasmin, and proteases from bacteria, macrophages, and tissues. Nonenzymatic cytotaxigens include antigen-antibody complexes, aggregrated immunoglobulins, and bacterial lipopolysaccharides.
   2. The neutrophils must phagocytize the bacteria.
      a. The phagocytosis of most pathogenic bacteria require serum factors, especially antibacterial antibody and complement, whereas most nonpathogenic bacteria are readily phagocytized in the absence of serum.
      b. Various opsonins can alter the surface of the bacterium so as to make it bind to the phagocyte. Opsonins present in

serum include natural antibody, immune antibody, and the C3b
fragment of complement, which bind to specific receptors on
phagocytic cells.

    c.   Natural antibody is predominantly IgM and is considered to
arise in response to repeated antigenic stimulation by the
intestinal microflora.

    d.   Immune antibody is primarily IgM and IgG and is specific to
the inducing bacterial antigens.

    e.   During bacterial infection the alternate complement pathway,
which can be activated by bacterial lipopolysaccharides,
provides a major source of C3b.

    f.   The phagocytosis of the bacteria occurs rapidly following
the attachment to the phagocyte cell membrane. The
phagosome is formed by the invagination of the plasma
membrane to surround the attached bacterium, followed by the
separation of the phagosome from the newly constituted
membrane of the phagocyte.

  3. The neutrophils must kill the phagocytized bacteria.

    a.   Neutrophils possess numerous bactericidal mechanisms, which
often operate simultaneously.

    b.   Neutrophils exert a metabolic burst during phagocytosis,
resulting in the production of hydrogen peroxide. Two
metabolic pathways produce the reduced coenzymes NADH and
NADPH, which are required to produce hydrogen peroxide.
The glycolytic pathway produces NADH, and the hexose
monophosphate shunt produces NADPH. The NADH is used
primarily to reduce pyruvic acid to lactic acid, but only a
small quantity is used in the formation of hydrogen
peroxide. The hexose monophosphate shunt produces large
amounts of NADPH for hydrogen peroxide production. The
hydrogen peroxide diffuses from the cytoplasm into the
phagolysosomes, where the myelperoxidase-halide system
produces hypochloride, a strong oxidizing agent that is
bactericidal for most pathogens.

    c.   Lysosomes contain numerous hydrolytic enzymes and
antibacterial compounds. Lysosomes fuse with phagosomes
containing bacteria and release their contents into the
newly formed phagolysosomes.

      (1) Basic proteins become attached to and inhibit the
multiplication of some bacterial species.

      (2) Lactoferrin, an iron-binding protein, is bacteriostatic
when not fully saturated with iron.

      (3) Lysozyme kills some bacteria by itself and collaborate
with antibody and complement in killing others.

III. HOST IMMUNE RESPONSES TO BACTERIAL INFECTIONS

  A. Humoral and cell-mediated immunity

    1. Most naturally acquired bacterial infections elicit both a
humoral and a cellular immune response; however, one or the other

predominates for different types of host-bacteria relationships.
   a. Pyogenic bacteria, which multiply extracellularly, are
       normally effectively dealt with by a humoral immune response
       in concert with polymorphonuclear leukocytes. Extracellular
       pyogenic bacteria induce purulent lesions.
   b. Facultative intracellular bacteria (e.g., *B. abortus*, *M.
       bovis*, and *S. typhimurium*) and obligate intracellular
       bacteria (e.g., *C. psittaci*) that are able to successfully
       parasitize host mononuclear phagocytes elicit a more
       prominent cellular immune response. These intracellular
       pathogens tend to induce granulomatous lesions.
       (1) Bacterial pathogens (e.g., *C. psittaci* and *M. bovis*)
           can inhibit fusion of the phagosome with lysosomes and
           are able to survive within unfused host phagosomes.
           Specific antibody to these bacterial pathogens
           promotes phagolysosomal fusion, possibly by
           neutralizing a surface component of the bacterial cell
           that inhibits fusion.
2. The immune response to bacteria represents a means by which the
   host is able to focus the inflammatory response to eliminate
   bacteria with minimum damage to host tissue; for many bacterial
   infections, however, the immune response produces tissue injury
   and the clinical manifestations of inflammatory disease.
   a. In many acute and chronic bacterial infections, the host
       immune responses are suppressed.
       (1) Anergy may occur in the terminal stages of
           tuberculosis.
B. Secretory immunity
   1. The antibacterial activity of sIgA on mucosal surfaces is the
       inhibition of bacterial adherence to epithelial surfaces.
       a. Much of the sIgA found on mucosal surfaces is synthesized
           locally in plasma cells located beneath the mucosal
           epithelium.
       b. Some serum IgA is actively exported as sIgA at various
           mucosal sites of the body.
C. Complement
   1. The classical complement pathway can be activated following
       attachment of IgM and selected subclasses of IgG antibody to
       bacteria.
   2. The alternate complement pathway can be activated by endotoxins
       of gram-negative bacteria.

IV. ACQUIRED RESISTANCE TO BACTERIAL INFECTIONS
A. Extracellular bacteria
   1. The acquired resistance to extracellular bacterial infections is
       primarily dependent on humoral antibodies. Three mechanisms are
       normally effective in providing protective immunity to these
       infections.
       a. Opsonizing antibodies enhance the phagocytosis of the

infective bacteria by neutrophils and macrophages.
b.   Toxin-neutralizing antibodies neutralize the biological effects of bacterial exotoxins but do not affect the growth of the bacteria.
c.   Specific antibodies to bacterial surface antigens are capable of fixing complement and killing the bacteria.
   (1) The attachment of both antibody and complement to bacteria provides optimal conditions for phagocytosis by leukocytes, particularly neutrophils and macrophages.
      (a) Some bacteria have cell walls that activate complement by the alternate pathway, allowing phagocytosis in the absence of antibody.
   (2) Most gram-negative bacterial pathogens are lysed by these complement-fixing antibodies, whereas gram-positive bacteria are seldom lysed.
B.   Facultative intracellular and obligate intracellular bacteria
   1.   The acquired resistance to bacterial pathogens that are capable of intracellular survival and proliferation within host cells is largely dependent on cell-mediated immunity.
     a.   Serum antibodies produced during the course of these infections merely indicates exposure to antigen but does not necessarily connote protective immunity.
   2.   Bacteria that are facultative intracellular pathogens include *Brucella*, *Listeria*, *Mycobacterium*, and *Salmonella*, while bacteria that are obligate intracellular pathogens include the genera in the families Chlamydiaceae and Rickettsiaceae.

V. HUMORAL IMMUNITY
  A.   Antibody responses to bacterial antigens
    1.   Thymus-independent bacterial antigens
      a.   The antibody responses to certain bacterial antigens, such as capsular polysaccharides and lipopolysaccharides of gram-negative bacteria, are thymus-independent. The primary antibody responses are in the IgM class.
    2.   Thymus-dependent bacterial antigens
      a.   The antibody responses to most protein bacterial antigens, such as outer membrane proteins and protein exotoxins, are thymus-dependent. The primary antibody responses are in the IgM and IgG classes.
    3.   Systemic and secretory antibodies (Table 5.1)
      a.   Systemic antibodies against bacterial infections include IgM, IgG, and IgA. The site of action of these immunoglobulin classes are all organs and tissues accessible to blood vascular fluids.
      b.   Secretory antibodies against bacterial infections include sIgA and sIgM. The site of action of these immunoglobulins are the external surfaces of mucous membranes, including the gastrointestinal, respiratory, and urogenital tracts.

Table 5.1. Protective mechanisms of systemic and secretory antibodies

Characteristic	Humoral Components	
	Systemic	Secretory
Major immunoglobulin classes	IgM, IgG	sIgA
Opsonization	+	+
Agglutination	+	+
Toxin neutralization	+	+
Prevents bacterial adherence to mucous membranes	-	+

4. Comparative in vivo activity of IgG and IgM
   a. The opsonization ability of IgM on a molar basis is approximately 500 to 1000 times more effective than IgG.
   b. The complement-mediated bacterial lytic activity of IgM on a molar basis is approximately 100 times more effective than IgG.
B. Serologic tests (Table 5.2)
C. Passive immunity
   1. Sources of serum antibodies (Table 5.3)
      a. Transplacentally acquired antibodies
         (1) The nature of the placental barrier determines the amount of IgG, if any, acquired by the in utero fetus.
      b. Colostrum-acquired antibodies
         (1) Newborn domestic animals can absorb IgG in the colostrum for 24 to 36 hours after parturition.

Table 5.2. Role of serum immunoglobulin classes in serologic tests

Immunoglobulin Kinetics	Immunoglobulin Classes		
	IgM	IgG	IgA
First appearance of detectable Ab after Ag exposure	2-5 days	3-7 days	3-7 days
Maximum titers attained	5-14 days	7-21 days	7-14 days
Serologic Tests			
Precipitation	+	+++	±
Agglutination	+++	+	+
Complement-fixation	+++	+	-
Neutralization	++	+	+

Note: - = no reaction; ± = negative or very slight reaction; + = weak reaction; ++ = moderate reaction; +++ = strong reaction.

Table 5.3. Placenta types and sources of passively acquired antibodies in domestic animals

Species	Placenta Type	Sources of Serum IgG[a]	
		Transplacental	Colostral
Bovine	Syndesmochorial	0	100
Canine	Endotheliochorial	5-10	90-95
Equine	Epitheliochorial	0	100
Feline	Endotheliochorial	5-10	90-95
Ovine	Syndesmochorial	0	100
Porcine	Epitheliochorial	0	100

[a]Percentage of total serum antibody.

2. Sources of intestinal antibodies (Table 5.4)
D. Active immunity
1. Active immunity is acquired by an animal as a result of its own
   response to pathogenic bacteria or their products, either through
   infection or immunization.

Table 5.4. Antibody composition of colostrum and milk in
domestic animals

Species	Colostrum[a]			Milk		
	IgM	IgG	sIgA	IgM	IgG	sIgA
Bovine	+	++++	++	±	++++	++++
Canine	+	++++	++	±	+[b]	++++
Equine	+	++++	++	±	+[b]	++++
Feline	+	++++	++	±	+[b]	++++
Ovine	+	++++	++	±	++++	+
Porcine	+	++++	++	±	+[b]	+

[a]Colostrum represents the accumulated secretions of
the mammary gland over the last few weeks of pregnancy.
The colostrum is generally nursed out by 48 hours after
parturition and is replaced by milk.
[b]In nonruminants, the IgG concentration drops
rapidly as lactation proceeds.

VI. CELL-MEDIATED IMMUNITY
A. Cellular or cell-mediated immune (CMI) reactions are mediated by T-
   lymphocytes independent of antibody and are especially important in
   providing protective immunity to facultative intracellular and
   obligate intracellular bacterial pathogens.
   1. These intracellular bacterial infections are characterized by
      host granulomatous reactions and/or bacterial multiplication
      within host mononuclear phagocytes.
B. Characteristics of acquired cellular resistance
   1. Immune granuloma formation is closely correlated with delayed-
      type hypersensitivity (DTH) reactions.
      a. The development of DTH in the host correlates with the onset
         of antibacterial processes in brucellosis, listeriosis,
         mycobacteriosis, and salmonellosis.
   2. The acquired resistance to these bacterial infections is a
      nonspecific expression of activated monocytes and macrophages
      with an increased bacterial activity despite an immunologically
      specific induction.
      a. The T-lymphocytes actively secrete lymphokines that recruit
         and activate mononuclear phagocytes. These stimulated
         monocytes and macrophages undergo a marked increase in
         bactericidal activity.
      b. The efficient induction of T-lymphocyte DTH occurs by
         challenge with living bacteria only.
   3. The passive transfer of specific resistance occurs only with
      immune T-lymphocytes, not with serum antibody.

VII. BACTERINS AND VACCINES

A. Four types of bacterial vaccines are used to induce protective immunity in domestic animals and man. The mode of action and protective immunogens of the different types of vaccines are based on a fundamental knowledge of the mechanisms of acquired resistance and an understanding of the pathogenesis of bacterial infections.

  1. Bacterins
  a. Bacterins composed of whole killed bacteria elicit a humoral immune response and are used for immunoprophylaxis and occasionally immunotherapy for bacterial infections in which serum antibody appears important for protection. The whole killed bacteria present a variety of antigenic stimuli to the immunized animal, but often only one or a few bacterial antigens are protective immunogens.
    (1) Clostridial bacterins, such as *Clostridium chauvoei* and *C. septicum*, provide almost 100 percent protection from blackleg and malignant edema in cattle and sheep.
    (2) *Campylobacter fetus* ss *venerealis* bacterins are used to immunize cows for bovine campylobacteriosis and *C. fetus* ss *fetus* bacterins to immunize ewes for ovine epizootic abortion.

  2. Live attenuated bacterial vaccines
  a. Parentally administered live attenuated bacterial vaccines elicit both cellular and humoral immune responses and are most frequently used for facultative intracellular pathogens, which survive and multiply within host mononuclear phagocytes. Cell-mediated immunity is required to eliminate facultative and obligate intracellular pathogens, and humoral immunity plays little, if any, protective role in these infections.
    (1) *B. abortus* strain 19 is used in the United States to immunize cows against bovine brucellosis.
    (2) The Bacillus Calmette-Guerin (BCG) strain of *M. bovis* is occasionally used in tuberculosis endemic areas to immunize humans against the tubercle bacilli.
  b. Oral administration of live bacterial vaccines to enteric pathogens are used to stimulate an effective secretory immune response on the mucosal surfaces of the intestine. The sIgA prevents the colonization of pathogenic strains of the bacterium.
    (1) Enterotoxigenic *Escherichia coli* strains with specific fimbrial adherence antigens are commonly used in swine.

  3. Toxoids
  a. Parental administration of inactivated bacterial exotoxins that are highly immunogenic has proven highly efficacious for diseases caused by systemic action of absorbed bacterial

exotoxins. Toxoids induce humoral antibodies, which are
capable of neutralizing the toxic effects of the toxins.
- (1) Tetanus and diphtheria toxoids induce specific serum
  antibodies that prevent the clinical manifestations of
  Clostridium tetani and *Corynebacterium diphtheriae*
  infections.
4. Component vaccines
   a. Surface components of bacterial pathogens are occasionally
      used as protective immunogens.
      - (1) Purified M protein antigens of *Streptococcus equi*, when
        administered parentally, will induce protective
        immunity in horses against strangles.
      - (2) A highly immunogenic capsular vaccine for *Haemophilus
        influenzae* type b induces protective immunity to
        systemic disease in children and adults, but
        unfortunately this polysaccharide antigen is a poor
        immunogen in infants.

SECTION III

Extracellular and Facultative Intracellular Bacteria

PART **1**	# Aerobic Gram-positive Cocci

6	## Genus *Micrococcus*

I. *MICROCOCCUS* SPECIES
   A.   Nonpathogens

Species	Hosts
Micrococcus species	Domestic animals, man

      1.   The micrococci are not pathogens of domestic animals or man.

II. HABITAT AND ECOLOGY
   A.   *Micrococcus* species are normal flora of mammalian skin.

III. CELLULAR, CULTURAL, AND BIOCHEMICAL CHARACTERISTICS
   A.   Cellular characteristics
      1.   Gram-positive cocci
      2.   All *Micrococcus* species are nonmotile except *M. agilis*, which has one or more flagella.
   B.   Cultural characteristics
      1.   All *Micrococcus* species are obligate aerobes except *M. kristinae*, which is a facultative anaerobe.
      2.   Growth on blood agar at 37°C
         a.   Colonies of micrococci are large, entire, convex, and nonhemolytic. Most species produce white colonies, but some form yellow-, pink-, orange-, or red-pigmented colonies. *M. luteus* forms yellow colonies and *M. roseus* pink colonies.
   C.   Biochemical characteristics
      1.   Catalase-positive
      2.   Respiratory metabolism

      a.   Some micrococci are asaccharolytic, but others can utilize glucose oxidatively.

IV. DISEASE OVERVIEW
    A.   In domestic animals, the *Micrococcus* species are not pathogenic but are commonly found as contaminates in clinical specimens. The micrococci must be distinguished from the pathogenic aerobic gram-positive cocci in the genera *Staphylococcus* and *Streptococcus*.

| 7 | Genus *Staphylococcus* |

I.   *STAPHYLOCOCCUS* SPECIES
    A.   Pathogens

Species	Hosts	Specific Diseases	Nonspecific Diseases
S. aureus	Bovine	Mastitis	suppurative
	Canine	Pyoderma	urinary tract
	Equine	Botryomycosis	arthritis, mastitis
	Feline		urinary tract
	Porcine		mastitis, metritis
S. hyicus	Porcine	Exudative epidermitis	
S. intermedius	Canine	Pyoderma	suppurative

      1.   The coagulase-positive species (*S. aureus* and *S. intermedius*) and the coagulase-variable species (*S. hyicus*) are associated with a number of suppurative disease processes in domestic animals.
    B.   Nonpathogens
      1.   The coagulase-negative species (*S. auricularis, S. capitis, S. caprae, S. carnosus, S. caseolyticus, S. cohnii, S. epidermidis, S. gallinarum, S. haemolyticus, S. hominis, S. lentus, S. saccharolyticus, S. saprophyticus, S. sciuri, S. simulans, S. warneri*, and *S. xylosus*) are occasionally isolated from clinical diseases of domestic animals, but in general are considered to be nonpathogenic.
    C.   Species differentiation
      1.   Differentiation of the *Staphylococcus* species is strongly based

on differences in their chromosomal DNA. Biochemical differences coincide with DNA divergence, and traditional microbiologic tests are used for their identification.

D. Cellular antigens
1. Group antigens
    a. Carbohydrate
        (1) The cell wall of *S. aureus* contains ribitol teichoic acid, whereas the cell walls of *S. hyicus* and *S. intermedius* contain glycerol teichoic acid.
    b. Protein A
        (1) Protein A is present in the cell wall of *S. aureus* but not in the cell walls of *S. hyicus* and *S. intermedius*.
2. Type antigens
    a. Proteins other than Protein A
        (1) There are innumerable serovars of staphylococci.
E. Three groups of virulence factors
1. Surface components
    a. Capsule
        (1) The polysaccharide capsule is antiphagocytic.
    b. Cell wall antigens
        (1) Outer layer
            (a) Protein A has four Fc-binding sites on each molecule, which are capable of binding to the Fc region of normal IgG. It has been postulated that this property imparts antiphagocytic activity by competing with leukocytes for the Fc portion of specific opsonins.
        (2) Inner layer
            (a) Teichoic acids are complexed with the mucopeptide. They have some antiphagocytic ability.
        (3) Acidic polysaccharides
            (a) They have some antiphagocytic ability.
2. Exotoxins
    a. Hemolysins
        (1) Some staphylococcal toxins cause hemolysis (Table 7.1).
        (2) The hemolysins are antigenically distinct.
    b. Leukotoxins
        (1) Staphylococcal toxins with leukocidal activity includes alpha and delta toxins and the Panton-Valentine leukocidin.

Table 7.1. Staphylococcal toxins that cause hemolysis

Toxin	Hemolysis Type
Alpha toxin	Complete
Beta toxin	Partial (hot-cold hemolysis)
Delta toxin	Complete
Epsilon toxin	Complete

        c. Enterotoxins
- (1) Enterotoxins are not produced by all strains and are seldom produced by animal strains. There are several antigenically distinct types of heat-stable enterotoxins.

        d. Exfoliative toxins
- (1) This protein exotoxin causes exfoliation and intraepidermal separation in human staphylococcal epidermal infections, but its role in animal skin infections has not been delineated.

    3. Extracellular enzymes

        a. Coagulase
- (1) Traditionally staphylococci have been classified as coagulase-positive or coagulase-negative on the basis of their ability to coagulate plasma.
  - (a) Animal strains may differ in regard to their ability to coagulate plasma from different animal species.
- (2) Coagulase-positive staphylococci (CPS) are usually considered to be significant pathogens when isolated from lesions. Coagulase-negative staphylococci (CNS) are generally considered to be nonpathogenic.
  - (a) The majority of the CPS produce both bound and free coagulase.

        b. Hyaluronidase
- (1) Hyaluronidase hydrolyzes hyaluronic acid, the mucoid ground substance of connective tissue.

        c. Nucleases
- (1) Deoxyribonucleases (DNAse) hydrolyze deoxyribonucleic acid (DNA), and ribonucleases (RNAse) hydrolyze ribonucleic acid (RNA). The source of the DNA and RNA can be either lysed host eucaryotic cells or procaryotic cells.
- (2) Most CPS strains hydrolyze DNA, but only a minority of CNS strains produce a DNAse.

        d. Fibrinolysin
- (1) Fibrinolysin, which is commonly referred to as staphylokinase, is an activator of the plasma system, leading to the breakdown of fibrin.

        e. Lipases and esterases
- (1) These enzymes can hydrolyze lipids.

        f. Lysozyme
- (1) Lysozyme hydrolyzes the peptidoglycan in the cell wall of many bacteria.

F. Intracellular survival

    1. Some staphylococci can survive intracellularly in phagocytes, but bacterial multiplication is very limited. The bacteria are able to outlive the phagocytic cell and to continue multiplication when released.

G. Bacteriophage typing
1. Strains of staphylococci often differ in their susceptibility to various bacteriophages and can be distinguished by the pattern of their susceptibility.
   a. Phage typing of strains of staphylococci is frequently done in epidemiologic investigations.
   b. Many strains of staphylococci isolated from domestic animals are not lysed by the set of phages used to type staphylococci isolated from man.
   c. Several hundred phage types of *S. aureus* have been recognized.

II. HABITAT AND ECOLOGY
A. *Staphylococcus* species are part of the normal flora of the external surfaces of the body.
1. Animals show very little, if any, resistance to superficial colonization by the staphylococci but have a high degree of resistance to deep invasion and progressive disease.

III. CELLULAR, CULTURAL, AND BIOCHEMICAL CHARACTERISTICS
A. Cellular characteristics
1. Gram-positive cocci
   a. Cells are arranged in grapelike clusters.
2. Nonmotile
B. Cultural characteristics
1. Facultative anaerobic
2. Growth on blood agar at 37°C
   a. Colonies of staphylococci are large, convex, opaque, and may be either white or yellow. Most CPS are hemolytic, producing either a zone of complete hemolysis or a double zone of hemolysis. The CNS are usually nonhemolytic.
C. Biochemical characteristics
1. Catalase-positive
2. Fermentative metabolism

IV. DISEASE OVERVIEW
A. *Staphylococcus* species infections
1. Infections in domestic animals
   a. Various animal species differ in their susceptibility to staphylococci.
   b. Staphylococci characteristically cause pyogenic infections of the body surfaces, respiratory tract, urinary tract, or mammary gland. Abscesses are a common sequelae.
      (1) Predisposing factors that reduce the innate resistance of the host are often present when disease occurs.
   c. Coagulase reactions of staphylococcal isolates are usually correlated with virulence. When a CPS is isolated from a clinical specimen, it usually has clinical significance. However, isolated CNS are generally not considered to be

significant pathogens since they are part of the normal flora and have a low virulence.

B.   *S. aureus* infections

    1.   Bovine mastitis

       a.   Infection of the udder with *S. aureus* occurs via the teat canal with organisms derived from the contaminated environment and particularly from the skin of the udder and teat.

    2.   Equine botryomycosis

       a.   Botryomycosis is an infection of the spermatic cord of horses. It is often a sequela to castration. The lesions are characterized by exuberant granulation tissue with many fistular abscesses.

C.   *S. hyicus* infections

    1.   Porcine exudative epidermitis

       a.   Exudative epidermitis is a generalized nonpruritic dermatitis of young pigs. The condition may involve the entire body and is characterized by excessive sebaceous secretion, exudation, and exfoliation. The disease is readily transmitted to susceptible pigs by contact.

          (1) In suckling pigs, the disease is acute and usually affects the entire body. The infections are responsible for high mortality, and the time from exposure to death is often only a few days.

          (2) In pigs 6 to 10 weeks of age, the disease tends to be subacute and the skin lesions are restricted with less copious exudation.

          (3) Different strains vary markedly in virulence, so various predisposing factors play a significant role when low-virulence strains are involved.

          (4) Herd immunity may develop after the initial outbreak, thus lowering the incidence of disease.

    2.   Opportunistic infections in domestic animals

       a.   *S. hyicus* also has been isolated from infections of cats, cattle, dogs, and horses.

D.   *S. intermedius* infections

    1.   Canine pyoderma

       a.   *S. intermedius* is isolated from approximately 90 percent of the canine staphylococcal dermatoses; *S. aureus* is isolated from the majority of the remaining 10 percent. From the normal skin flora, *S. intermedius* is the primary coagulase-positive species recovered, while *S. aureus* is only occasionally isolated.

          (1) Some *S. intermedius* isolates from dogs are coagulase-negative when tested with rabbit plasma but coagulase-positive when tested with dog plasma.

| 8 | Genus *Streptococcus* |

I. *STREPTOCOCCUS* SPECIES

A. Pathogens

Species	Hosts	Specific Diseases	Nonspecific Diseases
S. agalactiae	Bovine	Mastitis	
S. dysgalactiae	Bovine	Mastitis	
S. equi	Equine	STRANGLES	
S. equisimilis	Porcine	Arthritis	
	Domestic animals		suppurative
S. pneumoniae	Man	Pneumococcal pneumonia	
S. pyogenes	Domestic animals		suppurative
	Man	Rheumatic fever, glomerulonephritis	
S. suis	Porcine	Cervical lymphadenitis	
S. uberis	Bovine	Mastitis	
S. zooepidemicus	Equine	NEONATAL STREP-TOCOCCAL INFECTIONS	respiratory and genital tract
Enterococci	Domestic animals		valvular endocarditis
Other species	Domestic animals		suppurative

B. Types of hemolysis

1. Alpha hemolysis
   a. There is a partial zone of hemolysis around the colony. The area of partial hemolysis contains both lysed and intact red blood cells and a green reduced product of hemogloblin.
2. Beta hemolysis
   a. There is a complete zone of hemolysis around the colony in which no color remains.
   b. Two hemolysins, streptolysin S and streptolysin O, can produce beta hemolysis.
      (1) Streptolysin S is stable in the presence of atmospheric oxygen and produces hemolysis in both aerobic and anaerobic conditions. It is a small polypeptide of about 28 amino acid residues and is not antigenic.
      (2) Streptolysin O is inactivated in the presence of oxygen and only produces hemolysis under anaerobic conditions. It is antigenic, and a significant increase in anti-streptolysin O antibodies indicates a recent streptococcal infection.

    3. Gamma hemolysis

       a. There is no hemolysis around the colony.

C. Lancefield classification (Table 8.1)

    1. The 20 Lancefield groups, which are designated A to H and K to V, are based on a precipitation test of extractable group-specific carbohydrate cell wall antigens. These antigens are called C carbohydrates. To extract these soluble carbohydrate antigens, streptococci are placed in dilute acid (pH 2) and heated at $100^{\circ}C$ for 10 minutes.

Table 8.1. Examples of Lancefield groups

Group	Species
A	*Streptococcus pyogenes*
B	*S. agalactiae*
C	*S. equi, S. equisimilis,* and *S. zooepidemicus*
D	*S. faecalis* and *S. faecium* (enterococci)

D. Traditional classification of streptococci

    1. Hemolytic streptococci, Lancefield classification

       a. In the 1930s, Dr. Rebecca Lancefield classified the beta hemolytic streptococci. Since then many nonhemolytic and alpha hemolytic staphylococci also have been classified.

    2. Viridans streptococci, no Lancefield classification

       a. They are either alpha hemolytic or nonhemolytic. They do not have C carbohydrate and therefore are not part of the Lancefield classification system.

    3. Enterococci, Lancefield group D

       a. They are normal intestinal flora. Most enterococci are nonhemolytic. *S. faecalis* and *S. faecium* are commonly isolated enterococci.

    4. Lactic streptococci, Lancefield group N

       a. They are found in milk and dairy products and are nonhemolytic. *S. lactis* is referred to as a lactic streptococci.

E. Capsular and cell wall antigens

    1. Capsular antigens

       a. Capsular composition

          (1) Hyaluronic acid capsules are present in Lancefield groups A and C. Antibodies are not formed to hyaluronic acid, since it is a normal component of connective tissue.

          (2) Polysaccharide capsules are present in Lancefield groups B, E, and G. They are antigenic and antibodies to the polysaccharide capsule may be protective.

       b. Function

          (1) Antiphagocytic

        (a) The capsule helps the bacterium resist phagocytosis.

        (b) Nonencapsulated streptococci have a low virulence.

  2. Cell wall antigens

    a. Carbohydrate antigens are group-specific.

      (1) The majority of the pathogens of domestic animals are classified in Lancefield groups A, B, C, D, E, and G.

      (2) Antibodies to these carbohydrate antigens are not protective.

    b. Protein antigens are type-specific.

      (1) M protein antigens often play a significant role in staphylococcal infections.

        (a) M protein extends through the capsule to the outermost surfaces as hairlike fimbriae.

        (b) In some *Streptococcus* species, the M proteins serve as an antiphagocytic virulence factor and antibodies directed against these protein antigens are protective.

      (2) R and T proteins play little, if any, role in the pathogenesis of streptococcal infections.

F. Extracellular virulence factors

  1. Streptolysins S and O hemolyze erythrocytes and can lyse neutrophils, macrophages, and platelets in some animal species.

  2. Streptokinase is a protease that lyses fibrin by catalyzing the conversion of plasminogen to plasmin. By promoting the lysis of fibrin blood clots, streptokinase is, in part, responsible for the spread of streptococcal infections by preventing the formation of a fibrin barrier around the infection site.

    a. There are two immunological types of streptokinase, A and B.

  3. Streptodornase is a term to describe the four immunologically distinct types of deoxyribonucleases: A, B, C, and D. Type B is the most common. These enzymes degrade DNA.

  4. Hyaluronidase hydrolyzes hyaluronic acid and therefore is considered to play a role in the spread of streptococci through tissues.

II. HABITAT AND ECOLOGY

A. The streptococci are normal flora of the skin and mucous membranes of domestic animals and man. Many *Streptococcus* species are host-specific or have a very limited host range.

  1. The enterococci are normal intestinal flora.

III. CELLULAR, CULTURAL, AND BIOCHEMICAL CHARACTERISTICS

A. Cellular characteristics

  1. Gram-positive cocci

    a. The cells are arranged in pairs or chains.

      2. Streptococci are nonmotile except for some motile group D streptococci.
- B. Cultural characteristics
  1. Facultative anaerobic
     a. The best initial growth is in microaerophilic conditions.
  2. Growth on blood agar at 37°C
     a. Colonies of streptococci are small and transparent to semiopaque. Most pathogenic *Streptococcus* isolates produce a wide zone of complete (beta) hemolysis around the colony, but the pathogens in groups B and D are often either nonhemolytic or produce alpha hemolysis.
- C. Biochemical characteristics
  1. Catalase-negative
  2. Fermentative metabolism
     a. All species of *Streptococcus* are homofermentative organisms, producing lactic acid from glucose.

IV. DISEASE OVERVIEW
- A. Clinical importance of genus *Streptococcus*
  1. Streptococci are common pathogens of domestic animals and man.
  2. They are often associated with specific disease processes, particularly suppurative conditions.
  3. Most pathogenic streptococci are beta hemolytic.
     a. The hemolytic streptococci when isolated usually have a clinical significance.
     b. The nonhemolytic streptococci are not considered to be clinically significant, since they are part of the normal flora and have a very low virulence. However, the streptococci isolated from endocarditis and urinary tract infections are often nonhemolytic.
  4. Streptococcal diseases are characterized by febrile symptoms, alone or associated with symptoms of septicemia. Septicemia may result from hematogenous spread of primary infection.
  5. Local areas of infection exhibit suppurative inflammation, and abscesses form where drainage is prevented.
  6. Toxemia and allergy are common sequelae.
- B. Primary streptococcal infections
  1. Respiratory tract infections
     a. Infections of mucous membranes may be primary infections with virulent streptococci or secondary infections to other diseases.
     b. Virulent streptococci invade and spread to local lymph nodes where abscesses form (e.g., *S. equi*).
     c. These infections may become bacteremic and localize in other lymph nodes.
        (1) *S. equi* may spread and produce "bastard strangles" in horses.

        d.   In young animals, these infections may become septicemic and localize in various tissues.

  2. Reproductive tract infections

      a.   Infections of mucous membranes may result in metritis, infertility, and abortion.

         (1) Streptococcal infections are common in horses.

         (2) These infections may contribute to the metritis-mastitis-agalactia complex of swine.

  3. Umbilical cord infections

      a.   These infections may be localized with draining purulent material and abscesses, or they may become septicemic.

      b.   Complications of the septicemia may result in localization in the joints (arthritis, joint ill) and brain (meningitis). Some septicemias result in the death of the neonate.

  4. Mammary gland infections

      a.   Streptococcal mastitis is common in ruminants and occurs in other animals.

  5. Skin infections

      a.   Streptococci are commonly isolated from suppurative lesions of the skin.

C. Immunological complications of primary streptococcal infections

  1. *S. equi* infections or postvaccination reactions to *S. equi* bacterins

      a.   Purpura hemorrhagica is considered to be a poststreptococcal immune complex disease. Antibody to M protein is produced, and immune complexes localize in the capillary beds and activate complement. This results in an increased vascular permeability, which allows plasma components and cells to leak into the tissues. Clinical signs include subcutaneous edema of face, muzzle, and limbs. Petechial and ecchymotic hemorrhages develop on the skin and mucous membranes.

  2. *S. pyogenes* infections in man

      a.   Rheumatic fever and glomerulonephritis are common postinfection immunological complications.

D. *S. agalactiae*, *S. dysgalactiae*, and *S. uberis* infections

  1. Bovine mastitis

      a.   These *Streptococcus* species are called the mastitis streptococci because of their association with mastitis. Numerous other streptococci can also cause mastitis.

         (1) *S. agalactiae* is an obligate intramammary parasite that is highly contagious between cows.

      b.   Mastitis arises from the multiplication of streptococci in the teat sinus and extends into the ducts and secreting tissues of the mammary gland. Clinical signs of infection are detectable only after the lesions have become extensive. As the infection progresses, milk secretion will decrease.

E. *S. equi* infections
   1. Equine strangles (see Chap. 109)
      a. Strangles is an acute contagious disease of horses characterized by inflammation of the upper respiratory tract and abscessation in the regional lymph nodes.
         (1) *S. equi* can be introduced into a group of horses by clinically infected or carrier horses.
            (a) The bacterium is probably an obligate parasite on the upper respiratory tract mucous membranes.
         (2) The bacterium can invade the mucous membranes of the oral pharynx and upper respiratory tract without predisposing damage to the respiratory epithelium.
         (3) After an incubation period of 3 to 6 days, clinical symptoms are characterized as an acute pharyngitis accompanied by swelling and abscessation of the lymph nodes draining the head and neck.
         (4) Purpura hemorrhagica is a common sequela.

F. *S. equisimilis* infections
   1. Porcine arthritis
      a. The bacterium causes a suppurative, proliferative, and erosive arthritis in young pigs.
   2. Infections in domestic animals
      a. It is a pathogen of domestic animals.
      b. From horses, *S. equisimilis* has been isolated from various suppurative processes, neonatal septicemia and polyarthritis, enteritis in foals, endometritis, and as secondary invaders of viral respiratory tract infections.
         (1) The infectious processes caused by *S. equisimilis* are very similar to those caused by *S. zooepidemicus*.

G. *S. pyogenes* infections
   1. Infections in domestic animals
      a. *S. pyogenes* is a pathogen of domestic animals and is associated with suppurative lesions.

H. *S. suis* infections
   1. Porcine cervical lymphadenitis
      a. *S. suis* is a primary etiologic agent of cervical lymphadenitis and is frequently isolated from swine with pneumonia, septicemia, arthritis, endocarditis, meningitis, and reproductive tract infections.

I. *S. zooepidemicus* infections
   1. Equine neonatal streptococcal infections (see Chap. 108)
      a. It is the most common cause of bacterial infection of the horse and is especially common in young horses. The infections may be either primary or secondary to some other condition. The bacterium is commonly isolated from genital infections, respiratory infections, and foal diseases.

(1) *S. zooepidemicus* and *Klebsiella pneumoniae* are the two most common causes of chronic vaginitis, cervicitis, endometritis, and sterility in the mare. When an infected mare conceives, embryonic reabsorption and abortion in the first trimester of gestation are the most probable outcomes, but some abortions occur in the second and third trimesters.

J.   Enterococci infections

   1.   Infections in domestic animals

      a.   The enterococci are common isolates from vegetative endocarditis and urinary tract infections.

K.   *Streptococcus* species infections

   1.   Canine

      a.   *Streptococcus* species, particularly in groups C, D, and G, are isolated from a variety of canine infections. These streptococcal diseases include endocarditis, mastitis, metritis, otitis externa, neonatal puppy septicemia, pyoderma, and respiratory and urinary tract infections.

PART 2	Family Entero-bacteriaceae, Aerobic Gram-negative Rods

9	Family Enterobacteriaceae

I. GENERA
    A. Pathogens

Genera	Intestinal Diseases		Extraintestinal Diseases	
	Domestic animals	Man	Domestic animals	Man
Citrobacter	−	−	+	+
Edwardsiella	−	−	+	+
Enterobacter	−	−	++	+
Escherichia	+	+	+++	+
Klebsiella	−	−	++	+
Morganella	−	−	+	+
Proteus	−	−	+++	+
Providencia	−	−	++	+
Salmonella	+	+	+	+
Serratia	−	−	+	+
Shigella	−	+	−	−
Yersinia	−	+	++	+

Comparative incidence of genera in extraintestinal infections of domestic animals: +++ = commonly isolated; ++ = occasionally isolated; + = rarely isolated; − = not isolated.

    B. Nonpathogens
        1. The genera *Cedecea, Erwinia, Hafnia, Kluyvera, Obesumbacterium, Rahnella, Tatumella*, and *Xenorhabdus* do not have species that are pathogens of either domestic animals or man.

II. HABITAT AND ECOLOGY
    A. Pathogenic genera
        1. Most members of the family Enterobacteriaceae are normal inhabitants of the digestive tracts of domestic animals.
            a. Many species are found ubiquitously in the environment as

fecal contaminants and can survive for days or weeks under ideal conditions.

III. CELLULAR, CULTURAL, AND BIOCHEMICAL CHARACTERISTICS

A. Cellular characteristics
 1. Gram-negative rods
    a. The bacilli are approximately 1 um in diameter and 2 to 6 um in length.
 2. Motility
    a. The genera *Klebsiella* and *Shigella* are nonmotile. All species in the genera *Citrobacter, Edwardsiella, Enterobacter, Morganella, Proteus,* and *Providencia* are motile by means of peritrichous flagella. Some species, serovars, and/or strains in the genera *Escherichia, Salmonella,* and *Serratia* are motile.

B. Cultural characteristics
 1. Facultative anaerobic
 2. Growth on blood agar and MacConkey agar at 37°C
    a. Colonies of most genera are large, gray, and mucoid. A few species have characteristic colony morphologies.
    b. On blood agar, most pathogenic strains of *Escherichia coli* are beta hemolytic, but the majority of the other members of the family Enterobacteriaceae are nonhemolytic.
    c. On MacConkey agar, the lactose-positive genera *Citrobacter, Enterobacter, Escherichia, Klebsiella,* and *Serratia* form pink to red colonies, distinguishing them from the lactose-negative genera *Edwardsiella, Morganella, Proteus, Providencia, Salmonella, Shigella,* and *Yersinia,* which form colorless colonies.

C. Biochemical characteristics
 1. Oxidase-negative
 2. Metabolism is both respiratory and fermentative.
    a. All genera ferment glucose under anaerobic conditions and oxidize glucose under aerobic conditions.
    b. Mixed acid fermentations and butanediol fermentations are carried out by various members of the family Enterobacteriaceae. Bacteria in the genera *Escherichia* and *Salmonella* ferment sugars to acetic, formic, lactic, and succinic acids, whereas species in the genera *Enterobacter* and *Serratia* produce large amounts of acetoin and 2, 3-butanediol. The methyl red test is used to quantitate mixed acid fermentations, and the Voges-Proskauer test detects butanediol fermentation.
 3. Identification to species level of each pathogenic genus except *Salmonella* is based on biochemical criteria.
    a. Some species of the family Enterobacteriaceae exhibit very little biochemical variability (e.g., *Y. pseudotuberculosis*)

whereas other species contain hundreds of different biotypes
(e.g., *E. coli*).
b.   The enterobacteriae have the ability to acquire plasmids
that specify metabolic genes.
(1) A chromosomal gene for hydrogen sulfide production has
never been demonstrated in *E. coli*, nor have
chromosomal genes for lactose fermentation been
demonstrated in *S. typhimurium*. However, hydrogen
sulfide-producing strains of *E. coli* and lactose
fermenting stains of *S. typhimurium* have been
described in which these functions are mediated by
genes present on plasmids.
4.   Identification of the *Salmonella* serovars is based on serologic
criteria.

IV. DISEASE OVERVIEW
A.   Modes of infection in the gastrointestinal tract
1.   Extracellular bacteria
a.   Bacterial habitat is the lumen of the digestive tract
(e.g., enterotoxigenic *E. coli*).
2.   Intracellular bacteria
a.   Bacteria penetrate the epithelial lining of the digestive
tract and multiply in the host cells.
(1) Innate immune responses of the host protect the body
against common opportunistic pathogens. Phagocytosis
by neutrophils and macrophages quickly eliminates
saprophytes and slightly virulent bacteria.
(2) The advantages of intracellular parasitism are that
the bacteria are sheltered against the host defense
reactions and have a source of nutrition.
b.   Two groups of intracellular bacteria
(1) Intraepithelial
(a) The bacteria multiply almost without exception in
the epithelial cells of the intestinal mucosa.
The *Shigella* species, which cause bacillary
dysentery, and some strains of *E. coli*
demonstrate this mode of pathogenesis.
(2) Intramacrophage
(a) The bacteria multiply in the macrophages,
particularly within the intestinal submucosa.
Some *Salmonella* serovars and some strains of *E.
coli* demonstrate this mode of pathogenesis.
B.   Intestinal diseases in domestic animals
1.   *E. coli* infections
a.   Colibacillosis
(1) Colibacillosis is a group of diseases in which the

primary site of the *E. coli* infection is the small intestine.

(2) All species of domestic animals are affected. It is primarily a disease of the young.

(3) Different pathogenic mechanisms of *E. coli*

(a) Enterotoxigenic *E. coli* (ETEC) are capable of causing primary intestinal disease by the production of enterotoxin(s). The exotoxins cause a loss of fluid and electrolytes into the lumen of the small intestine by active hypersecretion and/or impaired absorption. The pathogenic mechanisms are similar to *Vibrio cholerae.*

(b) Enteropathogenic *E. coli* (EPEC) penetrate and multiply within the subepithelial tissues. The pathogenic mechanisms are similar to the salmonellae.

(c) Enteroinvasive *E. coli* (EIEC) penetrate and multiply within the mucosal epithelium. The pathogenic mechanisms are similar to the shigellae.

2. *Salmonella* infections

a. Salmonellosis

(1) Salmonellosis causes an enteritis of both the small and large intestine.

(2) It is transmitted by the oral ingestion of contaminated feed and water.

(3) The minimum infective dose for most serovars in the healthy animal is about 10^8 bacteria. Since many serovars tend to be host-specific, it takes a large dose of a serovar to infect an unusual host.

(4) Pathogenesis of intestinal infections

(a) Bacteria from the intestinal lumen penetrate into the epithelial cells, where they have very limited multiplication. Eventually the bacteria penetrate into the lamina propria, where many of the bacteria are phagocytized. Many of the bacteria phagocytized by neutrophils are killed, but often bacteria phagocytized by macrophages survive and multiply intracellularly. These bacteria are released when the macrophages lyse.

3. Other bacterial species

a. Enteritis

(1) Most bacterial species in the family Enterobacteriaceae seldom, if ever, cause disease in the digestive tracts of domestic animals because of

host immunity and the low virulence of these microorganims in the digestive tract. However, many species have the potential to produce disease under appropriate conditions and must be considered opportunistic.

C.   Extraintestinal diseases in domestic animals
1.   Bacterial species in the family Enterobacteriaceae are isolated from over 50 percent of the opportunistic infections of domestic animals.
a.   Because of fecal contamination, these bacteria may be involved in bacterial infections anywhere in the animal, including infections of the genital and respiratory tracts, mastitis, septicemias, and wounds.
2.   These infections may be primary or secondary to other disease-causing agents.
a.   Disease is dependent on the virulence of the species and strain of bacteria, the innate and specific immunological resistance of the host, and the particular organs and tissues involved.
b.   These infections may be caused by only one bacterial species, but many infections are polymicrobial. Bacterial species in the family Enterobacteriaceae are commonly found in mixed cultures with other facultative anaerobes and/or obligate anaerobic bacteria.

10 | Genus *Escherichia*

I. *ESCHERICHIA* SPECIES
A. Pathogens

Species	Hosts	Intestinal Diseases	Extraintestinal Diseases
E. coli	Porcine	COLIBACILLOSIS	opportunistic
	Domestic animals	Colibacillosis	opportunistic

1. *E. coli* is the only species in the genus that produces clinical disease in domestic animals.
B. Serovars and fimbrial antigens
1. Serovars are based on an antigenic formula for the different O (somatic), K (capsular), and H (flagellar) antigens. The O antigens are based on the antigenicity of the lipopolysaccharides. The K antigens are the capsular polysaccharides and are best considered as extensions of the O antigens. Three types of K antigens can be differentiated by their stability in various physical tests. In any one strain, only one K antigen (L, A, or B) is present. The K antigens are not always present. The H antigens are protein. The nonmotile strains are designated NM.
   a. The antigenic formula of a serovar is indicated as 026:K60(B6):H11 or 26:60(B6):11. If nonmotile, it is written as 26:60(B6):NM or 26:60(B6).
2. Fimbriae are protein antigens and are used for serologic classification of some pathogenic serovars. Fimbriae can function as virulence factors in both intestinal and extraintestinal diseases and can be both species-specific and organ-specific in their adhesive characteristics.
   a. Two types of fimbriae have been described based on their hemagglutinating ability.
      (1) Type 1 fimbriae are characterized by hemagglutination (HA) that is inhibited by mannose. The HA is mannose-sensitive. They are called F1 antigens.
      (2) Type 2 fimbriae are characterized by HA that is not inhibited by mannose. The HA is mannose-resistant. The K88 and the K99 fimbriae are now called F4 and F5, respectively.
3. Characteristics of *E. coli* antigens (Table 10.1)

Table 10.1. Characteristics of *Escherichia coli* antigens

Characteristic	Bacterial Antigens			
	O	K	H	Fimbrial
Chemistry	Lipopolysaccharide	Polysaccharide	Protein	Protein
Heat stability (100°C, 1 hr)	Stable	Stable	Labile	Labile
Genetic determination				
Chromosome	+	+	+	+
Plasmid	−	−	−	+

II. HABITAT AND ECOLOGY

A. *E. coli* is normal intestinal flora of animals.
1. The natural habitat of *E. coli* is the lower part of the intestine.
    a. From a few hours after birth throughout life, a succession of different *E. coli* strains inhabit the most distal part of the ileum and the whole of the colon.
    b. *E. coli* makes up 1 percent or less of the bacteria found in the colon; nevertheless, the bacterium is the most numerous facultative anaerobic species in the healthy gastrointestinal tracts of domestic animals.
        (1) The majority of the intestinal flora comprise obligate anaerobic bacteria.
2. *E. coli* is ubiquitous in the environment from fecal contamination.

III. CELLULAR, CULTURAL, AND BIOCHEMICAL CHARACTERISTICS

A. Cellular characteristics
1. Gram-negative rods
2. Most pathogenic *E. coli* are motile by peritrichous flagella; however, the enteroinvasive *E. coli* strains tend to be nonmotile.
B. Cultural characteristics
1. Facultative anaerobic
2. Growth on blood agar and MacConkey agar at 37°C
    a. Colonies of *E. coli* on blood agar, like most species in the family Enterobacteriaceae, are round, convex, gray, opaque, and somewhat mucoid. Most pathogenic *E. coli* are beta hemolytic.
    b. Lactose-positive
C. Biochemical characteristics
1. Oxidase-negative
2. Metabolism is both respiratory and fermentative.
    a. Identification to species level is based on biochemical criteria.

IV. DISEASE OVERVIEW

A. Intestinal diseases in domestic animals (colibacillosis)
1. Colibacillosis is a group of diseases in which the primary site of the *E. coli* infection is the small intestine (see Chap. 99).

2. All species and ages of animals are affected, but it is primarily a disease of the young.
3. *E. coli* strains have considerable variation with respect to pathogenic mechanisms.
   a. Enterotoxin production is determined by plasmids.
      (1) Two types of enterotoxins are described. One toxin is protein, heat-labile, and immunogenic; the other toxin is of low molecular weight, heat-stable, and nonimmunogenic. These enterotoxins cause a loss of fluid and electrolytes into the intestinal lumen.
   b. Bacteria penetrate and multiply within the mucosal epithelium.
   c. Bacteria penetrate the intestinal mucosa and multiply within subepithelial tissues.
4. Very little is known about the relative importance of the enteroinvasive (EIEC), enteropathogenic (EPEC), and enterotoxigenic (ETEC) strains of *E. coli* in most species of domestic animals.
   a. The serovars of *E. coli* involved in these conditions have not been studied extensively except the ETEC of cattle and swine.
B. Extraintestinal diseases in domestic animals
   1. Urinary tract infections
      a. Cystitis and pyelonephritis caused by *E. coli* are common in the dog and cat.
   2. Genital tract infections
      a. These infections are common in the dog and horse.
   3. Mammary gland infections
      a. *E. coli* causes mastitis in all domestic animals.
         (1) The bacterium can cause a severe mastitis in dairy cows and has been implicated as a major pathogen in the metritis-mastitis-agalactia syndrome in swine.
   4. Pneumonia
      a. *E. coli* is occasionally a secondary opportunistic pathogen in pneumonia.
   5. Wounds
      a. *E. coli* is frequently isolated from open wounds. The bacterium may be isolated in pure or mixed cultures.
C. Theories of *E. coli* in extraintestinal disease
   1. Prevalence theory
      a. The prevalence theory is based on the premise that the serogroups and serovars of *E. coli* frequently found in the various extraintestinal diseases are the same as those found to be most prevalent in the feces.
   2. Special pathogenicity theory
      a. The special pathogenicity theory is based on the premise that selected serogroups and serovars of *E. coli* have a special affinity to induce extraintestinal disease.
   3. Current data suggest some validity for each theory, depending on the particular disease condition.

11 | Genus *Salmonella*

I. *SALMONELLA* SEROVARS
  A. Pathogens

Serovars	Hosts	Intestinal Diseases	Extraintestinal Diseases
S. abortusbovis	Bovine		Abortion
S. abortusequi	Equine		Abortion
S. abortusovis	Ovine		Abortion
S. choleraesuis	Porcine		SEPTICEMIA
S. dublin	Bovine	Salmonellosis	Abortion
S. paratyphi	Man	Paratyphoid	
S. typhi	Man	Typhoid	
S. typhimurium	Domestic animals	Salmonellosis	
	Porcine	SALMONELLOSIS	
S. typhisuis	Porcine	SALMONELLOSIS	
Other serovars	Domestic animals	Salmonellosis	opportunistic

   1. Approximately 120 serovars have been isolated from intestinal
       disease in domestic animals. Commonly isolated serovars include
       S. agona, *S. anatum*, *S. derby*, and *S. newport*. *Salmonella*
       serovars may be strictly adapted to one particular host or may
       be found in a large number of animal species.
  B. Serovars
   1. The serovar is the basic taxon of the genus. There are over
       2,000 serovars. They are based on an antigenic formula for the
       different O (somatic), Vi (capsular), and H (flagella) antigens.
       The Vi antigens are restricted to a few serovars adapted to man
       (e.g., *S. typhi*) and are not used in the serotyping of isolates
       from domestic animals. The O antigens are designated by arabic
       numbers. The H phase 1 antigens are shared by only a few
       serovars and are designated by small letters. The H phase 2
       antigens are common to many different serovars and are designated
       by arabic numbers.
       a. For example, the antigenic formula of *S. choleraesuis* is 6,
           7:c:1,5. The O antigens are 6 and 7, the H phase 1 antigen
           is c, and the H phase 2 antigens are 1 and 5.
  C. Biovars
   1. Biovars are strains of the same serovar that have different
       biochemical characteristics.
       a. Most strains of *S. choleraesuis* are H_2S-negative, whereas *S.
           choleraesuis* biovar *kunzendors* is H_2S-positive.

II. HABITAT AND ECOLOGY

A. *Salmonella* serovars
  1. They are intestinal flora of animals.
      a. The presence of salmonellae in the intestinal flora of domestic animals may be a transient change in the bowel flora with no apparent illness, or at the other extreme, salmonellosis may be a persistent disease with high mortality.
      b. They are found in soil and water as fecal contaminants.

III. CELLULAR, CULTURAL, AND BIOCHEMICAL CHARACTERISTICS

A. Cellular characteristics
  1. Gram-negative rods
  2. All *Salmonella* serovars are motile except the avian host-adapted serovars *S. pullorum* and *S. gallinarium*.
B. Cultural characteristics
  1. Facultative anaerobic
  2. Growth on blood agar and MacConkey agar at 37^0C
      a. Nonhemolytic
      b. Lactose-negative
C. Biochemical characteristics
  1. Oxidase-negative
  2. Metabolism is both respiratory and fermentative.
      a. Identification to genus level is based on biochemical criteria.
      b. Identification of serovars is based on serologic criteria.
  3. The pathogenic salmonellae, except for *S. typhi*, produce acid and gas from carbohydrate fermentation, thus distinguishing them from the shigellae, which produce only acid.

IV. DISEASE OVERVIEW

A. Transmission
  1. Ingestion of fecal contaminated material, especially feed and water, is the primary mode of transmission.
      a. The two primary sources are clinically affected animals and nonclinical carrier animals. Carriers of *Salmonella* are very common in all mammalian species.
      b. Intraspecies transmission from adult animals to young animals is very common.
      c. The majority of *Salmonella* serovars are animal pathogens that only incidentally infect man.
          (1) Most human infections are acquired by the ingestion of salmonellae-contaminated animal products used for food.
B. Clinical forms of salmonellosis
  1. There are two clinical forms of salmonellosis, a gastroenteritis and an enteric fever.
      a. The gastroenteritis form is primarily an infection of the intestine characterized by the abrupt onset of fever,

vomiting, and diarrhea 8 to 24 hours after the ingestion of contaminated food and water. Clinically the enteritis may be presented as acute, subacute, or chronic. In these infections, the bacilli colonize the intestine, penetrate the columnar epithelial cells of the intestinal villi, and establish foci of infection in the lamina propria. However, dissemination of the bacilli to the bloodstream rarely occurs.

   b.   The enteric fever form is characterized by dissemination of bacilli via the lymphatic vessels and phagocytic cells to the bloodstream after penetration of the intestinal epithelium. These infections are characterized by septicemia, endotoxemia, and localization in internal organs, including the lymph nodes, spleen, liver, and uterus. Abortion is a common sequela to bacterial localization in the uterus and placenta.

C.   Pathogenesis

   1.   Colonization and invasion of intestinal mucosa

      a.   Colonization of the intestinal mucosa must occur and may involve adherence factors, chemotaxis, and mobility.

      b.   The salmonellae adhere to the brush border of the epithelial cells and penetrate the mucosa of the small and large intestine. The bacteria are usually found in membrane-bound vacuoles within the epithelial cells and eventually migrate to the base of the cells. Bacterial proliferation within the epithelial cells is very limited. The bacteria also are capable of passing between adjacent epithelial cells in their migration to the lamina propria, where the bacteria are phagocytized by either neutrophils or macrophages. Most of the bacteria phagocytized by neutrophils are killed, whereas bacteria phagocytized by macrophages may be killed or multiply intracellularly and eventually kill the macrophage.

   2.   Bacterial virulence factors

      a.   Lipopolysaccharides

         (1)   Surface O antigens may allow the bacteria to survive intracellularly. The loss of specific side chains decreases virulence, and variation in O antigens of a serovar can significantly change the virulence of a serovar.

         (2)   Endotoxins damage the intestinal mucosa and are responsible for intestinal hemorrhages and perforations.

         (3)   Endotoxemia and endotoxic shock are common manifestations in animals with septicemia.

      b.   Exotoxins

         (1)   Two protein toxins, enterotoxin and cytotoxin, have been shown to contribute to the intestinal pathology.

        (a) The enterotoxin is similar to the heat-labile enterotoxin of *Escherichia coli* and choleragen of *Vibrio cholerae*. It activates adenylate cyclase, causing an elevation of mucosal cAMP concentration. This toxin causes the hypersecretion of fluid and electrolytes from the intestinal epithelium.

        (b) The cytotoxin is similar to the shigellae cytotoxin. It inhibits protein synthesis in epithelial cells of the intestinal mucosa.

    (2) The enterotoxin and cytotoxin are produced in relatively low concentrations, so that the invasion of epithelial cells by salmonellae could provide an effective toxin delivery mechanism. Once the toxins are inside the intestinal epithelial cells, even trace amounts of these toxins could have a marked effect on fluid and electrolyte transport, as well as cell viability.

3. Host factors

    a. The type and severity of salmonellosis is largely determined by the age of the host, animal species affected, immunological status of host, and various types of stress.

4. Infective dose and serovar

    a. The minimum infective dose for most serovars in the healthy animal is about 10^8 bacteria. Since most serovars tend to be host-specific, it takes a larger dose of a serovar to infect an unusual host.

D. Salmonelloses (Table 11.1)

  1. Bovine salmonellosis

    a. *S. typhimurium* and *S. dublin* are the most common serovars.

    b. Most cases of salmonellosis are of the acute enterocolitis type. Blood and diarrhea may be present.

    c. Problem areas include feedlot cattle, especially calves that have been shipped.

  2. Canine salmonellosis

    a. Clinical salmonellosis occurs primarily in pups, where the

Table 11.1. Predominant types of salmonellosis

Species	Age	Enterocolitis Acute	Subacute	Chronic	Acute Septicemia	Carrier Status
Bovine	Calves	+			+	
	Adults	+				+
Canine	Pups	+			+	
	Adults		+			+
Equine	Foals	+			+	
	Adults		+	+		+
Feline	All ages					+
Ovine	Lambs	+			+	
	Adults		+			+
Porcine	All ages	+	+	+	+	+

disease is manifested as an acute or subacute enteritis. Canine salmonellosis is often associated with animals housed in overcrowded unsanitary conditions.

    b. Food poisoning-type infections are occasionally seen in adult dogs. These infections are usually self-limiting and are probably due to the eating habits of dogs.

3. Equine salmonellosis

    a. *S. typhimurium* is the most common serovar.

        (1) Salmonellae, especially *S. typhimurium*, *S. newport*, and *S. anatum*, cause outbreaks of enteritis with high mortality.

    b. The disease is often stress-related. Various stresses may induce the activation of a quiescent infection.

        (1) Stress reduces the minimum infective dose. Common types of stress include worming, general anesthesia, surgery, and transportation.

    c. Antibiotic-induced salmonellosis is common in horses.

        (1) Oral and systemic therapy with tetracyclines alters the normal bacterial flora, which antagonizes salmonellae, thus serving as the inciting cause.

    d. Salmonellosis in foals is commonly manifested as an acute enterocolitis and septicemia. Common sequelae are bacterial localization in joints, lungs, and brain.

    e. Abortions due to *S. abortusequi* occur late in gestation; foals born alive but infected will often die of a septicemia within a few days.

        (1) The mares may be either asymptomatic or exhibit a mild illness.

4. Feline salmonellosis

    a. Clinical salmonellosis is rarely observed, but when it occurs, it primarily affects kittens.

5. Ovine salmonellosis

    a. Clinical disease is similar to bovine salmonellosis.

    b. Abortion and neonatal death can occur due to *S. abortusovis*, as well as to several other *Salmonella* serovars.

6. Porcine salmonellosis (see Chap. 103)

    a. *S. cholerasuis* causes an acute septicemia, but clinical signs of an enteritis are seldom manifested.

    b. *S. typhimurium* causes a catarrhal to mucohemorrhagic necrotic enterocolitis that may become chronic. These infections have been linked to porcine rectal strictures when the pigs have a history of severe enteric disease 4 to 8 weeks prior to the appearance of the strictures.

    c. *S. typhisuis* causes a chronic necrotic enterocolitis.

12	Genus *Shigella*

I. *SHIGELLA* SPECIES
   A. Pathogens

Species	Host	Intestinal Disease
Shigella species	Man	Bacillary dysentery

      1. Four species (*S. boydii*, *S. dysenteriae*, *S. flexneri*, and *S. sonnei*) are etiologic agents of diarrhea and dysentery in man and subhuman primates.

II. HABITAT AND ECOLOGY
   A. *Shigella* species are intestinal flora of animals.
      1. The minimum infective dose of shigellae in man and primates is small.

III. CELLULAR, CULTURAL, AND BIOCHEMICAL CHARACTERISTICS
   A. Cellular characteristics
      1. Gram-negative rods
      2. Nonmotile
   B. Cultural characteristics
      1. Facultative anaerobic
      2. Growth on blood agar and MacConkey agar at 37^0C
         a. Nonhemolytic
         b. Lactose-negative
   C. Biochemical characteristics
      1. Oxidase-negative
      2. Metabolism is both respiratory and fermentative.
         a. The shigellae produce acid but no gas from carbohydrate fermentation.

IV. DISEASE OVERVIEW
   A. Human diarrhea and bacillary dysentery
      1. Man and subhuman primates are the only animals that develop clinical infections. They are infected orally and clinically exhibit either diarrhea or dysentery. All four *Shigella* species are capable of causing these two distinct types of intestinal infections. The two clinical forms are attributed to different pathogenic mechanisms and involve anatomically distinct parts of the gastrointestinal tract.

a. In the diarrhea form, the small intestine is involved, but there does not appear to be bacterial invasion of the intestinal epithelial cells. The watery diarrhea has been correlated with the secretion of electrolytes and water in the proximal jejunum. An enterotoxin produced by the shigellae has been posulated to be a primary virulence factor.

b. In bacillary dysentery, the infections are limited to the epithelial lining of the terminal ileum and large intestine. The capacity of the shigellae to invade intestinal epithelial cells and multiply therein has been demonstrated to be a critical virulence factor. Typical intestinal lesions are acute inflammation with ulceration limited to the epithelium. Shigellae rarely penetrate deeper than the lamina propria. A cytotoxin produced by the shigellae has been shown to inhibit cellular protein synthesis, which in turn leads to epithelial cell death. It has been postulated that cellular invasion is an effective mechanism to deliver the cytotoxin to the ribosomal protein synthetic site. Bacillary dysentery is manifested by frequent passage of bloody mucus-containing stools and is a more severe clinical syndrome than is the diarrhea form.

13 | Genus *Citrobacter*

I. *CITROBACTER* SPECIES
    A. Pathogens

Species	Hosts	Extraintestinal Diseases
Citrobacter species	Domestic animals	opportunistic

    1. *C. freundii* is the most commonly isolated species.

II. HABITAT AND ECOLOGY
    A. *Citrobacter* species are normal intestinal flora of domestic animals and also are found in soil and water.

III. CELLULAR, CULTURAL, AND BIOCHEMICAL CHARACTERISTICS
    A. Cellular characteristics
        1. Gram-negative rods
        2. Motile by peritrichous flagella
    B. Cultural characteristics
        1. Facultative anaerobic
        2. Growth on blood agar and MacConkey agar at 37°C
            a. Nonhemolytic
            b. Lactose-positive
    C. Biochemical characteristics
        1. Oxidase-negative
        2. Metabolism is both respiratory and fermentative.

IV. DISEASE OVERVIEW
    A. In domestic animals, *Citrobacter* species are opportunistic pathogens in a variety of extraintestinal infections. They are seldom isolated in pure culture from clinical infections. The *Citrobacter* species are not enteric pathogens.

14	Genus *Edwardsiella*

I. *EDWARDSIELLA* SPECIES
    A. Pathogens

Species	Hosts	Extraintestinal Diseases
Edwardsiella species	Domestic animals	opportunistic

    1. Most *Edwardsiella* species are fish pathogens.

II. HABITAT AND ECOLOGY
    A. The natural reservoir of *Edwardsiella* species appears to be the intestinal tracts of fish and various mammals.

III. CELLULAR, CULTURAL, AND BIOCHEMICAL CHARACTERISTICS
    A. Cellular characteristics
        1. Gram-negative rods
        2. Motile by peritrichous flagella
    B. Cultural characteristics
        1. Facultative anaerobic
        2. Growth on blood agar and MacConkey agar at 37°C
            a. Nonhemolytic
            b. Lactose-negative
    C. Biochemical characteristics
        1. Oxidase-negative
        2. Metabolism is both respiratory and fermentative.

IV. DISEASE OVERVIEW
    A. In domestic animals, *Edwardsiella* species are opportunistic pathogens but are rarely isolated from them.

15 | Genus *Enterobacter*

I. *ENTEROBACTER* SPECIES
   A. Pathogens

Species	Hosts	Extraintestinal Diseases
Enterobacter species	Domestic animals	opportunistic

      1. *E. cloacae* and *E. agglomerans* are the most commonly isolated species.

II. HABITAT AND ECOLOGY
   A. *Enterobacter* species are normal intestinal flora of domestic animals and also are found in soil and water.

III. CELLULAR, CULTURAL, AND BIOCHEMICAL CHARACTERISTICS
   A. Cellular characteristics
      1. Gram-negative rods
      2. Motile by peritrichous flagella
   B. Cultural characteristics
      1. Facultative anaerobic
      2. Growth on blood agar and MacConkey agar at 37^{0}C
         a. Nonhemolytic
         b. Lactose-positive
   C. Biochemical characteristics
      1. Oxidase-negative
      2. Metabolism is both respiratory and fermentative.

IV. DISEASE OVERVIEW
   A. In domestic animals, *Enterobacter* species are opportunistic pathogens in a variety of extraintestinal infections. *E. cloacae* can be isolated in pure culture; however, the other *Enterobacter* species are generally found in mixed culture. They are not considered to be enteric pathogens.

16 | Genus *Klebsiella*

I. *KLEBSIELLA* SPECIES
   A. Pathogens

Species	Hosts	Specific Disease	Nonspecific Diseases
K. pneumoniae	Equine	METRITIS	opportunistic
	Domestic animals		opportunistic
Other species	Domestic animals		opportunistic

       1. *K. pneumoniae* and *K. oxytoca* are the most commonly isolated species from domestic animals.

II. HABITAT AND ECOLOGY
   A. *Klebsiella* species occur naturally in soil and water and are normal intestinal flora of domestic animals.
   B. *K. pneumoniae* is commonly found in wood products.
       1. Many infections in domestic animals are acquired from wood products contaminated with *K. pneumoniae*.

III. CELLULAR, CULTURAL, AND BIOCHEMICAL CHARACTERISTICS
   A. Cellular characteristics
       1. Gram-negative rods
       2. Nonmotile
   B. Cultural characteristics
       1. Facultative anaerobic
       2. Growth on blood agar and MacConkey agar at $37^{0}C$
           a. The klebsiellae are nonhemolytic on blood agar and are lactose-positive on MacConkey agar.
           b. Colonies of *K. pneumoniae* are large, convex, mucoid, and tend to coalesce. On MacConkey agar, colonies are often pink due to slow lactose fermentation.
   C. Biochemical characteristics
       1. Oxidase-negative
       2. Metabolism is both respiratory and fermentative.

IV. DISEASE OVERVIEW
   A. *K. pneumoniae*
       1. Equine infections
           a. *K. pneumoniae* and *Streptococcus zooepidemicus* are the two most common causes of metritis in the mare.

2. Infections in domestic animals
   a. It can be a primary pathogen in a variety of infections.
     (1) Canine cystitis, mastitis, and metritis
     (2) Bovine mastitis
     (3) Porcine mastitis
   b. Because of the very potent endotoxin, endotoxemia and endotoxic shock are commonly observed in these infections.

---

17 | Genus *Morganella*

I. *MORGANELLA* SPECIES
   A. Pathogens

Species	Hosts	Extraintestinal Diseases
M. morganii	Domestic animals	opportunistic

     1. It is the only species in the genus.

II. HABITAT AND ECOLOGY
   A. *M. morganii* is normal intestinal flora of domestic animals.

III. CELLULAR, CULTURAL, AND BIOCHEMICAL CHARACTERISTICS
   A. Cellular characteristics
     1. Gram-negative rods
     2. Motile by peritrichous flagella
   B. Cultural characteristics
     1. Facultative anaerobic
     2. Growth on blood agar and MacConkey agar at $37^{\circ}C$
       a. Nonhemolytic
       b. Lactose-negative
   C. Biochemical characteristics
     1. Oxidase-negative
     2. Metabolism is both respiratory and fermentative.

IV. DISEASE OVERVIEW
   A. In domestic animals, *M. morganii* is an opportunistic pathogen and is most frequently isolated from wound and urinary tract infections. It is not an enteric pathogen.

18	Genus *Proteus*

I. *PROTEUS* SPECIES

A. Pathogens

Species	Hosts	Extraintestinal Diseases
Proteus species	Domestic animals	urinary tract, opportunistic

1. *P. mirabilis* and *P. vulgaris* are the most commonly isolated species.

II. HABITAT AND ECOLOGY

A. *Proteus* species are normal intestinal flora of domestic animals and also are found in soil and polluted water.

III. CELLULAR, CULTURAL, AND BIOCHEMICAL CHARACTERISTICS

A. Cellular characteristics
   1. Gram-negative rods
   2. Motile by peritrichous flagella
B. Cultural characteristics
   1. Facultative anaerobic
   2. Growth on blood agar and MacConkey agar at $37^{\circ}C$
      a. *Proteus* species often swarm or produce a thin bacterial film on the agar surface. They are nonhemolytic and lactose-negative.
C. Biochemical characteristics
   1. Oxidase-negative
   2. Metabolism is both respiratory and fermentative.

IV. DISEASE OVERVIEW

A. In domestic animals, *P. mirabilis* and *P. vulgaris* are seldom incriminated as enteric pathogens but are commonly found in a wide variety of extraintestinal infections. Urinary infections in dogs and cats are very common.

19 | Genus *Providencia*

I. *PROVIDENCIA* SPECIES
A. Pathogens

Species	Hosts	Extraintestinal Diseases
Providencia species	Domestic animals	opportunistic

    1. *P. rettgeri* and *P. stuartii* are the most commonly isolated species.

II. HABITAT AND ECOLOGY
A. *Providencia* species are normal intestinal flora of domestic animals.

III. CELLULAR, CULTURAL, AND BIOCHEMICAL CHARACTERISTICS
A. Cellular characteristics
    1. Gram-negative rods
    2. Motile by peritrichous flagella
B. Cultural characteristics
    1. Facultative anaerobic
    2. Growth on blood agar and MacConkey agar at $37^{o}C$
       a. Nonhemolytic
       b. Lactose-negative
C. Biochemical characteristics
    1. Oxidase-negative
    2. Metabolism is both respiratory and fermentative.

IV. DISEASE OVERVIEW
A. Infections in domestic animals
    1. *Providencia* species are opportunistic extraintestinal pathogens but do not cause enteric disease.
    2. *P. rettgeri* is frequently isolated in pure culture from urinary infections.

20	Genus *Serratia*

I. *SERRATIA* SPECIES
    A. Pathogens

Species	Hosts	Extraintestinal Diseases
Serratia species	Domestic animals	opportunistic

      1. *S. liquefaciens* and *S. marcescens* are the most commonly isolated species.

II. HABITAT AND ECOLOGY
    A. *Serratia* species are normal intestinal flora of domestic animals and also occur in soil and water.

III. CELLULAR, CULTURAL, AND BIOCHEMICAL CHARACTERISTICS
    A. Cellular characteristics
        1. Gram-negative rods
        2. *S. liquefaciens* and *S. marcescens* are motile by peritrichous flagella, but some *Serratia* species are nonmotile.
    B. Cultural characteristics
        1. Facultative anaerobic
        2. Growth on blood agar and MacConkey agar at 37°C
            a. Nonhemolytic
            b. Lactose-positive
            c. Colonies of *Serratia* species are white, pink, or red, and most are opaque. *S. marcescens* is readily identified in cultures because of the production of a deep red pigment.
    C. Biochemical characteristics
        1. Oxidase-negative
        2. Metabolism is both respiratory and fermentative.

IV. DISEASE OVERVIEW
    A. In domestic animals, *Serratia* species do not cause enteric disease but are occasionally found in extraintestinal infections, often in mixed culture with other bacterial species.

21	Genus *Yersinia*

I. *YERSINIA* SPECIES
   A. Pathogens

Species	Hosts	Intestinal Disease	Extraintestinal Diseases
Y. pestis	Man		Plague
Other species	Domestic animals	enteritis	opportunistic

   1. *Y. enterocolitica* and *Y. pseudotuberculosis* are the most
      commonly isolated species from domestic animals.

II. HABITAT AND ECOLOGY
   A. *Yersinia* species are normal intestinal flora of domestic animals.
   1. Some species are adapted to specific hosts.

III. CELLULAR, CULTURAL, AND BIOCHEMICAL CHARACTERISTICS
   A. Cellular characteristics
      1. Gram-negative rods
         a. Cells of *Yersinia* species are small coccobacilli.
      2. *Yersinia* species are motile by peritrichous flagella when grown
         below 30°C but nonmotile when grown at 37°C except *Y. pestis*,
         which is always nonmotile.
   B. Cultural characteristics
      1. Facultative anaerobic
      2. Growth on blood agar and MacConkey agar at 37°C
         a. Nonhemolytic
         b. On MacConkey agar, *Y. enterocolitica* and *Y.
            pseudotuberculosis* are lactose-negative. These yersinae are
            distinct from other pathogenic members of the family
            Enterobacteriaceae because of the paucity of growth after 24
            hours of aerobic incubation at 37°C. The colonies vary from
            barely perceptible to pinpoint in size.
   C. Biochemical characteristics
      1. Oxidase-negative
      2. Metabolism is both respiratory and fermentative.

IV. DISEASE OVERVIEW
   A. In some species of domestic animals, *Y. enterocolitica* and *Y.
      pseudotuberculosis* can cause diarrhea, mesenteric lymphadenitis, and
      septicemia.

1. These yersinae are facultative intracellular bacteria that favor localization in macrophages, where they exist within phagolysosomes and multiply extensively. These intracellular bacteria are apparently resistant to the oxidative and nonoxidative killing mechanisms of macrophages.

PART 3	Aerobic Gram-positive Rods

22	Genus *Corynebacterium*

I. *CORYNEBACTERIUM* SPECIES
  A. Pathogens

Species	Hosts	Specific Diseases	Nonspecific Diseases
C. diphtheriae	Man	Diphtheria	
C. pseudotuberculosis	Equine	Ulcerative lymphangitis	
	Ovine	CASEOUS LYMPH-ADENITIS	abortion, arthritis
C. renale	Bovine	PYELONEPHRITIS	
	Porcine		kidney abscesses
C. ulcerans	Bovine		mastitis

  B. Nonpathogens
    1. *C. bovis* is a commensal of the bovine mammary gland.

II. HABITAT AND ECOLOGY
  A. Many *Corynebacterium* species occur as commensals of the skin and mucous membranes of domestic animals.

III. CELLULAR, CULTURAL, AND BIOCHEMICAL CHARACTERISTICS
  A. Cellular characteristics
    1. Gram-positive rods
      a. The cellular morphologies of the different *Corynebacterium* species vary markedly. The term diphtheroid has traditionally been used to describe the cells of *C. diphtheriae*, which have a characteristic "Chinese letter" appearance, often showing "V," "L," or "Y" shapes with club-shaped swellings in the ends or middle. Most pathogenic corynebacteria have pleomorphic, often filamentous, cells.
    2. Nonmotile

B. Cultural characteristics
1. The pathogenic corynebacteria have a wide range of oxygen requirements and may be aerobic, microaerophilic, or facultative anaerobic.
2. Growth on blood agar at 37°C
   a. Colonies of *C. pseudotuberculosis* are small with a cream or orange color and may produce a slight hemolysis.
   b. Colonies of *C. renale* are small, ivory-colored, opaque, and nonhemolytic.
C. Biochemical characteristics
1. Catalase-positive
2. Fermentative metabolism
   a. Pathogenic species of domestic animals ferment glucose.

IV. DISEASE OVERVIEW
A. *C. pseudotuberculosis* infections
1. Equine ulcerative lymphangitis
   a. Occasionally, *C. pseudotuberculosis* will cause ulcerative lymphangitis and caseous abscesses in horses.
2. Ovine caseous lymphadenitis (see Chap. 91)
   a. Caseous lymphadenitis is a chronic infection of the lymph nodes. The lesions are characterized by caseous necrosis.
   (1) In rams, the bacterium has been associated with orchitis and epididymitis.
B. *C. renale* infections
1. Bovine contagious pyelonephritis (see Chap. 81)
   a. Bovine contagious pyelonephritis results from an ascending infection of *C. renale* that localizes in the ureter and kidney. Disease is most common in mature cows because of the shortness of the female urethra and is predisposed to by pregnancy and parturition. Contagious pyelonephritis is the most common cause of infectious renal disease in cattle.
C. *C. ulcerans* infections
1. Bovine mastitis
   a. *C. ulcerans* is occasionally found in bovine mastitis.

23 | Genus *Rhodococcus*

I. *RHODOCOCCUS* SPECIES
  A. Pathogens

Species	Hosts	Specific Disease	Nonspecific Diseases
R. equi	Equine	Foal pneumonia	
	Domestic animals		opportunistic

    1. *R. equi* was previously classified as *Corynebacterium equi*.

II. HABITAT AND ECOLOGY
  A. *R. equi* is normal fecal flora of horses and can persist for long periods on contaminated pasture. On horse farms, the organisms are usually sporadic but may become endemic on a premise.

III. CELLULAR, CULTURAL, AND BIOCHEMICAL CHARACTERISTICS
  A. Cellular characteristics
    1. Gram-positive rods
    2. Nonmotile
  B. Cultural characteristics
    1. Obligate aerobic
    2. Growth on blood agar at 37°C
      a. Colonies are round, smooth, and mucoid with a tendency to coalesce and are nonhemolytic. Colonial pigmentation has been described as yellowish, pink, tan, red, or salmon-colored.
  C. Biochemical characteristics
    1. Catalase-positive
    2. Respiratory metabolism
      a. Glucose is not utilized oxidatively.

IV. DISEASE OVERVIEW
  A. Equine foal pneumonia
    1. Clinical *R. equi* infections occur most frequently in foals from 1 to 6 months of age. Horses over 6 months of age rarely develop clinical signs of infection. The decline in colostral antibody, which occurs about 6 weeks of age, coincides with the peak age for disease.
      a. Foals with combined immunodeficiency disease are particularly susceptible to infection.

      b.   The infections in foals are usually sporadic, but outbreaks have occasionally been reported on farms where the disease is endemic.

  2.   Susceptible foals usually acquire the infection by ingestion. Other modes of transmission include by inhalation, congenital, via the umbilicus, and by migrating helminth larvae from the gastrointestinal tract.

  3.   Foal pneumonia is characterized as a pyogranulomatous bronchopneumonia with lung abscesses, often complicated by an ulcerative colitis with mesenteric lymphadenitis.

  4.   *R. equi* is considered to be a facultative intracellular pathogen with an affinity for macrophages. The bacterium produces an exotoxin termed equi factor that is considered to play a major role in the pathogenesis of the disease.

  B. Infections in domestic animals

    1.   *R. equi* infections also have been reported in cattle, sheep, swine, dogs, and cats.

| 24 | Genus *Dermatophilus* |

I. *DERMATOPHILUS* SPECIES
  A. Pathogens

Species	Hosts	Specific Disease
D. congolensis	Ovine	DERMATOPHILOSIS
	Domestic animals	Dermatophilosis

II. HABITAT AND ECOLOGY
  A. *D. congolensis*

    1.   The bacterium has only been isolated from the integument of animals. It probably has a saprophytic existence in soil; however, attempts to isolate it from the soil have been unsuccessful.

    2.   Dermatophilosis is ubiquitous among domestic herbivores and can exist in a quiescent form until exacerbation occurs when climatic conditions are favorable for its infectivity.

      a.   The disease has a worldwide distribution.

III. CELLULAR, CULTURAL, AND BIOCHEMICAL CHARACTERISTICS
   A. Cellular characteristics
      1. Gram-positive rods
         a. It has two characteristic morphologic forms, nonmotile filamentous hyphae and motile zoospores.
            (1) The filamentous form develops through the germination of motile zoospores. The branching filaments are 1 to 5 um in diameter.
            (2) The motile zoospores are approximately 1 um in diameter and can have 5 to more than 50 flagella.
            (3) The filaments fragment by both transverse and longitudinal septation into packets of coccoid cells. These packets of cells dissociate into motile zoospores.
   B. Cultural characteristics
      1. Facultative anaerobic
      2. Growth on blood agar at 37°C
         a. Colonies are generally bright orange or yellowish, but occasionally white to gray variants occur. The bacterium produces hemolysis on blood agar.
   C. Biochemical characteristics
      1. Catalase-positive
      2. Fermentative metabolism

IV. DISEASE OVERVIEW
   A. Infections in domestic animals
      1. Dermatophilosis is an acute or chronic bacterial infection of the epidermis characterized by exudative dermatitis with scab formation.
      2. The condition frequently affects cattle and sheep and occasionally horses but is rare in dogs, cats, and pigs.
      3. In cattle, the disease is commonly called cutaneous streptothricosis.
   B. Ovine dermatophilosis (see Chap. 92)
      1. In sheep, the condition is called "lumpy wool" when the wooled areas of the body are affected and "strawberry foot rot" when the distal portions of the limbs are affected.

25 | Genus *Erysipelothrix*

I. *ERYSIPELOTHRIX* SPECIES
   A. Pathogens

Species	Hosts	Specific Diseases
E. rhusiopathiae	Ovine	Polyarthritis
	Porcine	ERYSIPELAS
	Man	Erysipeloid

   1. *E. rhusiopathiae* is the only species in the genus.

II. HABITAT AND ECOLOGY
   A. *E. rhusiopathiae*
      1. The bacterium can survive in the intestinal tracts of nonporcine animals and immune pigs.
      2. The bacterium can live in soil for 20 days or longer. Alkaline soils with a high content of organic matter favor its survival.

III. CELLULAR, CULTURAL, AND BIOCHEMICAL CHARACTERISTICS
   A. Cellular characteristics
      1. Gram-positive rods
         a. Cells are slender and often filamentous.
      2. Nonmotile
   B. Cultural characteristics
      1. Facultative anaerobic
         a. On primary isolation, the bacterium grows best in a microaerophilic atmosphere.
      2. Growth on blood agar at 37°C
         a. Colonies of *E. rhusiopathiae* are small, translucent and produce a narrow zone of incomplete hemolysis.
   C. Biochemical characteristics
      1. Catalase-negative
      2. Fermentative metabolism
         a. The bacterium has only weak fermentative activity for carbohydrates.
         b. In triple sugar iron agar, *E. rhusiopathiae* produces H_2S and an acid slant and butt, distinguishing this bacterium from other nonsporeforming, aerobic, gram-positive bacilli.

IV. DISEASE OVERVIEW
   A. Ovine polyarthritis
      1. A polyarthritis caused by *E. rhusiopathiae* is occasionally diagnosed in sheep.
   B. Porcine erysipelas (see Chap. 102)
      1. Erysipelas occurs in pigs of all ages, but pigs from 2 months to 1 year of age tend to be the most susceptible to infection and clinical disease. Most infections are acquired by the ingestion of *E. rhusiopathiae*-contaminated feces and soil. The bacterium also may be maintained in a swine herd for years by asymptomatic carrier swine.
      2. Clinical erysipelas is generally recognized as acute, subacute, or chronic.
         a. The acute septicemia form is characterized by high fever, lameness, depression, and high mortality rates within the first 48 to 72 hours. Sudden deaths without premonitory signs are also common.
         b. The clinical signs of subacute erysipelas are similar but are often less intense than acute erysipelas. After 3 to 4 days, cutaneous lesions develop on the skin of the abdomen, ears, and extremities. These necrotic skin lesions are rhomboid-shaped and have a reddish purple color. These cutaneous lesions are pathognomonic for erysipelas.
         c. Chronic erysipelas is often a sequela to the acute and subacute forms of the disease. It is characterized by a chronic arthritis that is nonsuppurative, proliferative, and erosive and/or vegetative endocarditis.

26 | Genus *Listeria*

I. *LISTERIA* SPECIES
   A. Pathogens

Species	Hosts	Intestinal Diseases	Extraintestinal Diseases
L. monocytogenes	Bovine	INTESTINAL-VISCERAL	MENINGOENCEPHA-LITIS, SEPTICEMIA, ABORTION
	Domestic animals	Intestinal-visceral	Septicemia

   1. *L. monocytogenes* is the only species in the genus that produces clinical disease in domestic animals.

II. HABITAT AND ECOLOGY
   A. *L. monocytogenes*, which is ubiquitous in nature, is found in soil, vegetation, and feces. It prefers decaying vegetable matter with a neutral or alkaline pH.
      1. Feeding poor-quality silage with a high pH increases the opportunity for the bacterium to survive, multiply, and induce clinical disease.

III. CELLULAR, CULTURAL, AND BIOCHEMICAL CHARACTERISTICS
   A. Cellular characteristics
      1. Gram-positive rods
      2. Motility is temperature-dependent. The bacterium is motile by peritrichous flagella when grown at 20°C but nonmotile at 37°C.
   B. Cultural characteristics
      1. Facultative anaerobic
      2. Growth on blood agar at 37°C
         a. On blood agar, colonies are small, smooth, and grayish. A narrow zone of beta hemolysis is produced.
   C. Biochemical characteristics
      1. Catalase-positive
      2. Metabolism is both respiratory and fermentative.

IV. DISEASE OVERVIEW
   A. Pathogenic characteristics
      1. It is a facultative intracellular pathogen. The bacterium has a high infectivity but a low pathogenicity. Clinical disease is related to the number of bacteria ingested.

B. Infections in domestic animals (see Chap. 86)
1. Intestinal and visceral listeriosis
   a. Subclinical infections of the digestive tract are the most common form of infection.
2. Septicemic listeriosis
   a. Septicemic listeriosis occurs primarily in neonatal animals, principally in calves, lambs, piglets, and foals.
      (1) The principal clinical sign is septicemia, but gastroenteritis and meningitis may occur.
      (2) Lesions include focal necrosis of the liver, spleen, and gastrointestinal tract.
3. Abortion
   a. Listerial abortion is sporadic in cattle and sheep.
      (1) In pregnant animals, the ingested bacteria penetrate the mucous membranes, and a neutrophil-associated bacteremia disseminates the infection with subsequent bacterial localization in the placenta. There are placentitis and fetal septicemia. After fetal death, the fetus may be retained 24 to 72 hours before abortion, which occurs during the last trimester of pregnancy.
4. Neural listeriosis
   a. Neural listeriosis is a meningoencephalitis of cattle and sheep.
      (1) It is the most common type of clinical disease.
      (2) Ingested bacteria penetrate the mucous membranes of the oral and nasal cavities, then migrate along the cranial nerves, especially the trigeminal nerve to the brain stem. In the brain stem, there is unilateral bacterial localization with focal microabscess formation.
      (3) Typical clinical signs include directional circling, unilateral facial paralysis, and unilateral corneal opacity. Death is due to dehydration and starvation.

27 | Genus *Mycobacterium*

I. *MYCOBACTERIUM* SPECIES
   A. Pathogens

Species	Primary Hosts	Other Hosts	Specific Diseases
M. avium	Fowl		Tuberculosis
			TUBERCULOSIS
		Porcine	Tuberculosis,
			Mycobacteriosis
M. bovis	Bovine		TUBERCULOSIS
		Man	Tuberculosis
M. leprae	Man		Leprosy
M. paratuberculosis	Bovine		PARATUBER-
			CULOSIS
		Ovine	Paratuberculosis
M. tuberculosis	Man		Tuberculosis

   B. Nonpathogens
      1. Other mycobacteria
         a. Some members of *M. avium* complex and the atypical
            mycobacteria are considered to be soil saprophytes.
            Mycobacteriosis is primarily a disease of swine and
            occasionally of cattle and can be caused by select members
            of the *M. avium* complex and a few of the atypical
            mycobacteria.
   C. Classification
      1. *Mycobacterium* complexes
         a. Complex names are used for grouping closely related
            Mycobacterium species with a common pathogenic potential
            for which further speciation would be of little clinical
            value.
      2. *M. avium* complex
         a. The complex is composed of *M. avium*, which includes
            serovars 1, 2, and 3, and *M. intracellulare*, which includes
            serovars 4 to 28.
            (1) Some serovars cause avian tuberculosis and porcine
                tuberculosis, whereas others cause mycobacteriosis in
                domestic animals, particularly swine. The different
                serovars vary in host range and pathogenicity for fowl
                and domestic animals.
      3. Runyon classification schema (Table 27.1)
         a. The four Runyon groups (I, II, III, and IV) are based on
            pigment production and growth rate. This traditional

Table 27.1. Runyon classification based on colony pigmentation and growth rate

Group Designation	Colony Pigmentation	Growth Rate
I Photochromogens	Yellow-orange colonies in light	Slow
II Scotochromogens	Yellow-orange colonies in dark	Slow
III Nonchromogens	Buff-colored colonies	Slow
IV Rapid growers	Nonpigmented colonies	Rapid

classification is helpful in the presumptive identification of the various *Mycobacterium* species, complexes, and atypical mycobacteria.

   b. In the pigment production procedure, two slants of Lowenstein-Jensen medium are inoculated. One slant is exposed to light and one wrapped in foil. When colonies appear on the uncovered slant, the foil is removed from the covered slant and the presence or absence of pigment noted. If the culture is nonchromogenic, it is exposed to light for 1 hour. After exposure, the slant is covered and reincubated overnight. The presence or absence of pigment in a culture grown exposed to light, in total darkness, and exposed to light for a brief period will allow for its classification as a photochromogen, scotochromogen, or nonchromogen.

II. ECOLOGY AND HABITAT

  A. Some mycobacteria are host-adapted to various domestic animals, man, and birds. Others are soil saprophytes and opportunistic pathogens.

    1. Mycobacteria are highly resistant to the environment due to their waxy cell wall. These lipids give the mycobacteria a high level of resistance to environmental influences and to the action of disinfectants.

  B. *M. avium* complex

    1. Some serovars are highly host-adapted and cause avian tuberculosis and porcine tuberculosis.

      a. Serovars 1, 2, and 3 are usually pathogenic for birds; serovars 4 to 28, however, do not produce progressive disease in chickens.

      b. Avian tuberculosis is transmissible from infected birds to swine.

    2. Some serovars are soil saprophytes and cause mycobacteriosis in domestic animals, particularly swine.

      a. Mycobacteriosis is a noncommunicable disease.

  C. *M. bovis*

    1. Cattle are the primary hosts.

    2. Man is very susceptible to *M. bovis*.

  D. *M. leprae*

    1. Leprosy occurs as a natural disease in man and nine-banded armadillos.

a. The disease is transmitted from infected to susceptible
     humans, but some studies have suggested that man also can
     contract leprosy from handling infected armadillos.
E. *M. paratuberculosis*
    1. The bacterium is host-adapted to ruminants, particularly cattle.
F. *M. tuberculosis*
    1. The primary host is man.
    2. It is easily transmitted from infected or carrier humans to
        monkeys and apes.

III. CELLULAR, CULTURAL, AND BIOCHEMICAL CHARACTERISTICS
    A. Cellular characteristics
        1. Gram-positive rods
        2. Acid-fast
            a. The cell walls of these acid-fast bacteria contain
                approximately equal amounts of peptidoglycan, lipid, and an
                arabinogalactan polysaccharide. The high lipid content,
                which ranges from 20 to 40 percent of the dry cell weight,
                is largely responsible for the ability of these bacteria to
                resist decoloration with acidified organic solvents.
            b. The Ziehl-Neelsen method is commonly used to stain the
                mycobacteria. The smears are treated with concentrated
                carbol fuchsin, mordanted by heating, and then decolorized
                with a sulfuric acid and alcohol solution. Malachite green
                or methylene blue are commonly used counterstains. The
                acid-fast mycobacteria retain the carbol fuchsin dye and
                are bright red.
        3. Nonmotile
    B. Cultural characteristics
        1. Obligate aerobic
            a. Most mycobacteria grow best in an atmosphere of 3 to 10
                percent carbon dioxide.
        2. Fastidious growth requirements
            a. The mycobacteria have fastidious nutritional growth
                requirements and will not grow on blood agar. An egg base
                culture medium such as Lowenstein-Jensen medium, which is
                composed of coagulated eggs, glycerol, potato flour, and
                salts, is commonly used to cultivate the mycobacteria.
                Mycobactin is frequently added to the medium to support the
                growth of mycobactin-dependent species such as *M.
                paratuberculosis*.
                (1) All pathogenic mycobacteria produce mycobactins except
                     M. paratuberculosis.
                (2) *M. leprae* has not been cultured on artificial media.
            b. The generation time for most pathogenic species of domestic
                animals is 20 to 24 hours. The cultures are frequently
                incubated for 6 to 12 weeks to obtain visible growth.
            c. Presumptive identification of the mycobacteria is largely

based on determining the optimal temperature for growth, rate of growth, and pigmentation of colonies.

(1) Different species of mycobacteria show a striking dependence on temperature for optimal growth. The optimal temperature for *M. bovis*, *M. tuberculosis*, and *M. paratuberculosis* is 37°C and for *M. avium* is 42°C. These species are slow growing and nonchromogens. Colonies of *M. bovis*, *M. tuberculosis*, and *M. paratuberculosis* have a buff color. The colonies of *M. avium* are buff to lightly pigmented.

d. Definitive identification of species is largely based on biochemical criteria, including catalase production, niacin accumulation, reduction of nitrate to nitrite, Tween 80 hydrolysis, and urease and arylsulfatase reactions.

(1) *M. avium* is almost indistinguishable from *M. intracellulare*. The only known biochemical differences between the two species are in their rates of arylsulfatase and nitrate reduction.

e. Culture and identification procedures for the mycobacteria are complex and are usually only performed by reference state or federal microbiology laboratories.

C. Biochemical characteristics
   1. Catalase-positive
   2. Respiratory metabolism

IV. DISEASE OVERVIEW
   A. The pathogenic mycobacteria are facultative intracellular pathogens.
   B. Infections in domestic animals
      1. Tuberculosis is caused by *M. bovis*, *M. tuberculosis*, and some serovars of *M. avium*.
      2. Mycobacteriosis is caused by some serovars of *M. avium* and some atypical mycobacteria.
      3. Paratuberculosis in ruminants is caused by *M. paratuberculosis*.
   C. Tuberculosis (see Chaps. 90 and 104)
      1. The tubercle is the characteristic lesion.
         a. The core of the tubercle is composed of mycobacteria, epithelioid cells, and giant cells. A narrow band of lymphoid cells surround the core. The tubercle is encapsulated by fibrous connective tissue.
         b. Tubercles can form in any organ in which reticuloendothelial tissue is present.
      2. Infections induce a granulamatous tissue reaction.
         a. The mycobacteria are implanted in the tissues and phagocytized. Some phagocytized bacteria are killed; others survive, particularly if they are ingested by macrophages. The bacteria proliferate within the macrophages and are released when the host cells die and lyse. There is an influx of more macrophages to the focus

of infection, and this sequence continues as the tubercle enlarges. The center of the tubercle is composed of dead macrophages, killed bacteria, and live extracellular bacteria. The necrotic caseous center of the lesion enlarges as the blood clotting mechanism is activated and the capillaries, arterioles, and venules are thrombosed. Calcification of the tubercles occur in man and cattle but is seldom, if ever, observed in other species of domestic animals.

3. The lesions are disseminated.
    a. Macrophages laden with tubercle bacilli
        (1) Some macrophages that leave the lesion via the lymphatics contain tubercle bacilli, which they carry to the draining lymph nodes. In this location, another focus of infection may develop.
    b. Erosion of a primary lesion into a blood vessel
        (1) Miliary tuberculosis is characterized by multiple lesions in multiple organs. It results from the erosion of a primary lesion into a blood vessel with hematogenous dissemination.

4. Bacterial components contribute to the granulomatous inflammatory reaction.
    a. Tuberculoprotein induces a specific immunological inflammation.
    b. Wax D and cord factor induce nonimmunological inflammation and are required for maximal granulomatous inflammation.
        (1) Cord factor is present in both *M. bovis* and *M. tuberculosis* but not in *M. avium*.
            (a) Cord factor is a mycoside that contains two molecules of mycolic acid esterified to the disaccharide trehalose.

5. Delayed hypersensitivity plays a role in pathogenesis and immunity.
    a. Immunity to tuberculosis is largely dependent on the presence of activated macrophages, which in turn depends on the degree of delayed hypersensitivity developed by the host. This hypersensitivity is directed primarily against tuberculin.
    b. Humoral immunity apparently plays little, if any, role in the immunity to tuberculosis.

6. Tuberculin tests are used for antemortem diagnoses.
    a. A positive tuberculin reaction indicates either a past or present infection.
    b. Tuberculin is prepared from culture filtrates.
        (1) Old tuberculin (OT) is prepared from crude mycobacterial culture filtrates.
        (2) Purified protein derivative (PPD) is a semipurified culture filtrate.

(3) Three types of PPD are used in domestic animals and man: *M. avium* PPD, *M. bovis* PPD, and *M. tuberculosis* PPD.

c. Tuberculin tests measure delayed hypersensitivity.

(1) The tuberculin is administered intracutaneously, and the reactions are measured at 48 to 72 hours. The diameter of the lesions are measured in millimeters.

(a) Polymorphonuclear leukocytes are the first major elements of the cellular infiltrate to appear; they are seen during the initial 12 hours of a tuberculin reaction. After the first 12 hours, large mononuclear cells and lymphocytes become the major cellular components of the delayed-type hypersensitivity (DTH) reaction.

(b) In man, the standard test dose of *M. tuberculosis* PPD is five tuberculin units. A tuberculin unit's potency is determined by comparison with the international standard (PPD-S), which is measured on the basis of weight.

(2) Many diseased animals do not react to tuberculin testing due to poor cell-mediated responses.

D. Mycobacteriosis

1. Mycobacteriosis is characterized by tuberculosislike granulomatous lesions that are caused by acid-fast mycobacteria other than *M. avium*, *M. bovis*, and *M. tuberculosis*.

a. These saprophytic acid-fast bacteria are inhabitants of soil and water and occasionally infect domestic animals.

b. Mycobacteriosis is not communicable.

2. Mycobacteriosis causes diagnostic problems because the disease mimics tuberculosis and infected animals may react to tuberculin skin tests.

E. Paratuberculosis (see Chap. 87)

1. Paratuberculosis is a chronic enteric infection of ruminants. It primarily affects cattle and occasionally sheep and numerous other ruminant species. Clinically affected cattle have a chronic diarrhea and weight loss and generally are debilitated.

28	Genus *Nocardia*

I. *NOCARDIA* SPECIES
   A. Pathogens

Species	Hosts	Specific Diseases	Nonspecific Disease
N. asteroides	Bovine	Mastitis	
	Canine	Pulmonary nocardiosis	pyogranulomatous
	Domestic animals		pyogranulomatous
N. brasilensis	Domestic animals		pyogranulomatous

   1. *N. asteroides* is the principal species isolated from domestic
      animals.

II. HABITAT AND ECOLOGY
   A. The soil is the natural habitat of *Nocardia* species.

III. CELLULAR, CULTURAL, AND BIOCHEMICAL CHARACTERISTICS
   A. Cellular characteristics
      1. Gram-positive rods
         a. Nocardiae are pleomorphic and frequently appear as branched
            filaments ranging from 0.5 to 1.0 um in width and from 10
            to 30 um or more in length. Bacillary and coccobacillary
            forms result from the fragmentation of filaments.
      2. Partially acid-fast
      3. Nonmotile
   B. Cultural characteristics
      1. Obligate aerobic
      2. Growth on blood agar at 37°C
         a. Colonies of *N. asteroides* develop slowly on blood agar, are
            nonhemolytic, and adhere to the agar. After 24 hours,
            colonies are minute and have a chalk-white, cream, or tan
            color. After 48 hours, colonies are about 1 mm in
            diameter. When incubated 72 to 96 hours, colonies often
            develop a yellow-orange pigment.
   C. Biochemical characteristics
      1. Catalase-positive
      2. Respiratory metabolism
         a. Glucose is not utilized.

IV. DISEASE OVERVIEW
  A. Bovine mastitis
    1. Mammary gland infections are acquired from exogenous sources through the teat canal. The lesions are characterized by pyogranulomatous inflammation and diffuse abscesses.
  B. Canine pulmonary nocardiosis
    1. *N. asteroides* is the primary agent of pulmonary nocardiosis, a condition that is characterized by empyema and pleuritis. Clinically the condition is often indistinguishable from pulmonary actinomycosis. *Actinomyces viscosus* is a primary agent of canine pulmonary actinomycosis.
  C. Canine and feline infections
    1. In dogs and cats, nocardial infections are characterized as chronic pyogranulomatous lesions, often with draining fistulous tracts. The skin and subcutaneous tissues are commonly infected.
  D. Equine, ovine, and porcine infections
    1. The *Nocardia* species are rarely implicated in infections of the equine, ovine, and porcine.

<table>
<tr><td rowspan="3">PART 4</td><td>Aerobic and Anaerobic
Gram-positive
Sporeforming Rods</td></tr>
</table>

29	Genus *Bacillus*

I. *BACILLUS* SPECIES
 A. Pathogens

Species	Hosts	Specific Disease
B. anthracis	Bovine	ANTHRAX
	Other domestic animals	Anthrax

    1. *B. anthracis* is the only significant pathogenic species of domestic animals.
 B. Virulence factors
    1. Capsular antigens
        a. The D-glutamic acid polypeptide capsule is antiphagocytic.
        b. The role of the capsule appears to be limited to the establishment of the infection. Nonencapsulated mutants are avirulent.
    2. Exotoxin complex
        a. There are three antigenically distinct components, which are heat-labile proteins or lipoproteins (Table 29.1).

Table 29.1. Components of the exotoxin complex

Fraction	Name	Pathogenic Character
Factor I	Edema factor	Edema
Factor II	Protective factor	Antiphagocytic
Factor III	Lethal factor	Lethality

        b. Exotoxin factors must act in concert to cause pathology.
           (1) Factor I has the edema-producing activity of the toxin. It must be associated with factor II to produce edema.

(2) Factor II is an antiphagocytic factor. It is a good immunogen, and antibodies to factor II provide protective immunity. If factor II is neutralized, factors I and III are not manifested.

(3) Factor III is responsible for the lethal effects of the toxin. It must be associated with factor II to be lethal. Factor III alters the integrity of eucaryotic cell membranes, resulting in increased capillary permeability.

    c. The exotoxin plays a major role in the pathogenesis of the disease.

3. Plasmid-mediated virulence factors

    a. The genes coding for the polypeptide capsule and the exotoxin proteins are carried on plasmids.

II. HABITAT AND ECOLOGY

A. *B. anthracis* is associated with alkaline or calcarous soils, in which the spores can survive indefinitely.

1. Epidemic outbreaks of anthrax in domestic ruminants are often associated with extreme changes in the general climatic conditions of an area. These changes are believed responsible for germination of spores and proliferation of the bacterium.

    a. When soil conditions are favorable to the vegetative state, the spores germinate and a nonpathogenic life cycle may be maintained for years.

        (1) Survival of the organisms in soil is favored by a neutral or alkaline pH, an ambient temperature of $20^{\circ}C$ to $37^{\circ}C$, and a relative humidity of 60 percent or higher.

        (2) Anthrax is endemic in parts of the southwestern and western United States, where an animal-soil-animal cycle has been established.

B. Spores of *B. anthracis* may contaminate a large number of products derived from animals, including wool, hides, hair, bones, and animal feeds.

III. CELLULAR, CULTURAL, AND BIOCHEMICAL CHARACTERISTICS

A. Cellular characteristics

1. Gram-positive rods

    a. Cells of *B. anthracis* are large bacilli with square or concave ends. The cells measure 1 to 1.5 um in width by 3 to 10 um in length. The cells are frequently arranged in chains.

2. Sporeformers

    a. *B. anthracis* has ovoid subterminal spores.

    b. The spores produced by members of genus *Bacillus* seldom distend the vegetative cells, whereas the spores produced by the clostridia often distend the cells.

3. Motility
   a. *B. anthracis* is nonmotile, but most other *Bacillus* species are motile by peritrichous flagella.

B. Cultural characteristics
   1. Facultative anaerobic
      a. *B. anthracis* grows best aerobically.
      b. *Bacillus* species often form larger colonies on aerobically incubated media than on media incubated anaerobically. Aerotolerant clostridia grow better under anaerobic conditions and form larger colonies than on media incubated aerobically.
      c. Aerobic conditions are required for sporulation but not for germination.
   2. Growth on blood agar at 37°C
      a. Colonies of *B. anthracis* are large, flat, gray, and nonhemolytic. Virulent strains have a "Medusa head" appearance (i.e., the colony edge has a tangled mass morphology). When grown under 5 to 10 percent carbon dioxide on media containing 0.5 percent sodium bicarbonate or serum, virulent strains produce a capsule, which gives rise to the formation of smooth, convex, mucoid colonies with an entire edge.
      b. Colonies of *Bacillus* species, other than *B. anthracis*, produce either alpha or beta hemolysis on sheep blood agar.

C. Biochemical characteristics
   1. Catalase-positive
   2. Fermentative metabolism

IV. DISEASE OVERVIEW
A. Susceptibility of domestic animals to anthrax
   1. Considerable variation in the innate susceptibility to anthrax exists among domestic animals. Their resistance to anthrax appears to fall into two groups.
      a. Some animals are resistant to the establishment of infection, but once infection is established, are sensitive to the toxin. Other animals are susceptible to the establishment of infection but resistant to the toxin.
   2. The full expression of virulence of *B. anthracis* is dependent on both the capsule and exotoxin complex.
      a. Spores of *B. anthracis*, when ingested or inhaled, germinate within a few hours.
         (1) The capsule on vegetative cells inhibits opsonization and phagocytosis.
         (2) The exotoxin is responsible for the clinical manifestation of anthrax.

B. Infections in domestic animals
   1. Bovine and ovine infections (see Chap. 76)
      a. Peracute septicemia is characterized by death within 1 to 2

hours after clinical signs are first observed.
  b.   In acute septicemia, death occurs in 48 to 96 hours.
  c.   Chronic infections are rarely observed.
  2.   Equine and porcine infections
      a.   Acute pharyngitis is the most common syndrome.
      b.   Acute septicemia and death do occur but are very rare.
  3.   Canine and feline infections
      a.   Anthrax rarely occurs in dogs and cats.
C.   Pathogenesis of anthrax
  1.   Ingestion is the primary mode of transmission.
      a.   Common sources of *B. anthracis* are contaminated forages and
          the carcasses of infected animals.
  2.   Bacteria proliferate at the primary foci of infection.
      a.   Encapsulated bacteria proliferate and resist phagocytosis.
      b.   Animal species with leukocytes sensitive to the toxin tend
          to be more susceptible to the establishment of infection
          than are animal species with highly resistant leukocytes.
  3.   Bacteria spread to and multiply in regional lymph nodes.
      a.   In susceptible animal species, the bacterial multiplication
          exceeds the capacity of the lymph nodes to contain the
          infection. This results in the spread of the infection to
          other lymph nodes and a bacteremia.
  4.   Bacteria in the blood can either be cleared by the
       reticuloendothelial system or continue to proliferate and
       produce an overwhelming bacteremia and toxemia.
      a.   The level of lethal toxin increases rapidly late in the
          course of the disease.
  5.   The toxemia has pathophysiological effects.
      a.   Vascular permeability is increased, and capillary
          thrombosis leads to secondary shock and asphyxia.
      b.   The toxin has a direct effect on the central nervous system.
  6.   Acquired immunity to anthrax is provided by antibodies to the
       capsule and toxin.
      a.   The relative importance of these two forms of humoral
          immunity appears to vary widely in different animal
          species.

30 | Genus *Clostridium*

I. *CLOSTRIDIUM* SPECIES
   A. Pathogens

Species	Hosts	Specific Diseases	Nonspecific Diseases
C. botulinum	Domestic animals	Botulism	
C. chauvoei	Bovine	BLACKLEG	
	Ovine	Blackleg	
C. difficile	Man	Pseudomembranous colitis	
C. haemolyticum	Bovine	BACILLARY HEMO-GLOBINURIA	
C. novyi	Bovine	INFECTIOUS NECROTIC HEPATITIS	
	Ovine	Infectious necrotic hepatitis	
C. perfringens	Bovine	Enterotoxemia, Gas gangrene	
	Canine	Hemorrhagic gastroenteritis	
	Equine	Enterotoxemia	
	Ovine	ENTEROTOXEMIA	
	Porcine	Enterotoxemia	
C. septicum	Domestic animals	Malignant edema	
C. tetani	Domestic animals	Tetanus	
Other species	Domestic animals	Gas gangrene	cellulitis, myonecrosis

   1. Over 25 *Clostridium* species have been isolated from clinical specimens. *C. sordellii* and *C. histolyticum* are commonly isolated.
   B. Two methods of disease production
      1. Intoxication
         a. Disease is due to the ingestion of a preformed toxin or toxins elaborated from a localized lesion (e.g., *C. botulinum*, *C. haemolyticum*, *C. perfringens*, and *C. tetani*).
      2. Infection
         a. Disease is due to the infection of host tissues with subsequent toxin production (e.g., *C. chauvoei*, *C. novyi*, *C. perfringens*, *C. septicum*, and *C. sordellii*).
   C. Exotoxins
      1. Clostridia produce potent exotoxins that are the main mediators of pathological changes in the host (Table 30.1).
         a. The toxins are highly immunogenic.
         b. All pathogenic *Clostridium* species produce exotoxin(s).
            (1) Clostridial strains frequently lose their ability to produce toxin, and at least some of the toxins are bacteriophage-mediated, thus allowing the transfer of this property from one organism to another and even to another species.

Table 30.1. Lethal clostridial toxins

Clostridium Species	Designation	Mode of Action
C. botulinum	Neurotoxin	Prevents release of acetylcholine at motor end plate
C. chauvoei	Alpha	Lethal activity unknown, hemolytic
C. haemolyticum	Lecithinase C	Hemolytic, necrotizing, phospholipase
C. novyi	Alpha	Necrotizing
	Beta	Hemolytic, necrotizing, phospholipase
C. perfringens	Alpha	Hemolytic, necrotizing, phospholipase
	Beta	Necrotizing
	Epsilon	Necrotizing
	Iota	Necrotizing
	Enterotoxin	Diarrheal, erythemal
C. septicum	Alpha	Hemolytic, necrotizing, leukocidal
C. sordellii	None	Lethal activity unknown
C. tetani	Tetanospasmin	Neurotoxic
	Tetanolysin	Hemolytic, edema-inducing

2.   Three modes of toxin production are described.
   a.   Extracellular toxins
      (1)   The toxins readily diffuse out of the cell and are found in maximum amounts in the culture fluid shortly after the end of the log phase of growth.
      (2)   Almost all clostridial toxins are extracellular.
   b.   Protoplasmic toxins
      (1)   The toxins are released after cell lysis.
      (2)   *C. botulinum* (toxin types A to G), *C. novyi* (alpha toxin), and *C. tetani* (tetanospasmin) are examples of *Clostridium* species that produce protoplasmic toxins.
   c.   Sporulation toxins
      (1)   The toxin is formed intracellularly and is released only at the time of sporulation. The enteropathogenic strains of *C. perfringens* produce sporulation toxins.
3.   Toxin production and activation mechanisms are described.
   a.   Active toxins are fully active when synthesized.
   b.   Some toxins are synthesized as less active prototoxins and attain full toxicity only after exposure to certain proteolytic enzymes.
      (1)   In some bacteria, proteolytic enzymes also are synthesized by the bacteria producing the prototoxin and the activation is spontaneous.
4.   Toxin testing
   a.   The purpose of toxin testing is to identify selected *Clostridium* species and/or toxin types. Toxin testing is frequently used to identify *C. botulinum* types A to G, *C. novyi* types A and B, *C. perfringens* types A to E, and *C. tetani.*
   b.   To determine a toxin type within a *Clostridium* species, the toxin is identified by neutralization with type-specific antitoxin. Mice are commonly used in the toxin neutralization tests.

(1) The seven toxigenic types (A to G) of *C. botulinum* are tested in mice for identification of toxin in a culture of the suspect organism, animal's serum, or food sample by specific antitoxin. Mice inoculated with appropriate antitoxin survive, while mice inoculated with the toxin but not with an appropriate antitoxin become paralyzed and die.

(2) The five toxigenic types (A to E) of *C. perfringens* are identified on the basis of four major lethal toxins (alpha, beta, epsilon, and iota). These four toxins are produced in various proportions by the five types of *C. perfringens* (Table 30.2).

Table 30.2. Toxigenic types of *Clostridium perfringens*

Type	Major Lethal Toxins Produced			
	Alpha	Beta	Epsilon	Iota
A	++	–	–	–
B	+	++	+	–
C	+	++	–	–
D	+	–	++	–
E	+	–	–	++

Note: ++ = large amounts; + = small amounts; – = none produced.

(3) A culture filtrate of a suspected clostidial organism is injected into mice, some of which have been protected by previous inoculation of tetanus antitoxin. In a test positive for *C. tetani*, the unprotected animals die with typical tetanic spasms, while the mice protected with antitoxin survive.

D. Immunogens and immunization
1. Clostridial cells (vegetative) and toxins are highly immunogenic.
2. The three types of immunization products are antitoxins, bacterins, and toxoids (Table 30.3).
   a. Bacterins and toxoids are often combined in commercial products.

Table 30.3. Immunization products of *Clostridium* species

Species	Antitoxins	Bacterins	Toxoids
C. botulinum		+	+[a]
C. chauvoei		+	+
C. haemolyticum		+	
C. novyi		+	+
C. perfringens	+[b]	+	+[b]
C. septicum		+	+
C. sordellii		+	+
C. tetani	+		+

[a]Toxin type C.
[b]Toxin types B, C, and D.

II. ECOLOGY AND HABITAT

  A. The soil and intestinal tracts of domestic animals and man are major habitats of medically important *Clostridium* species.

    1. Clostridia isolated from soils become associated with disease either by direct contamination of wounds or as transient flora of the gastrointestinal tract.

      a. In general, clostridia cause disease only as opportunistic infections that are secondary to some primary injury or management problem.

III. CELLULAR, CULTURAL, AND BIOCHEMICAL CHARACTERISTICS

  A. Cellular characteristics

    1. Gram-positive rods

    2. Sporeformers

      a. Members of the genus *Clostridium* form spores under anaerobic conditions.

      b. The location and shape of the endospores are characteristic of some *Clostridium* species. The clostridia can be differentiated from the sporeformers in the genus *Bacillus* by the swollen area of the spore in the sporangium.

        (1) *C. tetani* is a long, thin bacillus with round terminal spores (a characteristic drumstick appearance).

    3. Most *Clostridium* species are motile by peritrichous flagella, but *C. perfringens* is nonmotile.

    4. *C. perfringens* has a capsule, unlike most clostridia.

  B. Cultural characteristics

    1. Obligate anaerobic

      a. Some clostridia are aerotolerant.

    2. Fastidious growth requirements

  C. Biochemical characteristics

    1. Catalase-negative

    2. Fermentative metabolism

      a. Clostridia are usually fermentative, proteolytic, or both, but some are asaccharolytic and nonproteolytic.

    3. Fluorescent antibody stains are used for the rapid identification of *C. chauvoei*, *C. septicum*, *C. sordellii*, and certain other clostridia.

IV. DISEASE OVERVIEW

  A. *C. botulinum* infections

    1. Botulism in domestic animals

      a. Disease

        (1) Botulism toxin(s) cause a flaccid paralysis with death due to asphyxiation. The toxin(s) depress the formation and/or release of acetylcholine at the myoneural junction.

      b. Ecology

        (1) *C. botulinum* is ubiquitous in the environment. The bacterium is found in soil, vegetation, and

occasionally in the intestinal contents of mammals, fish, and birds.

(2) Vegetative cells can multiply in any dead material under anaerobic conditions and produce toxin, which is released on autolysis of the bacterial cells.

c. Modes of infection

(1) Intoxication, in which preformed toxin(s) are ingested, is the most common mode of infection.

    (a) The breakdown of *C. botulinum* toxin(s) by gastrointestinal proteases to more readily absorbable lower molecular weight active fragments may play a significant role in contributing to toxicity by the oral route.

(2) Toxicoinfection, where *C. botulinum* causes an infection of the digestive tract or wounds with subsequent toxin absorption, is a rare mode of infection.

    (a) *C. botulinum* seldom invades living tissue or produces enough toxin in the intestine to cause disease.

d. Pathogenesis

(1) Botulism toxin(s) attaches to the presynaptic terminal of cholinergic nerves, where it blocks the release of acetylcholine. Toxin receptors in the presynaptic membrane contain gangliosides that bind the toxin. Once the toxin has become fixed at susceptible nerve endings it is not affected by antitoxins.

(2) Botulism toxin affects the peripheral autonomic nervous system, the peripheral motor nerves, and the central nervous system.

(3) Three general mechanisms of action have been attributed to botulinum toxin.

    (a) The toxin binds to a specific receptor on the cell surface.

    (b) The toxin is transported inside the cell. It has been suggested that botulinum toxin, like diphtheria toxin, can form channels in the eucaryotic cell membranes.

    (c) The toxin expresses an intracellular activity that results in the pharmacological response. The nature of the intracellular activity of the toxin, which blocks the release of the neurotransmitter, remains unknown.

e. Toxin characteristics

(1) The seven toxin types (A to G) are immunologically distinct, but the mode of action of each type is identical. All seven serotypes are proteins with MW 150,000. The toxins are synthesized by the bacteria

as single polypeptides but are nicked by proteases to produce chains with MW 50,000 and 100,000. The two nascent polypeptides are held together by an interchain disulfide linkage.

(a) Generally, a given strain of *C. botulinum* produces only one toxin serotype, although there are exceptions.

(b) The toxins of serotypes A, B, E, F, and G are carried on the bacterial chromosome, whereas the genes for serotypes C and D are carried by lysogenic bacteriophages. Therefore, it is possible to cure certain C- and D-producing strains, resulting in nontoxigenic *C. botulinum*, while reinfection with a bacteriophage restores toxigenicity. If a cured strain of *C. botulinum* is infected with a heterologous bacteriophage carrying a different toxin serotype, the new strain will produce a different toxin serotype.

(2) All toxins are heat-labile (100°C for 10 minutes) and are inactivated by the acidity of the gastric secretions.

f. Species susceptibility to botulism

(1) Each species of animal is susceptible to different toxin types (Table 30.4). This may be due to two causes. First, the antigenically different toxins are absorbed differently from the gastrointestinal tract by different animal species. Second, the toxin receptor sites of the different animal species may differ and prevent the attachment of toxins.

(2) Although clinical botulism is considered to be rare in domestic animals, it is probable that many cases are not diagnosed in ruminants and horses.

Table 30.4. Botulism toxin susceptibility by species

Species	Toxin Susceptibility[a]	Toxin Types[b]
Bovine	+	C, D
Canine	−	
Equine	+	B
Feline	−	
Ovine	+	D
Porcine	−	
Man[c]	+++	A, B, E, F
Fowl	++	C, E

[a] +++ = extremely susceptible; ++ = very susceptible; + = susceptible but disease is uncommon; − = not susceptible or disease extremely rare.

[b] The toxin types producing disease vary with the source and geographic location.

[c] Botulism toxin is the most potent toxin on a gram for gram basis known to produce intoxication in man.

g. Immunity
(1) Natural infection
(a) Clinical botulism does not induce demonstrable antibody because the amount of toxin sufficient to induce an immune response would be lethal.
(2) Passive immunity
(a) Antitoxins are not effective once symptoms are seen. Toxoids (type-specific) have been used successfully in the immunization of cattle in areas where the disease is endemic.
h. Diagnosis
(1) The initial diagnosis of botulism is based on the clinical symptoms.
(2) The diagnosis is confirmed by demonstrating the presence of the toxin in the serum or feces, isolation of the organism from the animal's feces, or isolation of the organism from the contaminated food or environment.
(a) The typing of *C. botulinum* found in serum, feces, or food is accomplished using the mouse assay in conjunction with specific antisera. Dilutions of the test sample are made and injected intraperitoneally into mice. Specific antisera are added to the samples before injection for determination of toxin type. The specific antiserum neutralizes the activity of its respective toxin and thus protects the animal from death.
(3) At present, supportive therapy is the only established efficacious treatment for the toxicosis.
B. *C. chauvoei* infections
1. Bovine blackleg (see Chap. 78)
a. Blackleg is a gangrenous myositis that principally affects young cattle (from 6 months to 2 years of age) in good nutritional condition.
(1) The infections are initiated by the activation of spores in muscle tissues, which germinate, proliferate, and produce exotoxins.
2. Ovine blackleg
a. Blackleg in sheep occurs mostly at the time of shearing and castration, at which time traumatized and devitalized tissues are contaminated with spores of *C. chauvoei*.
C. *C. haemolyticum* infections
1. Bovine bacillary hemoglobinuria (see Chap. 77)
a. Bacillary hemoglobinuria is an acute hemolytic anemia that is characterized by anemia, icterus, and hemoglobinuria.
D. *C. novyi* infections
1. Bovine infectious necrotic hepatitis (see Chap. 84)

a.   Infectious necrotic hepatitis is caused by *C. novyi* type B.

b.   Deaths occur rapidly, often without clinical signs having been observed.

E.   *C. perfringens* infections

1.   Gas gangrene in domestic animals

   a.   Cattle, sheep, horses, and pigs are highly susceptible to gas gangrene, but dogs and cats are rarely affected with this condition.

   b.   *C. perfringens* is the most commonly isolated agent from clostridial myonecrosis, which is characterized by muscle necrosis, gas production, and systemic toxicosis. Other commonly isolated clostridia are *C. chauvoei*, *C. novyi*, and *C. septicum.*

       (1)   Since gas gangrene frequently results from the contamination of an open wound with soil and feces, most infections have a mixed bacterial flora composed of one or more pathogenic clostridia acting alone or in combination with each other. A variety of facultative anaerobes and obligate anaerobes are often isolated with the *Clostridium* species.

   c.   The distinctive characteristics of gas gangrene are severe edema, the formation of gas (which causes crepitation), discoloration of the underlying skin, coldness of the affected area, profound toxemia with prostration, and sudden death.

       (1)   Animals often die within 24 hours of the onset of clinical signs.

2.   Bovine enterotoxemia

   a.   Neonatal enterotoxemia is caused by *C. perfringens* types B and C. It affects calves under 2 weeks of age and is characterized as a hemorrhagic necrotic enteritis.

   b.   Enterotoxemia in feedlot cattle is frequently caused by *C. perfringens* type D and occasionally by type C. This form of enterotoxemia generally affects cattle on full grain rations. The condition is often referred to as overeating disease.

3.   Canine hemorrhagic gastroenteritis

   a.   *C. perfringens* type A is considered to be a primary etiologic agent of canine hemorrhagic gastroenteritis. The condition is characterized by sudden onset of vomiting, an acute enteritis with bloody diarrhea and circulatory failure and shock and is almost always fatal within 24 hours from when clinical signs are manifested. Pathologic findings are usually confined to the lower small intestine. Frank hemorrhage is found in the lumen of the intestine, and the mucosal surface has a dark red or black color.

4.   Equine enterotoxemia

   a.   A *C. perfringens* associated enteritis and enterotoxemia has occasionally been observed in horses.

5. Ovine enterotoxemia (see Chap. 93)
    a. Neonatal enterotoxemia in lambs under 2 weeks of age is caused by *C. perfringens* type B. It is characterized as an acute hemorrhagic enteritis. This disease is often referred to as lamb dysentery.
    b. Enterotoxemia and pulpy kidney disease in feeder lambs and older sheep is caused by *C. perfringens* type D. Affected animals are frequently on full grain rations.
6. Porcine enterotoxemia
    a. Neonatal enterotoxemia of piglets is caused by *C. perfringens* type C.

F. *C. septicum* infections
1. Bovine and ovine malignant edema
    a. *C. septicum* is the most common cause of malignant edema in cattle and sheep. Occasionally other *Clostridium* species are implicated in the condition.
        (1) *C. septicum* is commonly found in the gastrointestinal tracts of domestic ruminants and has a saprophytic existence in the soil.
    b. Deep wounds contaminated with feces or soil that contain spores or vegetative cells of *C. septicum* are the primary mode of transmission. Malignant edema occurs sporadically in susceptible cattle and sheep of all ages.
        (1) Common types of wounds that predispose to the infection include castration, shearing, penetrating stake wounds, and injuries to the female genitalia during parturition.
    c. Malignant edema is characterized by edematous swelling of the subcutaneous tissue, but unlike blackleg, it is more typically a cellulitis, in which the inflammation is confined primarily to the fascial planes, than a myositis. Malignant edema, like blackleg, is a highly toxigenic and fulminating infection that is invariably fatal within 48 hours after symptoms appear. Spontaneous recovery is rare.
2. Porcine malignant edema
    a. *C. septicum* infections of swine are rare.

G. *C. tetani* infections
1. Tetanus in domestic animals
    a. Disease
        (1) Tetanus is an intoxication following an infection.
        (2) Tetanus is characterized by tonic muscular contractions of the face, neck, and other parts of body. The muscular spasms are provoked by the slightest stimulation, including noise, movement, and touch.
        (3) Clinical signs of tetanus spasms in response to stimuli are pathognomonic. The spasms are painful and

have a sudden onset. There is violent rigidity, and opisthotonus is extreme. Severe contractions may compromise respiration.

(a) The name "lockjaw" describes the muscular contractions that rigidly close or lock the jaws together.

b. Ecology
   (1) *C. tetani* is found in soil and is a normal inhabitat of intestines of horses and domestic ruminants. Tetanus spores are found where manure is used as a fertilizer.

c. Transmission
   (1) Three modes of infection can occur.
       (a) Parental infections occur when wounds are contaminated with spores.
       (b) Puerperal tetanus results from postpartum infections. This mode of infection occasionally occurs in cows and mares.
       (c) Newborn tetanus infections are often acquired through the umbilicus.

d. Pathogenesis
   (1) A wound is contaminated with spores of *C. tetani*, which germinate in the wound.
   (2) On cell lysis, the neurotoxin (tetanospasmin) is released from the bacteria as a prototoxin that is composed of two polypeptide chains. The prototoxin is activated by proteolytic enzymes.
   (3) The toxin reaches the central nervous system either by vascular spread in the blood or by neural spread.
       (a) Vascular spread produces a descending generalized tetanus that begins with the head and progressively involves the body below the head.
       (b) Neural spread produces an ascending localized tetanus. The toxin is transported by the axoplasmic route centripetally from the peripheral nerve endings to the central nervous system along the axons.
       (c) Tetanospasmin affects the motor cells within the cerebrospinal axis. The toxin fixes to a ganglioside and is avidly bound to gray matter. The main action of tetanus toxin is on the anterior horn cells of the spinal cord and on the brain stem. The spasmogenic effect of the toxin is due to its blocking action of spinal inhibitory synapses, resulting in hyperflexia and spasms of skeletal muscle. The tetanus toxin blocks the release of two inhibitory substances, glycine and gamma amino-butyric acid. Glycine

mediates postsynaptic inhibition, while gamma-amino-butyric acid mediates presynaptic inhibition.

e. Toxins

(1) Tetanospasmin is a protein with MW 150,000. There is only one antigenic type. Tetanospasmin is one of the most powerful toxins known.

(2) Tetanolysin is a hemolysin.

f. Species susceptibility to tetanus

(1) Tetanus has been reported in all domestic animals. The horse is extremely susceptible.

g. Immunity

(1) Clinical tetanus is a nonimmunizing disease. The amount of tetanospasmin needed to produce disease and cause death is too small to induce an immune response.

h. Tetanus prophylaxis

(1) Tetanus immune globulin (TIG) is used to provide passive immunity.

(a) TIG is effective in neutralizing unbound tetanus toxin but not in neutralizing tetanus toxin bound to gangliosides on nerve cells.

(b) TIG is frequently produced in hyperimmunized horses.

(2) Tetanus toxoid is used to induce active immunity.

(a) Tetanus toxoids use inactivated tetanospasmin as the immunogen. A culture filtrate of toxigenic *C. tetani* is detoxified and incorporated in an adjuvant. Formalin is frequently used to treat the toxin to form the toxoid. The concentration of a toxoid is usually expressed in Lf units, which is a measure of the immunizing potency of the vaccine.

i. Diagnosis

(1) The initial diagnosis of tetanus is based on the clinical symptoms, often with a history of a puncture wound contaminated with soil or feces.

(2) The isolation of *C. tetani* from infected animals is often very difficult because the organism is not invasive and the amount of toxin needed to produce clinical tetanus is so small that there may be no apparent infected wound site to sample.

PART **5**	Anaerobic Gram-positive and Gram-negative Cocci

31	Genus *Peptococcus*

I. *PEPTOCOCCUS* SPECIES
   A. Pathogens

Species	Hosts	Nonspecific Diseases
Peptococcus niger	Domestic animals	suppurative

      1. It is the only species in the genus.

II. HABITAT AND ECOLOGY
   A. *P. niger* is normal flora of skin, mucous membranes, and gastrointestinal tracts of domestic animals.

III. CELLULAR, CULTURAL, AND BIOCHEMICAL CHARACTERISTICS
   A. Cellular characteristics
      1. Gram-positive cocci
         a. Cells may occur singly, in pairs, or in grapelike clusters.
      2. Nonmotile
   B. Cultural characteristics
      1. Obligate anaerobic
      2. Fastidious growth requirements
         a. On blood agar, the colonies are small, black, and nonhemolytic.
   C. Biochemical characteristics
      1. The various strains of *P. niger* have weak or variable catalase reactions.
      2. Fermentative metabolism
         a. Carbohydrates are not fermented.

IV. DISEASE OVERVIEW
   A. In domestic animals, *P. niger* is not a significant pathogen.

32	Genus *Peptostreptococcus*

I. *PEPTOSTREPTOCOCCUS* SPECIES
   A. Pathogens

Species	Hosts	Nonspecific Diseases
Peptostreptococcus species	Domestic animals	suppurative

   1. *P. anaerobius*, *P. indolicus*, and *P. magnus* are the most commonly
       isolated species.

II. HABITAT AND ECOLOGY
   A. *Peptostreptococcus* species are normal flora of skin, mucous
       membranes, and gastrointestinal tracts of domestic animals.

III. CELLULAR, CULTURAL, AND BIOCHEMICAL CHARACTERISTICS
   A. Cellular characteristics
       1. Gram-positive cocci
           a. Cells may occur in pairs, chains, or grapelike clusters.
       2. Nonmotile
   B. Cultural characteristics
       1. Obligate anaerobic
           a. It is often difficult to distinguish the peptostreptococci
               from the microaerophilic- and carbon dioxide-requiring
               staphylococci and streptococci, which are often incorrectly
               considered to be anaerobic.
               (1) The anaerobic peptostreptococci are sensitive to
                    metronidiazole, whereas the aerobic gram-positive
                    cocci are resistant.
       2. Fastidious growth requirements
           a. In general, the peptostreptococci lack characteristic
               colonial features, and most species are nonhemolytic.
   C. Biochemical characteristics
       1. Catalase reactions vary with the species.
       2. Fermentative metabolism
           a. Some *Peptostreptococcus* species have the ability to ferment
               glucose, but others are asaccharolytic and utilize peptones
               and amino acids as a source of energy.

IV. DISEASE OVERVIEW
   A. In domestic animals, *Peptostreptococcus* species are usually isolated from suppurative lesions. Peptostreptococci can be isolated in pure culture but are usually isolated in mixed culture with other obligate anaerobes and/or facultative anaerobes.

33	Genus *Veillonella*

I. *VEILLONELLA* SPECIES
   A. Pathogens

Species	Hosts	Nonspecific Diseases
Veillonella species	Domestic animals	opportunistic

   1. *V. parvula* is the most commonly isolated species.

II. HABITAT AND ECOLOGY
   A. *Veillonella* species are normal flora of mucous membranes and gastrointestinal tracts of domestic animals.

III. CELLULAR, CULTURAL, AND BIOCHEMICAL CHARACTERISTICS
   A. Cellular characteristics
      1. Gram-negative cocci
      2. Nonmotile
   B. Cultural characteristics
      1. Obligate anaerobic
      2. Fastidious growth requirements
   C. Biochemical characteristics
      1. Oxidase-negative
      2. Fermentative metabolism
         a. Carbohydrates are not fermented, but lactate and pyruvate can be metabolized.

IV. DISEASE OVERVIEW
   A. *Veillonella* species have a low virulence and are always found in mixed culture with other obligate anaerobes and/or facultative anaerobes.

PART 6	Anaerobic Gram-positive Rods

34	Genus *Actinomyces*

I. *ACTINOMYCES* SPECIES
    A. Pathogens

Species	Hosts	Specific Diseases	Nonspecific Diseases
A. bovis	Bovine	ACTINOMYCOSIS	
	Equine	Fistulous withers, Poll evil	
	Domestic animals		granulomatous
A. israelii	Man	Actinomycosis	
A. naeslundii	Domestic animals		granulomatous
A. pyogenes	Domestic animals		suppurative
	Ovine	INFECTIVE BULBAR NECROSIS	
A. viscosus	Canine	Pulmonary actinomycosis	granulomatous

    1. *A. pyogenes* was previously classified as *Corynebacterium pyogenes*.

II. HABITAT AND ECOLOGY
    A. The soil is the natural habitat of many *Actinomyces* species.
    B. The pathogenic species of domestic animals occur as commensals on the mucous membranes of the genital tract and the oral and nasal cavities.

III. CELLULAR, CULTURAL, AND BIOCHEMICAL CHARACTERISTICS
    A. Cellular characteristics
        1. Gram-positive rods
            a. The cellular morphologies of the different *Actinomyces* species vary markedly. Most pathogenic species have pleomorphic often filamentous cells, but the cells of *A. pyogenes* have a coccobacillary shape.
            b. Branching of *A. bovis* and *A. israelii* is usually present in

vivo but is often hard to demonstrate in vitro.
   (1) These species form sulfur granules in vivo but not in vitro.
   2. Nonmotile
B. Cultural characteristics
   1. The *Actinomyces* species that are pathogens of domestic animals and man have marked differences in their atmospheric requirements for growth, but the genus has been classified as facultative anaerobic. Carbon dioxide concentrations of 3 to 8 percent are required for maximum growth of most species.
      a. *A. bovis*, *A. israelii*, and *A. naeslundii* prefer an anaerobic environment for growth, whereas *A. viscosus* grows best under microaerophilic conditions.
         (1) Traditionally the genus *Actinomyces* had been classified as obligate anerobic, and techniques used to culture and identify obligate anerobic bacteria have been used for these *Actinomyces* species.
      b. *A. pyogenes* is a facultative anaerobe, and procedures used to culture and identify aerobic bacteria are employed in the identification of this bacterium.
   2. All pathogenic *Actinomyces* species have fastidious growth requirements except *A. pyogenes*, which will grow on blood agar incubated aerobically at 37°C.
C. Biochemical characteristics
   1. Catalase-negative except *A. viscosus*, which is catalase-positive.
   2. Fermentative metabolism
      a. The anaerobic species ferment carbohydrates with acid production but no gas. The major volatile fatty acids produced by glucose fermentation are formic and acetic acids, and the major nonvolatile fatty acids are lactic and succinic acids. These species are nonproteolytic.

IV. DISEASE OVERVIEW
A. *Actinomyces* species infections
   1. Infections in domestic animals
      a. Actinomycotic infections cause chronic granulomatous or pyogranulomatous tissue reactions.
         (1) In the bovine lesions caused by *A. bovis*, sulfur granules are formed that are 1 to 3 mm in diameter and composed of a bacterial colony in a hyaline matrix. The hyaline matrix helps protect the bacteria from host defense mechanisms, allowing the infection to persist within the host tissues.
B. *A. bovis* infections
   1. Bovine actinomycosis (see Chap. 74)
      a. Bovine actinomycosis (lumpy jaw) is a chronic proliferative osteomyelitis of the mandible or maxilla.

    b. Occasionally soft tissue granulomatous lesions and abscesses develop.

   2. Equine fistulous withers and poll evil

    a. *A. bovis* is a common cause of fistulous withers and poll evil.

     (1) *Brucella abortus* is also an etiologic agent of equine fistulous withers and poll evil.

C. *A. pyogenes* infections

   1. Ovine infective bulbar necrosis (see Chap. 96)

    a. Infective bulbar necrosis (heel abscess) is caused by a synergistic infection of *A. pyogenes* and *Fusobacterium necrophorum*, an obligate anaerobic gram-negative bacterium.

   2. Porcine cervical lymphadenitis

    a. *A. pyogenes* is an etiologic agent of porcine jowl abscesses.

     (1) In boars, the bacterium has been associated with orchitis and epididymitis.

   3. Infections in domestic animals

    a. *A. pyogenes* is found in various suppurative lesions and abscesses. The bacterium is frequently found in mixed infections with *F. necrophorum*.

D. *A. viscosus* infections

   1. Canine pulmonary actinomycosis

    a. *A. viscosus* is the primary etiologic agent. The bacterium may be recovered in pure culture, or in mixed culture with other facultative anaerobes and/or obligate anaerobes.

     (1) *Nocardia asteroides*, an obligate aerobic gram-positive filamentous bacterium, is the primary etiologic agent of canine pulmonary nocardiosis, which is clinically indistinguishable from pulmonary actinomycosis. Both infections are characterized by pleuritis and empyema.

35 | Genus *Bifidobacterium*

I. *BIFIDOBACTERIUM* SPECIES
   A. Pathogens

Species	Hosts	Nonspecific Diseases
Bifidobacterium species	Domestic animals	suppurative

II. HABITAT AND ECOLOGY
   A. *Bifidobacterium* species are normal intestinal flora of domestic animals.

III. CELLULAR, CULTURAL, AND BIOCHEMICAL CHARACTERISTICS
   A. Cellular characteristics
      1. Gram-positive rods
         a. These pleomorphic gram-positive bacilli are characterized by club-shaped rods and branching forms.
      2. Nonmotile
   B. Cultural characteristics
      1. Obligate anaerobic
      2. Fastidious growth requirements
   C. Biochemical characteristics
      1. Catalase-negative
      2. Fermentative metabolism

IV. DISEASE OVERVIEW
   A. In domestic animals, *Bifidobacterium* species are seldom pathogenic.

36 | Genus *Eubacterium*

I. *EUBACTERIUM* SPECIES
 A. Pathogens

Species	Hosts	Specific Diseases	Nonspecific Diseases
E. suis	Porcine	Cystitis, Pyelonephritis	
Other species	Domestic animals		suppurative

  1. *E. suis* was formerly classified as *Corynebacterium suis*.
  2. *E. lentum* is the most commonly isolated species from domestic animals.

II. HABITAT AND ECOLOGY
 A. *Eubacterium* species are normal intestinal flora of domestic animals.

III. CELLULAR, CULTURAL, AND BIOCHEMICAL CHARACTERISTICS
 A. Cellular characteristics
  1. Gram-positive rods
  2. Most *Eubacterium* species are nonmotile, including *E. suis*. A few species are motile.
 B. Cultural characteristics
  1. Obligate anaerobic
  2. Fastidious growth requirements
 C. Biochemical characteristics
  1. The eubacteria have negative or weak positive catalase reactions.
  2. Fermentative metabolism

IV. DISEASE OVERVIEW
 A. *E. suis* infections
  1. Porcine cystitis and pyelonephritis
   a. *E. suis* causes cystitis and pyelonephritis in swine. The infection can be transmitted during coitus.
    (1) *E. suis* is commonly found in the prepuce and preputial diverticulum of healthy boars, which are carriers of the disease, but it is rarely found in the lower urogenital tract of healthy sows.
 B. Other *Eubacterium* species infections
  1. In domestic animals, *Eubacterium* species are seldom pathogenic.

37 | Genus *Propionibacterium*

I. *PROPIONIBACTERIUM* SPECIES
A. Pathogens

Species	Hosts	Nonspecific Diseases
Propionibacterium species	Domestic animals	suppurative

    1. *P. acnes* is the most commonly isolated species.

II. HABITAT AND ECOLOGY
A. *Propionibacterium* species are normal flora of skin, mucous membranes, and gastrointestinal tracts of domestic animals.

III. CELLULAR, CULTURAL, AND BIOCHEMICAL CHARACTERISTICS
A. Cellular characteristics
1. Gram-positive rods
2. Nonmotile
B. Cultural characteristics
1. Obligate anaerobic
2. Fastidious growth requirements
C. Biochemical characteristics
1. Catalase-positive
2. Fermentative metabolism
    a. *Propionibacterium* species produce propionic acid as a major breakdown product of carbohydrate fermentation, which can be detected by gas liquid chromatography.
        (1) This metabolic characteristic is a differential feature used to distinguish members of genus *Propionibacterium* from other genera of anaerobic gram-positive bacilli.

IV. DISEASE OVERVIEW
A. In domestic animals, the *Propionibacterium* species are occasionally found in mixed culture with other obligate anaerobes and/or facultative anaerobes. They are rarely incriminated as pathogens in extraintestinal infections.

| PART 7 | Anaerobic Gram-negative Rods |

| 38 | Genus *Bacteroides* |

I. *BACTEROIDES* SPECIES
   A. Pathogens

Species	Hosts	Specific Diseases	Nonspecific Diseases
B. melaninogenicus	Bovine	FOOT ROT	suppurative
	Domestic animals		suppurative
B. nodosus	Bovine	Interdigital dermatitis	
	Ovine	CONTAGIOUS FOOT ROT	
Other species	Domestic animals		suppurative

   1. *B. fragilis*, *B. thetaiotaomicron*, and *B. vulgatus* are commonly isolated other species.

II. HABITAT AND ECOLOGY
   A. *B. nodosus*
      1. It is an obligate parasite of the digital epidermis of sheep.
         a. Under normal climatic conditions, *B. nodosus* will not survive on pasture for more than a few weeks.
      2. Although cattle can be infected with *B. nodosus*, their role as a reservoir for the bacterium is not clearly delineated.
   B. Other *Bacteroides* species
      1. The various *Bacteroides* species, other than *B. nodosus*, can be normal inhibitants of the skin, mucous membranes, and gastrointestinal tracts of domestic animals. These organisms occur in the environment as fecal contaminants.

III. CELLULAR, CULTURAL, AND BIOCHEMICAL CHARACTERISTICS
   A. Cellular characteristics
      1. Gram-negative rods
         a. *B. nodosus* is a large bacterium with a characteristic barbell or club shape.

2. The pathogenic *Bacteroides* species of domestic animals are nonmotile. Motile species have peritrichous flagella.
B. Cultural characteristics
   1. Obligate anaerobic
   2. Fastidious growth requirements
      a. Most bacteroides, like fusobacteria, require media enriched with blood or hemin and menadione. The addition of 10 percent carbon dioxide to the anaerobic atmosphere enhances the growth of most species.
   3. Colony characteristics
      a. Colonies of *B. fragilis*, *B. thetaiotaomicron*, and *B. vulgatus* are light gray, translucent, and 1 to 2 mm in diameter after 48 hours of anaerobic incubation at 37°C.
      b. *B. melaninogenicus* characteristically produces brown- or black-pigmented colonies with hemolysis on blood agar.
      c. Colonies of *B. nodosus* after 48 hours of anaerobic incubation at 37°C are circular, entire, convex, translucent, and nonhemolytic. Freshly isolated fimbriated strains may pit the agar surface.
C. Biochemical characteristics
   1. All pathogenic *Bacteroides* species of domestic animals are catalase-negative except *B. fragilis*, which is catalase-positive.
   2. Fermentative metabolism
      a. All pathogenic *Bacteroides* species of domestic animals will ferment glucose except *B. nodosus*.
         (1) Most bacteroides, like the fusobacteria, can be identified to generic level by examination of gram-stained smears and by gas chromatographical analysis of volatile and nonvolatile fatty acid end products of glucose metabolism.

IV. DISEASE OVERVIEW
   A. *B. melaninogenicus* infections
      1. Bovine foot rot (see Chap. 82)
         a. Bovine foot rot is caused by a synergistic infection of *B. melaninogenicus* and *Fusobacterium necrophorum*, both obligate anaerobic bacteria.
      2. Infections in domestic animals
         a. *B. melaninogenicus* is a commonly isolated *Bacteroides* species from domestic animals.
   B. *B. nodosus* infections
      1. Bovine contagious interdigital dermatitis
         a. Bovine contagious interdigital dermatitis (BCID) is caused by a mixed or synergistic infection of *B. nodosus* and *F. necrophorum*.
            (1) Cattle and sheep are the two principal domestic animals affected with *B. nodosus*, an obligate parasite

of the digital epidermis. Cattle are readily infected with cattle isolates, and sheep with sheep isolates. However, sheep isolates do not readily infect cattle, and cattle isolates cause only transient interdigital skin infections in sheep.

(2) *F. necrophorum* is a normal inhabitant of the bovine digestive tract and occurs in the environment as a fecal contaminant.

(3) Transmission of BCID has been demonstrated following environmental contact between affected and nonaffected cattle.

b. The primary sites of infection are the epidermal cells of the interdigital skin, characterized by inflammation of the interdigital skin with variable amounts of hyperemia and erosion. A thin, gray surface exudate is usually present.

(1) The interdigital infections are usually initiated when the feet are subjected to prolonged wetness with subsequent maceration of the interdigital skin, which allows the bacteria present in the feces-contaminated environment to colonize the interdigital lesions and initiate a bacterial dermatitis.

c. Some of the interdigital skin infections will spread to the bulb of the heel, where the bacteria produce characteristic pits and linear black grooves in the heel horn.

(1) As the epidermal infection spreads from the skin to the horn, the pits in the heel horn may be the only early evidence of this ongoing process. Eventually the pits in the bulbar epidermis may coalesce to form larger erosions and undermine the horn of the bulb of the heel and ultimately the wall and sole of the hooves.

d. Lameness is the principal clinical sign when there is heel horn erosion, but affected cattle with only interdigital lesions are usually asymptomatic although a slight tenderness may be exhibited when the interdigital lesion is palpated. An affected animal may not be lame at all times, and the only way to detect every case is to examine all the feet of each animal.

(1) All ages and breeds of cattle can be affected with BCID, but the condition is most prevalent in housed dairy cattle. The hind feet, especially the lateral claws, tend to be more frequently involved than the front feet.

(2) Sequelae to the interdigital dermatitis/heel horn erosion syndrome include pododermatitis circumscripta (sole ulcer), sole abscess, verrucose dermatitis, foot rot, white line disease, and complete heel horn erosion. Deep sepsis also may occur affecting the

coffin joint, navicular bone, navicular bursa, and/or flexor tendon sheaths.

e. Clinical diagnosis is based on a herd history of lameness, interdigital skin lesions, and characteristic pits and linear black grooves in the horn of the bulbs of the heel.

2. Ovine contagious foot rot (see Chap. 97)

a. Ovine contagious foot rot is caused by a synergistic infection of *B. nodosus* and *F. necrophorum*.

(1) In the initial interdigital dermatitis lesions, *F. necrophorum* is the primary pathogen, and *B. nodosus* is the primary pathogen in the hoof matrix. *Actinomyces pyogenes* and motile fusiforms are commonly found in the lesions and probably contribute to the severity of the condition but do not play a primary role in the pathogenesis of the condition.

C. *Bacteroides* species infections

1. Infections in domestic animals

a. The *Bacteroides* species, except *B. nodosus*, are frequently isolated from a variety of localized suppurative infections. Most of these infections are polymicrobial and have from 2 to 5 bacterial species of facultative anaerobic and/or obligate anaerobic bacteria.

39	Genus *Fusobacterium*

I. *FUSOBACTERIUM* SPECIES
   A. Pathogens

Species	Hosts	Specific Diseases	Nonspecific Diseases
F. necrophorum	Bovine	FOOT ROT	diphtheria
		Interdigital dermatitis	
		RUMENITIS-LIVER	suppurative
		ABSCESS COMPLEX	
	Ovine	CONTAGIOUS FOOT ROT	suppurative
		INFECTIVE BULBAR	
		NECROSIS	
Other species	Domestic animals		suppurative

   1. *F. necrophorum*, *F. nucleatum*, and *F. varium* are the most
       commonly isolated species.

II. HABITAT AND ECOLOGY
   A. The *Fusobacterium* species are normal inhabitants of the
       gastrointestinal tracts of domestic animals and occur in the
       environment as fecal contaminants.

III. CELLULAR, CULTURAL, AND BIOCHEMICAL CHARACTERISTICS
   A. Cellular characteristics
       1. Gram-negative rods
           a. The term fusiform is used to describe thin, gram-negative
               bacilli with pointed ends. All fusiform-shaped bacteria
               are not members of the genus *Fusobacterium*, and all
               fusobacteria are not fusiform-shaped.
           b. The cellular morphologies of the different *Fusobacterium*
               species are highly variable.
               (1) The cells of *F. necrophorum* are highly pleomorphic
                    with rounded ends.
               (2) *F. nucleatum* has fusiform-shaped cells, while the
                    cells of *F. varium* are coccobacillary to bacillary
                    with rounded ends.
       2. Nonmotile
   B. Cultural characteristics
       1. Obligate anaerobic
       2. Fastidious growth requirements
   C. Biochemical characteristics
       1. Oxidase-negative

   2. Fermentative metabolism
      a. Most *Fusobacterium* species, including *F. necrophorum*, will ferment glucose, but a few species are asaccharolytic.
      b. The fusobacteria produce large amounts of butyric acid from glucose, thus distinguishing them from the bacteroides.

IV. DISEASE OVERVIEW
   A. *F. necrophorum* infections
      1. Bovine rumenitis-liver abscess complex (see Chap. 88)
         a. Ruminal lesions are the primary foci of infection and liver abscesses the secondary foci.
         b. *F. necrophorum* is a component of the normal rumen microflora and the primary etiologic agent of liver abscesses.
      2. Bovine foot rot (see Chap. 82)
         a. Bovine foot rot is caused by a synergistic infection of *F. necrophorum* and *Bacteroides melaninogenicus*.
         b. Acute foot rot lesions are characterized by a suppurative necrosis of the subcutaneous tissues. The lesions can extend from the interdigital space to the fetlock.
      3. Bovine contagious interdigital dermatitis
         a. Bovine contagious interdigital dermatitis is probably caused by a synergistic infection of *F. necrophorum* and *B. nodosus*, both obligate anaerobic bacteria. The pathogenesis of this condition has been postulated to be similar to ovine contagious foot rot.
      4. Bovine diphtheria
         a. *F. necrophorum* is frequently isolated from necrotic infections of the larynx. It has been postulated that a prior infection of *Haemophilus somnus* damages the laryngeal mucosa, which predisposes the larynx to a subsequent infection with *F. necrophorum*.
         b. This necrotic laryngitis can occur in calves up to 2 years of age.
      5. Ovine contagious foot rot (see Chap. 97)
         a. Ovine foot rot is caused by a synergistic infection of *F. necrophorum* and *B. nodosus*.
      6. Ovine infective bulbar necrosis (see Chap. 96)
         a. Ovine infective bulbar necrosis (heel abscess) is caused by a synergistic infection of *F. necrophorum* and *Actinomyces pyogenes*.
         b. Heel abscesses are a complication of ovine interdigital dermatitis. The clinical signs are manifested 1 to 4 weeks following the primary interdigital dermatitis.
   B. *Fusobacterium* species infections
      1. Infections in domestic animals
         a. The *Fusobacterium* species are commonly isolated from a wide variety of clinical infections in domestic animals. The

infections are usually localized suppurative infections. Most infestions are polymicrobial with two or more species of facultative anaerobic and/or obligate anaerobic bacteria.

b. *F. necrophorum* is both the most virulent and most commonly isolated species. Frequently, the bacterium is isolated in pure culture from lesions that are characterized by a suppurative necrosis.

| PART **8** | # Aerobic and Anaerobic Spirochetes |

| 40 | ## Genus *Borrelia* |

I. *BORRELIA* SPECIES
A. Pathogens

Species	Hosts	Specific Diseases
B. anserina	Birds	Avian borreliosis
B. burgdorferi	Canine	Canine borreliosis
	Man	Lyme disease
B. recurrentis	Man	Louseborne relapsing fever
B. theileri	Bovine	Bovine borreliosis
	Equine	Equine borreliosis
Other species	Man	Tickborne relapsing fever

B. Classification
  1. Traditionally the borreliae have been classified into species according to their biological arthropod vectors.

II. HABITAT AND ECOLOGY
A. Arthropod vectors
  1. The geographical distribution of the borrelia-induced diseases of domestic animals and man is restricted by the location of their biological arthropod vectors.
    a. Canine borreliosis
      (1) *Ixodes dammini* is a primary tick vector of *B. burgdorferi*. The tick is found along the Atlantic Coast from Delaware to Massachusetts and also in Minnesota and Wisconsin. *I. dammini* has been found on several domestic animals, including cats, dogs, and horses.
      (2) Other ticks also have been found to be infected with *B. burgdorferi*. Their role in the transmission of canine borreliosis has not been clearly delineated.

   b. Bovine and equine borreliosis
       (1) *Rhipicephalus decoloratus* is a primary tick vector of
            B. theileri.
       (2) These diseases do not occur in the United States but
            are found in Australia and Africa.

III. CELLULAR, CULTURAL, AND BIOCHEMICAL CHARACTERISTICS

A. Cellular characteristics
   1. Gram-negative helical cells
      a. The borreliae are loosely coiled spirochetes that measure
          0.2 to 0.5 um in width and 3 to 20 um in length. These
          bacteria stain poorly with the Gram stain but well with
          Giemsa stain.
   2. Motile
      a. The cells are motile by means of 15 to 20 periplasmic
          flagella. The flagella of the borreliae, like those of the
          leptospires, are located between the peptidoglycan layer
          and the outer membrane and are attached subterminally to
          opposite ends of the protoplasmic cylinder.
B. Culture characteristics
   1. Borreliae are aerobes.
      a. Some *Borrelia* species that have been cultivated in vitro
          grow best under microaerophilic conditions.
   2. Fastidious growth requirements
      a. *B. burgdorferi* and *B. theileri* have not been cultivated in
          vitro.
      b. The *Borrelia* species that have been cultivated in vitro
          have fastidious nutritional requirements.
C. Biochemical characteristics
   1. The inability to cultivate many *Borrelia* species has limited
      their biochemical characterization.
   2. Some species will ferment glucose.

IV. DISEASE OVERVIEW

A. Canine borreliosis
   1. *B. burgdorferi* is transmitted by the bite of infected ticks,
      particularly *I. dammini*. The spirochetes migrate from the site
      of the tick bite into the blooodstream, where the organisms
      multiply. Most canine infections are asymptomatic, but some
      dogs are febrile and develop an arthritis.
   2. Clinical diagnoses of canine borreliosis are made on the basis
      of clinical symptoms and the presence of the tick vector in an
      endemic area. Most infections occur in the temperate climates
      of the United States from April through October, when the ticks
      are most active and feeding.

41	Genus *Leptospira*

I. *LEPTOSPIRA* SPECIES

A. Pathogens are in the species *L. interrogans.*

		Hosts with Clinical Leptospirosis						
Serovars	Reservoir Hosts	Bovine	Canine	Equine	Feline	Ovine	Porcine	Man
L. canicola	Canine	+	+	+	-	-	-	+
L. grippotyphosa	Wild animals	+	+	+	-	-	+	-
L. hardjo	Bovine	+	-	-	-	-	-	-
L. icterohaemorrhagiae	Rodents	+	+	+	-	-	+	+
L. pomona	Bovine, wild animals	+	-	-	-	+	+	-
L. szwajizak	Bovine	+	-	-	-	+	-	-

    1. There are over 200 serovars in the species *L. interrogans.* Six are responsible for most of the clinical leptospirosis in domestic animals in the United States. Other serovars are occasionally incriminated.

B. Nonpathogens are in the species *L. biflexa.*

C. Serogroups and serovars

    1. The serovar is the basic taxon of the leptospires.

    2. The pathogenic leptospires in the species *L. interrogans* are arranged into serogroups and serovars based on their antigenic composition.

        a. The identification of a leptospiral isolate as to serogroup and serovar is accomplished by microscopic agglutination and agglutinin adsorption test procedures. The leptospiral isolate to be identified is first screened against antisera to serovars representative of recognized serogroups. If the isolate is agglutinated at high titers, the isolate is considered to belong in the serogroup represented by that antiserum. After the serogroup of the isolate has been determined, it is reacted with antisera to the serovars in the serogroup to establish additional antigenic relationships. Reciprocal agglutination adsorption tests are used to determine the specific serovar.

        b. Cross reactions are common among the various serovars. The serovars within the same serogroup are very closely related antigenically.

    3. The six most common *Leptospira* serovars of domestic animals are classified in six different serogroups as follows: *L. canicola,* Canicola; *L. grippotyphosa,* Grippotyphosa; *L. hardjo,* Sejroe; *L. icterohaemorrhagiae,* Icterohaemorrhagiae; *L. pomona,* Pomona; and *L. szwajizak,* Hebdomadis.

    D. Serologic diagnostic tests
        1. Most diagnoses are based on serologic comparison of paired acute and convalescent serum samples.
            a. Serum antibodies induced with pathogenic serovars are often demonstrable after 1 week of infection, attain maximum levels in 3 or 4 weeks, and then slowly decline over the course of months or years. A 4-fold increase in titers of paired acute and convalescent sera taken 2 to 6 weeks apart is diagnostically significant.
        2. The macroscopic and microscopic agglutination tests are commonly used for the serologic diagnosis of leptospirosis.
            a. The macroscopic slide agglutination test uses killed leptospira antigens, which are commercially available. This test is less specific than the microscopic agglutination test.
            b. The microscopic agglutination test uses live leptospira cultures of the antigen. This test is the standard reference method for leptospira serology.

II. HABITAT AND ECOLOGY

    A. *L. interrogans*
        1. The reservoirs of the various serovars are rodents and other feral or domestic animals. Many serovars occur predominantly in selected mammalian hosts, but the distribution of a specific serovar in a select host is not exclusive.
            a. Pathogenic leptospires can survive in cool alkaline waters for 3 months or longer but do not persist in acid waters.
            b. Urine contaminated with leptospires is the primary source of environmental contamination. The persistence of leptospiruria may vary with the host and with the serovar causing the infection.
               (1) Leptospiruria in cattle, dogs, and swine may occur for only a few months after infection and is usually sparse or absent after 6 months.
               (2) In domestic animals, leptospires may be found in the urine after 1 week of disease.
    B. *L. biflexa*
        1. These nonpathogens are free-living and can be found in moist soil and fresh surface waters.

III. CELLULAR, CULTURAL, AND BIOCHEMICAL CHARACTERISTICS

    A. Cellular characteristics
        1. Gram-negative helical rods
            a. The pathogenic leptospires are 0.1 um in diameter and 6 to 20 um in length and are tightly coiled with 18 or more coils per cell. The cells have a hook or bend at one or both ends.
            b. Leptospiras are difficult to stain and are best observed by

darkfield microscopy. Silver impregnation stains are
commonly used.
2. Motile
    a. The pathogenic leptospires are motile by means of two
        periplasmic flagella (Fig. 41.1).

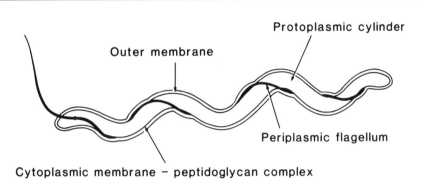

Fig. 41.1. A leptospira showing a periplasmic flagellum wound around the
protoplasmic cylinder and located between the cytoplasmic membrane-
peptidoglycan complex and the outer membrane. The two periplasmic flagella are
inserted subterminally at opposite ends of the cell.

B. Cultural characteristics
    1. Obligate aerobic
    2. Fastidious growth requirements
        a. The pathogenic leptospiras in *L. interrogans* are lipolytic
            bacteria with fatty acids serving as their source of carbon
            and energy. Culture media usually contain serum albumin,
            or serum plus a variety of long chain fatty acids, and has
            a pH between 6.8 and 7.8. These obligate aerobic bacteria
            have a generation time of 6 to 16 hours and usually require
            several days to a month or more to obtain visible growth.
            The optimal growth temperature is about 30°C.
            (1) Long chain fatty acids containing at least 15 carbon
                atoms are required for growth, since the leptospires
                are incapable of synthesizing fatty acids. Short
                chain fatty acids can be utilized if sufficient long
                chain fatty acids are not available.
            (2) Carbohydrates and amino acids are utilized only to a
                limited extent.
        b. Culture and serologic diagnostic procedures for leptospires
            are complex and usually only performed by reference
            veterinary microbiology laboratories.

C. Biochemical characteristics
  1. Oxidase-positive
  2. Respiratory metabolism

IV. DISEASE OVERVIEW
  A. Pathogenesis of leptospirosis
    1. The primary mode of transmission is direct contact with infected animals or through contact with urine-contaminated soil and water. The leptospires can penetrate intact mucous membranes and skin but produce no lesion at the point of infection. The leptospires spread from the lesion to establish a bacteremia of variable duration. The hematogenous leptospires localize and persist in the kidneys and liver, and some serovars show a marked affinity for the pregnant uterus.
      a. The incubation period in domestic animals is usually 10 to 12 days but ranges from 3 to 30 days.
      b. Leptospiremia occurs at the time of disease onset and persists for approximately 1 week.
    2. The clinical manifestations of leptospirosis are dependent on the serovar and the host tissues affected.
      a. Anemia and icterus commonly occur in acute infections.
        (1) The anemia is initially due to the action of hemolysins on the erythrocytes of susceptible animals and later by hemagglutinating antibodies produced by the host, which causes an intravascular type of hemolytic anemia.
          (a) Some pathogenic serovars produce hemolysins, and other serovars do not.
        (2) Icterus is a common manifestation of acute leptospirosis and results from both the intravascular hemolysis and the hepatocellular injury caused by some serovars.
          (a) *L. icterohaemorrhagiae* infections in dogs causes a marked hepatic necrosis and dissociation of the cords of hepatic cells. Other serovars localize and proliferate in the hepatic parenchyma but cause negligible damage.
      b. Nephritis occurs in all leptospiral infections.
        (1) The leptospires enter the kidneys hematogenously, penetrate the vascular endothelium, and then penetrate into the lumen of the proximal convoluted tubules, where they proliferate and are shed in the urine. The initial localization in the renal cortex causes a focal or diffuse interstitial nephritis characterized by interstitial edema, leukocyte infiltration, and focal tubular necrosis. Some serovars may progress to a chronic interstitial nephritis characterized by atrophy of the nephrons, mononuclear cell infiltration, and interstitial fibrosis.

      (a) Leptospiruria in domestic animals may last from a few weeks to several years. Adult animals are more likely to become renal carriers than are young animals. Leptospiruric animals may be seronegative.

      (b) Carnivores usually have urine with an acid pH and are not efficient transmitters of leptospirosis.

      (c) Herbivores have a neutral to slightly alkaline urine, which prolongs the survival of the leptospires and significantly contributes to the transmission of the disease.

  c. Abortions, stillbirths, and weak neonates commonly occur in cattle infected with *L. hardjo* and in swine infected with *L. pomona*. Uterine and fetal infections that result in abortions are relatively rare in dogs, cats, horses, and sheep.

  3. Domestic animals have marked differences in their susceptibility to leptospirosis.

    a. The bovine, canine, and porcine are susceptible to serious clinical disease.

    b. The equine and ovine are relatively resistant to acute clinical disease.

    c. The feline is susceptible to pathogenic leptospira infections but is very resistant to clinical disease.

B. Bovine leptospirosis (see Chap. 85)

  1. *L. hardjo* and *L. pomona* are the most common causes of clinical leptospirosis in cattle.

    a. *L. hardjo* is a major cause of abortion in cattle, but affected cattle seldom present other clinical signs.

    b. *L. pomona* in acute disease causes a hemolytic anemia, icterus, and occasionally abortion.

  2. Other *Leptospira* serovars that are occasionally incriminated include *L. canicola*, *L. grippotyphosa*, *L. icterohaemorrhagiae*, and *L. swajizak*.

C. Canine leptospirosis

  1. *L. canicola* and *L. icterohaemorrhagiae* cause most of the clinical leptospirosis. Dogs of all ages may be affected, but the majority of the clinical infections occur in dogs from 1 to 3 years of age.

    a. Both *L. canicola* and *L. icterohaemorrhagiae* can produce an acute severe hemolytic anemia with icterus.

    b. *L. canicola* causes a more severe diffuse interstitial nephritis, whereas *L. icterohaemorrhagiae* produces more hepatic necrosis.

  2. Dogs are the reservoir host of *L. canicola*, while rats are the principal reservoir host of *L. icterohaemorrhagiae*. Water contaminated with urine from infected reservoir hosts is the primary source of infection.

D. Equine leptospirosis
  1. Several *Leptospira* serovars can infect horses but rarely produce clinical signs of leptospirosis.
  2. Recurrent ophthalmitis has been postulated to result from antileptospira antibodies.
E. Feline leptospirosis
  1. Cats infected with pathogenic leptospires rarely, if ever, exhibit clinical disease.
F. Ovine leptospirosis
  1. *L. hardjo* and *L. pomona* are the two most common serovars isolated from sheep.
    a. *L. hardjo* produces an acute hemolytic anemia and an interstitial nephritis in lambs.
    b. *L. pomona* causes hemolytic anemia and abortion in ewes.
G. Porcine leptospirosis
  1. Most leptospiral infections are mild or asymptomatic. Infective serovars include *L. canicola*, *L. grippotyphosa*, *L. icterohaemorrhagiae*, and *L. pomona*.
  2. Abortions during the last trimester of gestation are often the only evidence of *L. pomona* infections.

---

42 | Genus *Treponema*

I. *TREPONEMA* SPECIES
  A. Pathogens

Species	Hosts	Specific Diseases
T. hyodysenteriae	Porcine	Swine dysentery
T. pallidum ss *pallidum*	Man	Syphilis
T. pallidum ss *pertenue*	Man	Yaws

  B. Nonpathogens
  1. *T. innocens* is normal intestinal flora of swine.

II. HABITAT AND ECOLOGY
  A. *T. hyodysenteriae* and *T. innocens* are intestinal flora of swine.
  1. These organisms can survive for extended periods in organic matter and anaerobic lagoons.

III. CELLULAR, CULTURAL, AND BIOCHEMICAL CHARACTERISTICS
  A. Cellular characteristics
    1. Gram-negative helical rods
        a. Cells of *T. hyodysenteriae* and *T. innocens* are large, tightly coiled spirochetes that measure 0.3 to 0.4 um in width and 6 to 30 um in length. These treponemas stain poorly with the Gram stain.
    2. Motile
        a. *T. hyodysenteriae* and *T. innocens* are motile by means of several periplasmic flagella.
  B. Cultural characteristics
    1. Obligate anaerobic
    2. Fastidious growth requirements
        a. On blood agar incubated anaerobically, colonies of *T. hyodysenteriae* are small, translucent, and produce a strong beta hemolytic reaction. The colonies of *T. innocens* are weakly beta hemolytic. Both species grow at both 37°C and 42°C.
            (1) Trypticase soy blood agar containing spectinomycin is commonly used as a selective medium when incubated anaerobically at 42°C. This procedure is used to isolate treponemas from swine feces.
        b. *T. pallidum* ss *pallidum* has not been successfully cultivated on artificial media or in tissue culture.
  C. Biochemical characteristics
    1. Oxidase-negative
    2. Fermentative metabolism

IV. DISEASE OVERVIEW
  A. *T. hyodysenteriae* infections
    1. Porcine swine dysentery
        a. Swine dysentery is a disease of the large intestine characterized by a mucohemorrhagic diarrhea.
            (1) Oral ingestion of feces from clinically ill and carrier swine is the primary mode of transmission.
        b. *T. hyodysenteriae* is considered to be a primary pathogen; however, pure cultures of *T. hyodysenteriae* do not cause swine dysentery in gnotobiotic pigs.

PART 9 | Aerobic Gram-negative Helical Rods

43 | Genus *Campylobacter*

I. *CAMPYLOBACTER* SPECIES
   A. Pathogens

Species	Hosts	Specific Diseases
C. fetus ss fetus	Bovine	Abortion
	Ovine	EPIZOOTIC ABORTION
C. fetus ss venerealis	Bovine	CAMPYLOBAC-TERIOSIS
C. jejuni	Domestic animals, man	Enteritis
C. sputorum ss mucosalis	Porcine	Proliferative enteritis

   B. Nonpathogens
      1. *C. coli* is normal intestinal flora of domestic animals.
      2. *C. sputorum* ss *bubulus* is normal genital tract flora of cattle and sheep.
      3. *C. sputorum* ss *sputorum* is normal intestinal flora of swine.

II. HABITAT AND ECOLOGY
   A. The various *Campylobacter* species are found in the reproductive organs, intestinal tracts, and oral cavities of animals and man.
      1. *C. fetus* ss *venerealis* is an obligate parasite of the bovine reproductive tract.

III. CELLULAR, CULTURAL, AND BIOCHEMICAL CHARACTERISTICS
   A. Cellular characteristics
      1. Gram-negative rods
         a. The cells are slender curved rods and often form spiral chains.

      2. Motile
          a. Campylobacters are motile with a characteristic corkscrewlike motion by means of a single polar flagellum at one or both ends of the cell.
  B. Cultural characteristics
      1. Campylobacters are microaerophilic, requiring an oxygen concentration of 3 to 15 percent and a carbon dioxide concentration of 3 to 5 percent. Some species can grow under anaerobic conditions.
      2. Fastidious growth requirements
          a. *Campylobacter* species will generally grow on blood agar, and all pathogens of domestic animals are nonhemolytic except *C. sputorum* ss *mucosalis*, which may produce a slight hemolysis. Some campylobacters will grow in a candlejar, some in a gas mixture of 10 percent carbon dioxide and 90 percent nitrogen, and others in a mixture of 5 percent oxygen, 10 percent carbon dioxide, and 85 percent nitrogen. Some species will grow better at $42^{\circ}C$ than at $37^{\circ}C$.
             (1) A variety of selective agar media, particular blood agar supplement with various antibiotics, are utilized to isolate campylobacters from clinical specimens.
  C. Biochemical characteristics
      1. Oxidase-positive
      2. Respiratory metabolism
          a. *Campylobacter* species do not utilize carbohydrates.

IV. DISEASE OVERVIEW
  A. *C. fetus* ss *fetus* infections
      1. Bovine abortion
          a. The bacterium is associated with sporadic abortion in cattle.
      2. Ovine epizootic abortion (see Chap. 95)
          a. The bacterium is the etiologic agent of ovine epizootic abortion.
  B. *C. fetus* ss *venerealis* infections
      1. Bovine campylobacteriosis (see Chap. 80)
          a. Bovine campylobacteriosis (vibriosis) is characterized clinically as temporary infertility with occasional abortions.
  C. *C. jejuni* infections
      1. Enteritis in domestic animals
          a. An enteritis believed to be caused by *C. jejuni* has been reported in dogs. The condition is commonly reported in man.
          b. Affected dogs exhibit a febrile enteritis with diarrhea and shed the organism in their feces. The infections are probably acquired by ingesting food and water contaminated by feces from carrier animals and man.

    c. *C. jejuni* produces at least two exotoxins, a cytotoxin and a heat-labile enterotoxin. The bacterium lacks fimbriae but may produce other adhesins.

D. *C. sputorum* ss *mucosalis* infections

    1. Porcine proliferative enteritis

        a. *C. sputorum* ss *mucosalis* has been isolated from the intestinal tracts of pigs with porcine intestinal adenomatosis, necrotic enteritis, regional ileitis, and proliferative enteritis. However, attempts to experimentally reproduce these diseases with pure cultures of the bacterium in gnotobiotic pigs have been unsuccessful.

           (1) Porcine intestinal adenomatosis develops as a progressive proliferation of immature epithelial cells infected with intracellular campylobacters, where the affected cells are not shed into the lumen of the bowel, resulting in glandular proliferation resembling adenomatous change. The condition usually involves the lower part of the small intestine and the upper part of the large intestine.

               (a) In pig herds with endemic disease, pigs from 6 to 20 weeks of age are most commonly affected and most pigs recover from 4 to 6 weeks after the onset of clinical signs.

           (2) Proliferative enteritis varies in severity from peracute to chronic and occurs in weaned and adult pigs.

44 | Genus *Vibrio*

I. *VIBRIO* SPECIES
   A. Pathogens

Species	Host	Specific Disease
V. cholerae	Man	Cholera

   B. Nonpathogens
      1. Other species
   C. Classification
      1. Domestic animal pathogens that were formerly classified in genus *Vibrio* are now classified in genus *Campylobacter*.

II. HABITAT AND ECOLOGY
   A. *Vibrio* species are found in aquatic habitats.

III. CELLULAR, CULTURAL, AND BIOCHEMICAL CHARACTERISTICS
   A. Cellular characteristics
      1. Gram-negative rods
         a. Cells are curved rods or in spiral chains.
      2. They are motile with a characteristic corkscrewlike motion by means of monotrichous or multitrichous polar flagella.
   B. Cultural characteristics
      1. Facultative anaerobic
      2. Growth on blood agar and/or MacConkey agar at 37^{0}C
   C. Biochemical characteristics
      1. Most *Vibrio* species are oxidase-positive.
      2. Metabolism is both respiratory and fermentative.
         a. The *Vibrio* species utilize carbohydrates, which distinguishes them from the asaccharolytic *Campylobacter* species.

IV. DISEASE OVERVIEW
   A. Currently classified *Vibrio* species are seldom incriminated as pathogens of domestic animals.

PART **10**	# Family Mycoplasmataceae, Aerobic Cell Wall–free Bacteria

45	## Genus *Mycoplasma*

I. *MYCOPLASMA* SPECIES
   A. Pathogens

Species	Hosts	Specific Diseases	Nonspecific Diseases
M. agalactiae	Ovine	Contagious agalactia	arthritis, vulvovaginitis
M. bovigenitalium	Bovine	Mastitis	
M. bovis	Bovine	Mastitis	
M. bovoculi	Bovine		keratoconjunctivitis
M. californicum	Bovine	Mastitis	
M. capricolum	Ovine	Contagious agalactia	
M. conjunctivae	Ovine	Keratoconjunctivitis	
M. dispar	Bovine	Mastitis	pneumonia
M. felis	Feline	Conjunctivitis	
M. hyopneumoniae	Porcine	ENZOOTIC PNEUMONIA	
M. hyorhinis	Porcine	Polyserositis-Polyarthritis	
M. hyosynoviae	Porcine	Arthritis	
M. mycoides ss *capri*	Ovine	Contagious pleuropneumonia	
M. mycoides ss *mycoides*	Bovine	Contagious pleuropneumonia	
M. ovipneumoniae	Ovine	Atypical pneumonia	
M. pneumoniae	Man	Atypical pneumonia	

1. This is a partial list of *Mycoplasma* species that are either primary etiologic agents of specific diseases, or have been associated with various diseases of domestic animals. The pathogenic significance of some species that have been isolated from various clinical diseases has not been clearly delineated. Many species are facultative pathogens that probably elicit pathological changes under natural conditions only when the defense mechanisms of the hosts are compromised.

II. HABITAT AND ECOLOGY
   A. The primary habitat of the animal mycoplasmas are the mucous membranes of the respiratory and urogenital tracts.

     1. The host range of most species is limited to one or only a few animal species.

III. CELLULAR, CULTURAL, AND BIOCHEMICAL CHARACTERISTICS

  A. Cellular characteristics
     1. Gram-negative pleomorphic cells
        a. Mycoplasmas lack a cell wall and are enclosed by a cytoplasmic membrane. The cells range in size from 0.3 to 0.8 um in diameter.
        b. The mycoplasmas are classified as gram-negative but stain poorly with the Gram stain.
     2. Nonmotile
  B. Cultural characteristics
     1. Facultative anaerobic
     2. Fastidious growth requirements
        a. Sterols are required for the growth of mycoplasmas, which are generally cultured on enriched agar media containing serum and yeast extract and incubated aerobically at $37^{o}C$. Some species also may require additional nutritional supplements and/or 5 to 10 percent carbon dioxide.
        b. After several days incubation, the colonies are flat, translucent, grow into the medium, and often have a "fried egg" appearance, where the central portion of the colony is embedded in the agar and the periphery is on the agar surface. Agar plates are usually incubated for 2 to 10 days before colonial growth is apparent, even then the colonies are rarely big enough to be seen with the naked eye.
            (1) Dienes' stained colony preparations are used for microscopic examination of the colonies. Dienes' stain, which contains both methylene blue and Azur II dyes, is used to stain one surface of a glass coverslip and allowed to dry. A block of agar bearing suspected mycoplasma colonies is then cut from the plate and placed face up on a glass microscope slide, and the stained coverslip is placed on the agar. The colonies stain a deep blue at the center, where the colony is embedded in the agar, and light blue at the periphery of the colony. Nonviable organisms either do not stain or assume a pinkish to violet hue.
        c. *Mycoplasma* species are often identified by inhibition of growth adjacent to disks impregnated with specific antisera.
            (1) The paper disk growth-inhibition technique is both simple to perform and highly specific. This method will generally serve to identify an isolate to the species level. Cross reactions between *Mycoplasma* species of domestic animals seldom, if ever, occur.

    C. Biochemical characteristics
        1. Mycoplasmas are both oxidase-negative and catalase-negative.
        2. Respiratory metabolism
            a. Most *Mycoplasma* species utilize glucose or arginine as the principal source of energy but seldom both.

IV. DISEASE OVERVIEW
    A. General concepts of mycoplasmal disease
        1. The mycoplasmas are most frequently associated with diseases of the respiratory tract, urogenital tract, and occasionally the joints.
            a. The organisms colonize and firmly adhere to the mucosal epithelium. This provides an environment in which local concentrations of toxic substances excreted by the organisms can accumulate and cause tissue damage.
            b. An exchange of antigens may occur between host and mycoplasma membranes. This exchange of antigens may trigger immunologic responses with serious consequences to the host.
        2. The pathogenic effects of mycoplasmas have been recorded for numerous mammalian and avian species, but the most severe and economically significant infections of domestic animals occur in cattle and sheep.
    B. *M. agalactiae* infections
        1. Ovine contagious agalactia
            a. In ewes, contagious agalactia frequently follows a transient mycoplasmemia and often occurs shortly after lambing. The condition is manifested as a total and permanent agalactia of the affected gland, frequently complicated by a nonsuppurative arthritis and keratoconjunctivitis.
            b. In rams, arthritis is the predominant manifestation of the disease.
    C. *M. bovigenitalium* infections
        1. Bovine mastitis
            a. *M. bovigenitalium* has been associated with outbreaks of mastitis and with genital tract infections.
    D. *M. bovis* infections
        1. Bovine mastitis
            a. *M. bovis* can cause severe mastitis and has been incriminated in infertility and abortion.
    E. *M. bovoculi* infections
        1. Bovine keratoconjunctivitis
            a. *M. bovoculi* has been incriminated as an etiologic agent of bovine keratoconjunctivitis. The symptoms are mild, compared with the clinical disease caused by *Moraxella bovis*.

F. *M. californicum* infections
   1. Bovine mastitis
      a. *M. californicum* causes an acute mastitis that results in either a marked reduction of milk flow or agalactia.
G. *M. capricolum* infections
   1. Ovine contagious agalactia
      a. *M. capricolum* causes a mastitis in ewes that results in a decrease or cessation of lactation. It also can cause fibrinopurulent polyarthritis and conjunctivitis.
H. *M. conjunctivae* infections
   1. Ovine keratoconjunctivitis
      a. *M. conjunctivae* can cause a keratoconjunctivitis in sheep.
I. *M. dispar* infections
   1. Bovine pneumonia
      a. *M. dispar* is primarily a respiratory tract pathogen and has been isolated from cattle with pneumonia. It also has been incriminated as a cause of mastitis.
J. *M. felis* infections
   1. Feline conjunctivitis
      a. *M. felis* is a relatively common inhabitant of the upper respiratory and lower genital tracts of cats. The bacterium causes conjunctivitis.
K. *M. hyopneumoniae* infections
   1. Porcine enzootic pneumonia (see Chap. 100)
      a. *M. hyopneumoniae* causes a chronic, nonresolving pneumonia that persists for many months or even years and has been considered to be the most economically important disease of swine in the United States.
      b. The bacterium induces a lobar pneumonia characterized by well-demarcated plum-colored or grayish pneumonic areas in the apical and cardiac areas of the lung. An uncomplicated case shows little or no clinical disease, but affected swine have a chronic nonproductive cough. Epidemics of acute bacterial pneumonia secondary to the primary mycoplasmal infection are common. Secondary bacterial pathogens include *Bordetella bronchiseptica*, *Pasteurella multocida*, *P. haemolytica*, *Haemophilus* species, and *Mycoplasma hyorhinis*.
L. *M. hyorhinis* infections
   1. Porcine polyserositis and polyarthritis
      a. *M. hyorhinis* can be isolated from 50 to 70 percent of the nasal cavities of healthy swine and from 50 percent of the pneumonic lungs of swine. The bacterium appears to be highly host-adapted to swine.
      b. The polyserositis due to *M. hyorhinis* occurs primarily in 3- to 10-week-old pigs and is characterized by a

serofibrinous pericarditis, pleuritis, and polyarthritis.
The arthritis is chronic and progressive with persistent
mycoplasmas. The disease in older pigs commonly occurs in
swine undergoing stress, and chronic arthritis is the
primary clinical sign. Young breeding boars introduced
into chronically infected herds may develop a severe
polyserositis that is often fatal.

    c.   A similar type of polyserositis may be caused by *H.*
parasuis.

M.   *M. hyosynoviae* infections
    1.   Porcine arthritis
        a.   Acute disease occurs primarily in pigs over 80 lb and
affects the stifle, elbow, and hip joint. The arthritis is
nonsuppurative, nonproliferative, and nonerosive. The
inflammatory changes are similar to *M. hyorhinis* but are
milder and regress spontaneously after a few weeks.

N.   *M. mycoides* ss *capri* infections
    1.   Ovine contagious pleuropneumonia
        a.   This disease has been diagnosed in sheep in the western
United States, although the bacterium is considered to be
primarily a pathogen of goats.
        b.   The condition is an acute serofibrinous pleurisy and
pneumonia that may involve the entire lung. A severe
arthritis may be a sequela of the bacteremia.

O.   *M. mycoides* ss *mycoides* infections
    1.   Bovine contagious pleuropneumonia
        a.   The characteristic lesions of contagious pleuropneumonia
are a fibrinonecrotic pneumonia with abundant serofibrinous
exudation in the pleural cavity.
           (1)   The bacterium is transmitted by inhalation of infected
droplets from the lungs of clinically ill animals.
The clinical signs are those of a febrile
pleuropneumonia with a normal duration of 2 to 8 weeks
ending in death or slow recovery. Some mild and
asymptomatic cases occur, as well as peracute cases
where the affected cattle die in less than 1 week.
           (2)   The disease was first observed in the United States in
1843 but was eradicated prior to 1900 by slaughtering
all infected cattle. The disease is still endemic in
much of the world.

P.   *M. ovipneumoniae* infections
    1.   Ovine atypical pneumonia
        a.   *M. ovipneumoniae* causes a chronic catarrhal bronchitis and
a proliferative interstitial pneumonia. It is one of the
most commonly isolated bacterial species from the ovine
respiratory tract.

46 | Genus *Ureaplasma*

I. *UREAPLASMA* SPECIES
  A. Pathogens

Species	Hosts	Nonspecific Diseases
Ureaplasma species	Domestic animals	respiratory and urogenital tract

  1. There are only two species in the genus, *U. diversum* and *U. urealyticum.*
  2. Most strains isolated from the respiratory tracts and genital tracts of domestic animals have not been given a species designation.

II. HABITAT AND ECOLOGY
  A. The primary habitat of *Ureaplasma* species is the mucous membranes of the mouth, respiratory tract, and urogenital tract.
    1. Most strains tend to be host-specific.

III. CELLULAR, CULTURAL, AND BIOCHEMICAL CHARACTERISTICS
  A. Cellular characteristics
    1. Gram-negative pleomorphic cells
      a. Ureaplasmas lack a cell wall and are enclosed by a cytoplasmic membrane. The cells range in size from 0.3 to 0.8 um in diameter.
    2. Nonmotile
  B. Cultural characteristics
    1. Microaerophilic
    2. Fastidious growth requirements
      a. Growth requirements, incubation conditions, and colony characteristics are similar to the genus *Mycoplasma*; however, the ureaplasmas produce smaller colonies than do the mycoplasmas. Colonies are 15 to 60 um in diameter and often lack the "fried egg" appearance of the mycoplasmas. Originally the ureaplasmas were called "T strains" (T for tiny) or "T mycoplasmas" because of the very small colonies.
  C. Biochemical characteristics
    1. The ureaplasmas, like the mycoplasmas, are both oxidase-negative and catalase-negative.
    2. Respiratory metabolism

a. Glucose is not utilized as a source of carbon.
3. Ureaplasmas hydrolyze urea, distinguishing them from the mycoplasmas, which lack the enzyme urease.

IV. DISEASE OVERVIEW
   A. *U. diversum* infections
      1. Bovine infections
         a. *U. diversum* has been associated with mastitis, respiratory infections, and urogenital infections in cattle.
   B. *Ureaplasma* species infections
      1. Infections in domestic animals
         a. Ureaplasmas are serologically heterogenous, and most have not been identified to the species level.
         b. The clinical significance of most ureaplasmas is vague at best.

PART **11**	Aerobic Gram-negative Cocci and Rods

47	Genus *Acinetobacter*

I. *ACINETOBACTER* SPECIES
   A. Pathogens

Species	Hosts	Nonspecific Diseases
A. calcoaceticus	Domestic animals	opportunistic

      1. It is the only species in the genus.

II. HABITAT AND ECOLOGY
   A. *A. calcoaceticus* occurs naturally in soil and water.

III. CELLULAR, CULTURAL, AND BIOCHEMICAL CHARACTERISTICS
   A. Cellular characteristics
      1. Gram-negative rods
         a. The cells are medium-sized coccobacilli.
      2. Nonmotile
   B. Cultural characteristics
      1. Obligate aerobic
      2. Growth on blood agar and MacConkey agar at $37^{\circ}C$
         a. On blood agar, some strains cause a strong hemolysis because of phospholipase C hemolysin activity. The colonies are circular, convex, glossy, grayish white to cream-colored, and opaque. The colonies are mucoid when the cells are encapsulated. After incubation for several days, the colonies often produce a marked depression in the agar surface and become surrounded by peripheral spreading zones.
         b. On MacConkey agar, the colonies are lactose-negative.

C. Biochemical characteristics
1. Oxidase-negative
2. Respiratory metabolism
a. Some strains of *A. calcoaceticus* can utilize glucose oxidatively as a carbon source for growth, but most do not use this substrate.

IV. DISEASE OVERVIEW
A. *A. calcoaceticus* is an opportunistic pathogen of domestic animals. It is commonly found in mixed infections with other bacterial species.

---

48 | Genus *Actinobacillus*

I. *ACTINOBACILLUS* SPECIES
A. Pathogens

Species	Hosts	Specific Diseases	Nonspecific Diseases
A. actinomycetemcomitans	Domestic animals		opportunistic
A. equuli	Equine	ACTINOBACIL-LOSIS	
	Porcine		arthritis, purulent nephritis
A. lignieresii	Bovine	ACTINOBACIL-LOSIS	
	Domestic animals		granulomatous, abscesses
A. pleuropneumoniae	Porcine	Pleuropneumonia	
A. seminis	Ovine	Epididymitis	arthritis, mastitis
A. suis	Porcine		arthritis, pneumonia, septicemia

II. HABITAT AND ECOLOGY
A. Most *Actinobacillus* species occur as commensals of the mouth and upper respiratory tract of their domestic animal hosts, but some may also be recovered from the mucous membranes of the alimentary tract and genitals. Some species are almost ubiquitous on the different mucous membranes of their specific host, whereas others have very specific etiological preferences.

1. All the *Actinobacillus* species are regarded as opportunistic pathogens of their respective hosts.
2. Diseases caused by the actinobacilli are usually of a sporadic nature, but groups of animals can be simultaneously infected.

III. CELLULAR, CULTURAL, AND BIOCHEMICAL CHARACTERISTICS
   A. Cellular characteristics
      1. Gram-negative rods
         a. Cells of actinobacilli are pleomorphic and vary from rod-shaped to filamentous forms. There is considerable variability of the cellular morphology of the different *Actinobacillus* species.
      2. Nonmotile
   B. Cultural characteristics
      1. Facultative anaerobic
      2. Growth on blood agar and/or MacConkey agar at 37°C
         a. Colonies of actinobacilli tend to be sticky on primary isolation; however, this characteristic is often lost on repeated subculture. Most species produce white colonies, but *A. suis* produces colonies with a creamy yellow color.
         b. On blood agar, *A. actinomycetemcomitans, A. lignieresii,* and *A. seminis* are nonhemolytic, but *A. pleuropneumoniae, A. suis,* and many *A. equuli* strains produce beta hemolysis.
            (1) The growth of *A. seminis* is greatly enhanced in 10 percent carbon dioxide.
         c. *A. equuli, A. lignieresii,* and *A. suis* will grow on MacConkey agar and are lactose-positive. *A. actinomycetemcomitans, A. pleuropneumoniae,* and *A. seminis* will not grow on MacConkey agar.
   C. Biochemical characteristics
      1. Oxidase-positive
      2. Fermentative metabolism
      3. Fastidious growth requirements
         a. *A. pleuropneumoniae,* which was previously classified as *Haemophilus pleuropneumoniae,* requires factor V (NAD) for growth but not factor X (hemin).

IV. DISEASE OVERVIEW
   A. *A. actinomycetemcomitans* infections
      1. Ovine epididymitis
         a. In rams, the bacterium is occasionally isolated from epididymitis lesions.
   B. *A. equuli* infections
      1. Equine actinobacillosis (see Chap. 105)
         a. The clinical manifestations of the infections are determined primarily by the age of the affected animals.
            (1) Acute septicemic infection in foals within the first few days of life is the most common syndrome. Chronic

infections cause a purulent nephritis and arthritis. The onset is rapid, and mortality is high. In older foals, *A. equuli* may be involved in respiratory disease.

    (2) In adult horses, *A. equuli* may be found in association with purulent nephritis, meningitis, and abortion. Septicemia is rare.

2. Porcine infections

    a. Clinical disease caused by *A. equuli* occasionally occurs in piglets and is manifested as a septicemia, arthritis, and purulent nephritis.

C. *A. lignieresii* infections

    1. Bovine actinobacillosis (see Chap. 73)

        a. The classic disease in cattle caused by *A. lignieresii* is wooden tongue, a chronic granulomatous lesion affecting the tongue and other soft tissues of the head and neck.

        b. The granules formed in *A. lignieresii* infections are grayish white and less than 1 mm in diameter. They are significantly smaller than the granules formed by *Actinomyces bovis*.

D. *A. pleuropneumoniae* infections

    1. Porcine pleuropneumonia

        a. *A. pleuropneumoniae* is not a normal inhabitant of the porcine respiratory tract. The disease is highly contagious, and healthy carriers that have survived the infection serve to perpetuate the disease during interepidemic periods.

        b. Porcine pleuropneumonia is primarily an infection of the respiratory tract causing a very severe fibrinous lobar pneumonia with fibrinous pleuritis. The disease tends to affect swine over 3 months of age. The onset is rapid, and both morbidity and mortality are high.

E. *A. seminis* infections

    1. Ovine epididymitis

        a. In rams, *A. seminis* is a primary etiologic agent of epididymitis. The condition is clinically indistinguishable from the epididymitis induced by *Brucella ovis*.

        b. In ewes, *A. seminis* will occasionally cause mastitis.

F. *A. suis* infections

    1. Porcine infections

        a. The bacterium is found in swine of all ages. The infections can cause an acute septicemia, pneumonia, nephritis, or a more chronic form with arthritis.

49 | Genus *Aeromonas*

I. *AEROMONAS* SPECIES
  A. Pathogens

Species	Hosts	Nonspecific Diseases
Aeromonas species	Domestic animals	opportunistic

  1. *A. hydrophila* is the most common aeromonad that causes disease in domestic animals.

II. HABITAT AND ECOLOGY
  A. Water is the natural habitat of *Aeromonas* species.

III. CELLULAR, CULTURAL, AND BIOCHEMICAL CHARACTERISTICS
  A. Cellular characteristics
    1. Gram-negative rods
    2. All *Aeromonas* species are motile by a single polar flagellum except *A. salmonicida*, which is nonmotile.
  B. Culture characteristics
    1. Facultative anaerobic
    2. Growth on blood agar and/or MacConkey agar
      a. The motile *Aeromonas* species will grow on blood agar, and many strains will grow on MacConkey agar. The optimal incubation temperature is 28°C.
        (1) On blood agar, the colonies are smooth, entire, and buff-colored, and many strains produce zones of beta hemolysis.
        (2) On MacConkey agar, the colonies may indicate that they are either lactose-positive or lactose-negative.
  C. Biochemical characteristics
    1. Oxidase-positive
    2. Metabolism is both respiratory and fermentative.

IV. DISEASE OVERVIEW
  A. The *Aeromonas* species are primarily pathogens of fish, reptiles, and amphibians but rarely cause disease in animals. Infections in animals and man usually occur when wounds are exposed to water contaminated with motile aeromonads.

50 | Genus *Alcaligenes*

I. *ALCALIGENES* SPECIES
    A. Pathogens

Species	Hosts	Nonspecific Diseases
Alcaligenes species	Domestic animals	opportunistic

    1. *A. faecalis* is the most commonly isolated species from domestic animals.

II. HABITAT AND ECOLOGY
    A. Most *Alcaligenes* species are intestinal tract flora of vertebrates and also occur in soil and water.

III. CELLULAR, CULTURAL, AND BIOCHEMICAL CHARACTERISTICS
    A. Cellular characteristics
        1. Gram-negative rods
        2. Motile by peritrichous flagella
    B. Cultural characteristics
        1. Obligate aerobic
        2. Growth on blood agar and MacConkey agar at 37°C
            a. *A. faecalis* is nonhemolytic on blood agar. The colonies are flat, nonpigmented, and translucent to opaque.
    C. Biochemical characteristics
        1. Oxidase-positive
        2. Respiratory metabolism
            a. Glucose is not utilized oxidatively.

IV. DISEASE OVERVIEW
    A. In domestic animals, *Alcaligenes* species are opportunistic pathogens. They are often isolated in pure culture.

51	Genus *Bordetella*

I. *BORDETELLA* SPECIES
A. Pathogens

Species	Hosts	Specific Diseases	Nonspecific Diseases
B. bronchiseptica	Canine	Tracheobronchitis	pneumonia
	Porcine	ATROPHIC RHINITIS	pneumonia
	Domestic animals		pneumonia
B. parapertussis	Man	Parapertussis	pneumonia
B. pertussis	Man	Pertussis	

II. HABITAT AND ECOLOGY
A. *B. bronchiseptica* is an obligate pathogen of animals and is highly communicable. The bacterium is often isolated from the respiratory tract of normal animals.

III. CELLULAR, CULTURAL, AND BIOCHEMICAL CHARACTERISTICS
A. Cellular characteristics
   1. Gram-negative rods
      a. Bordetellae are small coccobacilli.
   2. *B. bronchiseptica* is motile by peritrichous flagella, but the other *Bordetella* species are nonmotile.
B. Cultural characteristics
   1. Obligate aerobic
   2. Growth on blood agar and MacConkey agar at 37°C
      a. Colonies of *B. bronchiseptica* are smooth, convex, glistening, nearly transparent, and surrounded by a zone of hemolysis.
C. Biochemical characteristics
   1. Oxidase-positive
   2. Respiratory metabolism
      a. *B. bronchiseptica* does not utilize glucose.

IV. DISEASE OVERVIEW
A. *B. bronchiseptica* infections
   1. Canine tracheobronchitis
      a. The bacteria localize and multiply among the cilia of the epithelial cells of the trachea and bronchi. They do not invade the underlying tissues.
      b. In tracheobronchitis (kennel cough), *B. bronchiseptica* can

   be the primary etiologic agent or secondary to an upper
   respiratory viral infection.

   c.   The bacterium is a common isolate from bronchopneumonias.
   It is frequently a secondary bacterial pathogen to a
   primary respiratory viral infection, particularly canine
   distemper.

2.   Feline pneumonia

   a.   *B. bronchiseptica* will occasionally cause a
   bronchopneumonia as a sequela to a primary viral
   respiratory infection.

3.   Porcine atrophic rhinitis (see Chap. 98)

   a.   In piglets less than 8 weeks of age, the bacteria colonize
   the mucous membranes of the nasal cavity with subsequent
   hypoplasia of the nasal turbinates.

   b.   In older pigs, the infection causes no permanent damage
   to the nasal turbinates. Infected swine may exhibit a mild
   rhinitis due to the inflammation of mucous membranes of the
   nasal cavity, or they may be asymptomatic carriers.

   c.   Pneumonia is a common sequela to atrophic rhinitis, since
   the nasal turbinates have a reduced capacity to filter
   microorganisms from the inhaled air. Bordetellae are
   commonly isolated from pneumonias of swine with atrophic
   rhinitis.

52	Genus *Brucella*

I. *BRUCELLA* SPECIES
A. Pathogens

	Hosts		Diseases	
Species	Primary	Incidental	Reproductive Tract	Other
B. abortus	Bovine		ABORTION, ORCHITIS	
		Canine	Abortion	
		Equine		Fistulous withers
B. canis	Canine		Abortion, Orchitis	
B. melitensis	Ovine		Abortion, Orchitis	
		Bovine		
B. ovis	Ovine		Epididymitis, Abortion	
B. suis	Porcine		Abortion	

B. Nonpathogens
1. *B. neotomae* was initially isolated from the desert wood rat. The bacterium is not a pathogen for either domestic animals or man.

II. HABITAT AND ECOLOGY
A. The *Brucella* species are obligate parasites but can survive for 6 months in the environment if conditions are ideal.
B. Their distribution is worldwide, apart from the countries from which brucellae have been eradicated.
   1. *B. melitensis* has been eradicated from the United States.
C. The prevalence of the different species and biovars in domestic animals varies considerably.
   1. There are nine recognized biovars in the species *B. abortus*, four in *B. suis*, and three in *B. melitensis*. The biovars within a species do not differ markedly from one another.
   2. *B. abortus* is most prevalent in the southeastern and southwestern United States.
      a. Of the nine *B. abortus* biovars, only biovars 1, 2, and 4 are found in the United States. Biovar 1 is the most prevalent, followed by biovars 2 and 4, respectively. The biovars are often used in epidemiological investigations.
   3. *B. canis* was first recognized in the United States in the 1960s but is now widely distributed in the domestic canine population.

4. *B. ovis* is found predominantly in the sheep-raising areas of the western United States.
5. *B. suis* is found sporadically in swine-producing areas throughout the United States.

III. CELLULAR, CULTURAL, AND BIOCHEMICAL CHARACTERISTICS

A. Cellular characteristics
1. Gram-negative rods
a. Brucellae are small coccobacilli.
2. Nonmotile
B. Cultural characteristics
1. Obligate aerobic
2. Fastidious growth requirements
a. Some brucellae will grow on blood agar when incubated aerobically but are nonhemolytic. The growth of many brucellae is enhanced by serum, and some brucellae require 5 to 10 percent carbon dioxide for growth. These organisms are frequently cultured on a basal medium of trypicase agar or tryptose agar supplemented with 5 percent bovine serum and incubated under 5 to 10 percent carbon dioxide at 37°C. On primary isolation, most *Brucella* strains are slow growing, and colonies at 48 hours are usually from 0.5 to 1.0 mm in diameter, raised, and convex with an entire edge. Colonies may be smooth, mucoid, or rough.
b. The *Brucella* species and their biovars are presumptively identified based on their growth requirements for carbon dioxide, hydrogen sulfide production, urease activity, and selective inhibition of bacterial growth on agar media containing various concentrations of basic fuchsin and thionin dyes (Table 52.1).
c. Monospecific *B. abortus* (A) and monospecific *B. melitensis* (M) antisera will agglutinate the three smooth species (*B.*

Table 52.1. Differential characteristics of selected *Brucella* species and biovars that cause disease in domestic animals in the United States

Species	Strains	Biovars	CO_2 Required	H_2S	Urease	Basic Fuchsin II	Basic Fuchsin III	Thionin I	Thionin II	Thionin III	A	M	R
						Growth on Dyes[a]					Agglutination Reacti		
						Basic Fuchsin		Thionin			Type of Antisera[b]		
B. abortus[c]		1	±	+	+	+	+	−	−	−	+	−	−
		2	+	+	+	−	−	−	−	−	+	−	−
		4	±	+	+	+	+	−	−	−	+	−	−
	19	1	−	+	+	+	+	−	−	−	+	−	−
B. suis		1	−	+	+	−	−	+	+	+	+	−	−
		2	−	−	+	−	−	−	+	+	+	−	−
		3	−	−	+	+	+	+	+	+	+	−	−
		4	−	−	+	+	+	+	+	+	+	+	−
B. canis			−	−	+	−	−	−	−	−	−	−	+
B. ovis			+	−	−	+	+	+	+	+	−	−	+

[a]Dye concentrations in agar media: I = 1:25,000; II = 1:50,000; III = 1:100,000.
[b]Types of antisera: A = monospecific *B. abortus* antiserum; M = monospecific *B. melitensis* antiseru R = antirough serum.
[c]Only biovars 1, 2, and 4 occur in the United States.

abortus, *B. melitensis*, and *B. suis*) and is used to help distinguish their biovars. The antirough (R) serum will agglutinate the two rough species (*B. canis* and *B. ovis*).

(1) Agglutination by monospecific A and M antisera

    (a) Smooth *Brucella* species share surface antigens A and M and cross react serologically; however, the relative proportion of each antigen varies from one species or biovar to another.

    (b) The smooth colony species do not cross react with the rough colony species.

(2) Agglutination by antirough serum

    (a) Rough *Brucella* species cross react serologically but do not cross react with the smooth colony species.

  d. Definitive diagnosis of *Brucella* species is usually carried out in a state or federal microbiology laboratory.

C. Biochemical characteristics

  1. The pathogenic *Brucella* species are oxidase-positive except *B. ovis*, which is oxidase-negative.

  2. Respiratory metabolism

    a. Glucose is oxidized by all *Brucella* species except *B. ovis*.

IV. DISEASE OVERVIEW

A. General concepts

  1. Brucellae are facultative intracellular pathogens. Their growth is primarily intracellular, where they proliferate in monocytes and macrophages. This intimate and protected habitat within the host provides the brucellae with a means of intrahost transportation, a source of nutrients, and a site protected from host immune mechanisms.

  2. The severity of infection varies considerably and depends on both the species of brucellae and the host.

    a. In man, the severity of infections vary with the *Brucella* species. *B. melitensis* causes the most severe clinical manifestations, followed by *B. suis*, *B. abortus*, and *B. canis*, respectively.

    b. Brucellae infections in their natural hosts are rarely lethal and are often mild, with clinical manifestations occurring mainly in the pregnant animal.

  3. Ingestion of material contaminated with brucellae, particularly aborted fetuses, placentas, and milk, is the primary mode of transmission.

    a. The organisms are highly invasive and can penetrate intact mucous membranes.

  4. Following ingestion, generalized infections can occur with a bacteremic phase followed by localization in the reticuloendothelial system and in the reproductive organs.

    a. Infections in pregnant animals often lead to placental and fetal infections that can result in either abortion or birth of weak neonates.

       b.   The organisms may localize in the mammary tissue and be excreted in the milk.

   5.   Infection is accompanied by the production of specific antibodies, which do not provide protective immunity.

       a.   Serologic tests are available for the smooth species and the rough species.

          (1)   Diagnoses of brucellae infections are often based on serologic test results.

B.   *B. abortus* infections

   1.   Bovine brucellosis (see Chap. 79)

       a.   *B. abortus* causes no overt disease other than abortion and orchitis.

          (1)   In heifers and cows, the bacterium grows slowly in vivo except in the gravid uterus after the fifth month of gestation. In the placenta, fetal fluids, and chorion, the brucellae multiply very rapidly due to the presence of erythritol, which stimulates its growth. Abortion occurs after the fifth month of gestation; however, infected females may have a normal or weak calf and shed *B. abortus* after parturition. Common sequelae include retained placenta and metritis.

          (2)   In bulls, orchitis and epididymitis will occur occasionally.

       b.   Many diagnoses of bovine brucellosis are based on serologic test results.

          (1)   Commonly used serologic tests include the brucellosis card, standard tube agglutination, 2-mercaptoethanol, rivanol, and complement-fixation.

   2.   Canine infections

       a.   Ingestion of brucellae-contaminated placentas and aborted fetuses from infected cows is the primary mode of transmission.

          (1)   The incidence of *B. abortus* infections in dogs is directly related to the incidence of bovine brucellosis.

       b.   Most infected dogs never exhibit clinical signs, but infections acquired during pregnancy may result in abortion. Orchitis and epididymitis are occasionally observed in males.

          (1)   Aborted fetuses, fetal membranes, and vaginal discharges from bitches contain large numbers of brucellae, which are a potential source of infection for other animals as well as man.

       c.   Serologic tests used for bovine brucellosis are commonly employed in the diagnosis of *B. abortus* infections in dogs.

(1) The serologic tests that are used for diagnosing *B. canis* infections will not detect antibodies to *B. abortus*.

3. Equine brucellosis
   a. Ingestion of *B. abortus*-contaminated feed, water, and placentas and aborted fetuses from infected cows is the primary mode of transmission.
      (1) The incidence of equine brucellosis appears to be directly related to the frequency of contact with infected cattle.
   b. The brucellae localize in the bursae, tendons, and joints.
      (1) Fistulous withers and poll evil are characterized as chronic draining lesions. The affected bursae in poll evil are those between the nuchal ligament and the atlas and axis, and the bursae in fistulous withers are between the nuchal ligament and the dorsal spines of the thoracic vertebrae.
   c. Abortion is rare.
   d. Serologic tests used for bovine brucellosis are commonly employed in the diagnosis of *B. abortus* infections in horses.

C. *B. canis* infections
   1. Canine brucellosis
      a. Ingestion of brucellae-contaminated urogenital discharges, including vaginal discharges, placentas, and fetuses, is the primary mode of transmission. Vaginal discharges may be infective for 4 to 6 weeks.
      b. Venereal transmission may occur during coitus, when *B. canis* in the seminal fluids of an infected male are transferred to a susceptible female during coitus.
      c. Infected dogs are afebrile and exhibit discospondylitis, recurrent anterior uveitis, generalized lymphadenopathy, and splenitis.
         (1) In females, abortion in the last trimester of pregnancy is the primary clinical sign. Prolonged vaginal discharge after abortion is common. Females may have normal litters after one to three abortions, but infertility after abortion is common.
         (2) In males, clinical signs and lesions include epididymitis and orchitis with scrotal dermatitis and swelling. Infertility is common, but testicular atrophy is often unilateral.
      d. Serologic tests, using *B. canis* or *B. ovis* antigens, are commonly employed in the diagnosis of canine brucellosis.

D. *B. ovis* infections
   1. Ovine epididymitis and abortion
      a. In rams, *B. ovis* causes an epididymitis and orchitis that results in lowered sperm quality and infertility. Rams

transmit the infection to ewes during coitus. On palpation the epididymal lesions cannot be distinguished from those caused by *Actinobacillus seminis*.

    (1) *B. ovis* infections are diagnosed by semen cultures or by serologic diagnoses, using either the complement-fixation test or the ELISA test.

  b. In ewes, *B. ovis* will occasionally cause a placentitis and abortion, but most infections are subclinical. The role of ewes in the transmission of *B. ovis* is poorly understood.

  c. The disease is effectively controlled by the elimination of infected rams. Infected rams frequently transmit the disease to susceptible rams during homosexual episodes.

    (1) Vaccination with *B. ovis* bacterins has been used successfully to prevent rams from becoming infected.

E. *B. suis* infections

  1. Porcine brucellosis

    a. The two primary modes of transmission are the ingestion of brucellae-contaminated discharges from the female genital tract and venereal transmission from infected boars to susceptible gilts and sows.

      (1) Sows that abort may shed brucellae from their uterus for 1 or 2 years.

      (2) Boars with lesions in the testes and accessory genitalia often shed brucellae in the semen for life.

      (3) Brucellae also may be shed in the urine of infected swine.

    b. Most infections are subclinical even though the bacteremia may persist for months or even years.

      (1) Brucellae localization may occur in any organ, including the skeleton, joints, spleen, liver, kidney, urinary bladder, lymph nodes, and the male and female genitalia. *B. suis* produces focal granulomatous lesions with coagulation necrosis.

    c. In females, clinical signs are abortions, which occur during the second and third month of gestation, and the birth of weak or stillborn piglets. Retention of the placenta may occur. Abortions in a herd are usually sporadic, and abortion storms are rare. Herd infertility is common, with the sows and gilts coming into heat 30 to 45 days after first breeding. Part of a herd may be immune so only a few animals abort or are repeat breeders.

    d. In boars, orchitis is common but usually subclinical. Infected boars occasionally exhibit a reduced fertility and libido. Boars often have persistent infections that may last 3 to 4 years.

    e. Serologic tests used for bovine brucellosis are often employed for *B. suis* infections in swine.

53 | Genus *Francisella*

I. *FRANCISELLA* SPECIES
   A. Pathogens

Species	Hosts	Clinical Disease	Subclinical Infections
F. tularensis	Man	Tularemia	
	Domestic animals		+

       1. There are two biovars, *tularensis* and *palaearctica*.
   B. Nonpathogens
       1. *F. novicida* is not a pathogen of domestic animals or man.

II. HABITAT AND ECOLOGY
   A. *F. tularensis* is widely distributed in nature and has been isolated from domestic animals, birds, and biting insects, as well as from approximately 100 species of wildlife. The organism also has been isolated from natural waters in areas where the disease is endemic in wildlife.
       1. The two biovars of *F. tularensis*, which vary in virulence, are found in the United States.

III. CELLULAR, CULTURAL, AND BIOCHEMICAL CHARACTERISTICS
   A. Cellular characteristics
       1. Gram-negative rods
          a. Cells are small coccobacilli.
       2. Nonmotile
   B. Cultural characteristics
       1. Obligate aerobic
       2. Fastidious growth requirements
          a. *F. tularensis* requires cysteine for growth. The bacterium will grow on blood agar supplemented with cysteine when incubated aerobically at $37^{0}C$. The colonies are smooth, gray, and surrounded by a green zone of discoloration.
          b. *F. novicida* will grow on blood agar.
   C. Biochemical characteristics
       1. Oxidase-negative
       2. Respiratory metabolism
          a. Glucose is utilized oxidatively.

IV. DISEASE OVERVIEW
- A. Infections in domestic animals
  1. Although some domestic animals may become subclinically infected with *F. tularensis*, they are not considered to be a significant source of infection for man.
- B. Tularemia in man
  1. Tularemia is an acute febrile granulomatous infection. The incubation period ranges from 2 to 10 days dependent primarily on dose. *F. tularensis* biovar *tularensis* produces more severe infections than does *F. tularensis* biovar *palaearctica*.
  2. *F. tularensis* has great invasive ability. The bacterium is able to penetrate the unbroken skin and frequently is acquired from handling infected animal carcasses. The wild rabbit is the primary reservoir for man in the United States. Other common wildlife reservoirs are beavers and muskrats. Tularemia also may be contracted from insect bites, ingestion of improperly cooked meat or contaminated water, or inhalation of airborne organisms from excretions of infected animals.

54	Genus *Haemophilus*

I. *HAEMOPHILUS* SPECIES
- A. Pathogens

Species	Hosts	Specific Diseases	Nonspecific Diseases
H. agni	Ovine	Polyarthritis	septicemia, meningitis, pneumonia
H. ducreyi	Man	Chancroid	
H. influenzae	Man	Pneumonia	
H. parasuis	Porcine	Polyserositis	respiratory disease
H. somnus	Bovine	TEME	respiratory disease

- B. Special growth factors
  1. Most *Haemophilus* species require factors X and/or V for in vitro growth.
     a. The X factor, hemin, is used by the bacteria as a prosthetic group in the iron-containing respiratory cytochromes and in heme enzymes such as catalase and peroxidase. Factor X is heat-stable.

    b. The V factor is nicotinamide adenine dinucleotide (NAD), which serves as a coenzyme for pyridine-linked dehydrogenases, a class of oxidation reduction enzymes. Factor V is heat-labile.

2. Growth characteristics of some *Haemophilus* species
    a. A species may require both X and V factors, only X or V factor, or neither (Table 54.1).

Table 54.1. Growth requirements of selected *Haemophilus* species for factors X and V

Species	Require X	Require V
H. agni	-	-
H. ducreyi	+	-
H. influenzae	+	+
H. parasuis	-	+
H. somnus	-	-

II. HABITAT AND ECOLOGY

    A. The pathogenic *Haemophilus* species are obligate parasites on the mucous membranes of a variety of animal species. Most *Haemophilus* species tend to be host-specific.

III. CELLULAR, CULTURAL, AND BIOCHEMICAL CHARACTERISTICS

    A. Cellular characteristics
        1. Gram-negative rods
            a. The cells are small coccobacilli.
        2. Nonmotile
    B. Cultural characteristics
        1. The pathogenic *Haemophilus* species of domestic animals are facultative anaerobic.
        2. *H. agni*, *H. parasuis*, and *H. somnus* are nonhemolytic.
        3. Fastidious growth requirements
            a. Many *Haemophilus* species require factors X and V and increased carbon dioxide for growth.
            b. Sources of factors X and V are described.
                (1) Chocolate agar contains both factors X and V. It is prepared by heating molten blood agar medium to a temperature of approximately 80°C, which is high enough to lyse the red blood cells and release factor X but not to inactivate the heat-labile factor V. If the medium is overheated during preparation, factor V is inactivated and the medium will not support *Haemophilus* species, which require NAD for growth.
                (2) The satellite phenomenon of blood agar treated with *Staphylococcus aureus* provides both factors X and V.
                    (a) The hemolytic staphylococci lyse the red blood cells, causing the release of factor X and

producing an excess of factor V, which diffuses into the agar medium.

    (b) The specimen from which a species of *Haemophilus* is to be recovered is heavily streaked on the surfaces of a blood agar plate, and then a single streak of *S. aureus* is made through the area where the specimen had been inoculated. After 18 to 24 hours incubation under 5 to 10 percent carbon dioxide at $37^\circ C$, the colonies of haemophili may be observed within the hemolytic zone adjacent to the *S. aureus* colonies. This growth is referred to as the satellite phenomenon.

  (3) Paper disks impregnated with factors X and V are commonly used to determine the X and V growth requirements.

    (a) The organism to be tested is streaked on a medium deficient in factors X and V, such as trypticase soy agar, and then the disks are applied to the surface of the agar. After 18 to 24 hours incubation under 5 to 10 percent carbon dioxide at $37^\circ C$, the growth patterns around the disks are observed. Bacterial growth is limited to the vicinity of the disks impregnated with factors required for growth (Fig. 54.1.).

  C. Biochemical characteristics

    1. Oxidase reactions vary with species.

      a. *H. parasuis* is oxidase-negative, but *H. agni* and *H. somnus* are oxidase-positive.

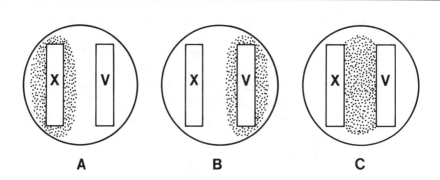

Fig. 54.1. Paper disks impregnated with factors X and V placed on the surface of agar plates inoculated with various *Haemophilus* species. The presence of visible growth around the disks indicates the species growth requirements for factor X (*A*), factor V (*B*), or both factors X and V (*C*).

      2. Fermentative metabolism

D. Presumptive identification procedures

      1. Three characteristics are used to provide presumptive identification of *Haemophilus* species: (1) their requirements for factors X and V; (2) their hemolytic reactions on blood agar, which will often vary with the species of animal from which the blood is obtained; (3) and their fermentation patterns of various carbohydrate substrates.

IV. DISEASE OVERVIEW

A. Infections in domestic animals

      1. Various *Haemophilus* species have been recovered at one time or another from all domestic animal species; however, only clinical *Haemophilus* infections with consistent clinical signs and pathologic lesions have been observed in cattle, sheep, and swine.

B. *H. agni* infections

      1. Ovine septicemia and polyarthritis

          a. *H. agni* causes septicemia and occasionally polyarthritis, pneumonia, and meningitis.

          b. Epidemic infections have been reported in feeder lambs on a high plane of nutrition. Acutely affected animals are febrile and depressed and often die within a day or two of first being observed ill. In surviving animals, a fibrinopurulent arthritis develops and the lambs are stiff and reluctant to move.

          c. Gross pathology lesions include necrotic foci on the liver, fibrinopurulent polyarthritis, meningitis, and ecchymotic hemorrhages on serous membranes in subcutaneous tissues and muscles. Microscopic lesions are characterized by a bacterial thrombosis and a necrotizing vasculitis.

C. *H. parasuis* infections

      1. Porcine polyserositis

          a. *H. parasuis* was described in 1931 by R. E. Shope, who first described both swine influenza and *H. (influenza) suis*.

          b. *H. parasuis* is a normal inhabitant of the porcine respiratory tract and a potential pathogen, particularly in animals under some sort of stress like weaning, weather changes, or movement to new quarters. The clinical condition in which *H. parasuis* is most frequently encountered is polyserositis, commonly called Glasser's disease. It is primarily a disease of pigs from 2 to 4 months of age. The systemic infection produces a fibrinous inflammation of the membranes lining the large body cavities, joints, and meninges, resulting in polyarthritis, pericarditis, peritonitis, pleuritis, and occasionally meningitis. The polyserositis lesions are very similar to those caused by porcine mycoplasmas such as *M. hyorhinis*.

     c. The clinical presentation in affected swine herds largely depends on the level of herd immunity. In swine herds lacking immunity to *H. parasuis*, the animals are fully susceptible. If the infection is introduced, the disease will spread rapidly and produce acute clinical infections in all age groups. The morbidity rate is often as high as 50 percent with up to 75 percent mortality of the affected pigs. One month after an acute outbreak practically all the surviving animals will have developed high CF titers and protective humoral immunity. The herd is then considered to be chronically infected, and clinical disease is not observed unless susceptible swine are introduced. In chronically infected herds, sporadic disease occurs in newly introduced susceptible weaner pigs, but the infection rarely assumes epidemic proportions. Most immune animals will retain low CF titers.

D. *H. somnus* infections

   1. Bovine thromboembolic meningoencephalitis (TEME) (see Chap. 89)

     a. TEME was first described in Colorado feedlot cattle in 1956. It is the classical disease associated with *H. somnus*. It is manifested as an encephalitis, and pathognomonic lesions in the brain are characterized by multiple foci of hemorrhage and necrosis.

     b. It is a sequela to septicemia and is usually associated with prior respiratory infection.

55	Genus *Taylorella*

I. *TAYLORELLA* SPECIES
A. Pathogens

Species	Host	Specific Disease
T. equigenitalis	Equine	CONTAGIOUS EQUINE METRITIS

    1. It is the only species in the genus. Previously the bacterium was called *Haemophilus equigenitalis*.

II. HABITAT AND ECOLOGY
A. *T. equigenitalis* is an obligate parasite of the equine genital tract.

III. CELLULAR, CULTURAL, AND BIOCHEMICAL CHARACTERISTICS
A. Cellular characteristics
    1. Gram-negative rods
    2. Nonmotile
B. Cultural characteristics
    1. Facultative anaerobic
    2. Fastidious growth requirements
        a. Good growth is attained on chocolate agar when incubated under 5 to 10 percent carbon dioxide. After 48 to 72 hours, colonies are pinpoint, raised, smooth, and gray. The bacterium grows poorly when incubated in air or anaerobically. On blood agar, the growth is scant and no hemolysis is produced. There is no growth on MacConkey agar.
C. Biochemical characteristics
    1. Oxidase-positive
    2. Fermentative metabolism

IV. DISEASE OVERVIEW
A. *T. equigenitalis* infections
    1. Equine contagious equine metritis (see Chap. 106)
        a. It is a venereal disease of horses that is transmitted during coitus.
        b. In mares, acute infections are characterized by vaginitis, cervicitis, and endometritis with copious production of a mucopurulent exudate. Infected mares either fail to conceive or abort during the first 60 days of gestation.
        c. In stallions, there are no clinical signs.

56 | Genus *Legionella*

I. *LEGIONELLA* SPECIES
  A. Pathogens

Species	Host	Specific Disease
Legionella species	Man	Legionellosis

  1. There are six species in the genus.
  2. The term legionellosis is used to indicate all infections caused by *Legionella* species.

II. HABITAT AND ECOLOGY
  A. *Legionella* species are isolated from water, mud, and thermally polluted lakes and streams.

III. CELLULAR, CULTURAL, AND BIOCHEMICAL CHARACTERISTICS
  A. Cellular characteristics
    1. Gram-negative rods
    2. Motile by monotrichous or multitrichous polar flagella
  B. Cultural characteristics
    1. Obligate aerobic
    2. Fastidious growth requirements
      a. L-cysteine and iron salts are required for growth.
  C. Biochemical characteristics
    1. Oxidase-negative or very weak positive reactions
    2. Respiratory metabolism
      a. Glucose is not utilized.

IV. DISEASE OVERVIEW
  A. Legionellosis in man
    1. Legionellosis is manifested as either a pneumonia with a high fatality rate or an acute, febrile illness with a low mortality rate.
  B. Infections in domestic animals
    1. Attempts to induce clinical disease experimentally in various domestic animals have been unsuccessful.

57 | Genus *Moraxella*

I. *MORAXELLA* SPECIES
   A. Pathogens

Species	Hosts	Specific Disease	Nonspecific Diseases
M. bovis	Bovine	INFECTIOUS KERATO-CONJUNCTIVITIS	
Other species	Domestic animals		opportunistic

II. HABITAT AND ECOLOGY
   A. Most *Moraxella* species are considered to be part of normal mucous membrane flora of domestic animals.

III. CELLULAR, CULTURAL, AND BIOCHEMICAL CHARACTERISTICS
   A. Cellular characteristics
   1. Gram-negative rods
      a. Cells of *M. bovis* are coccobacilli, usually occurring in pairs.
   2. Nonmotile
   B. Culture characteristics
   1. Obligate aerobic
   2. Growth on blood agar at 37°C
      a. Of the *Moraxella* species, only *M. bovis* produces hemolysis.
      b. Most bovine strains of *M. bovis* are hemolytic. Virulent fimbriated strains form small, flat colonies that corrode the agar. The nonfimbriated variants form larger, convex, noncorroding colonies.
   C. Biochemical characteristics
   1. Oxidase-positive
   2. Respiratory metabolism
      a. *M. bovis* does not utilize glucose.

IV. DISEASE OVERVIEW
   A. *M. bovis* infections
   1. Infectious bovine keratoconjunctivitis (see Chap. 83)
      a. This is a localized infection of the eye characterized by conjunctivitis, keratitis, corneal opacity, and ulceration. The condition is commonly called pinkeye.

B. Other *Moraxella* species infections
    1. Infections in domestic animals
        a. *Moraxella* species are opportunistic pathogens and have
            been implicated in a variety of conditions in all species
            of animals. They are frequently found in mixed bacterial
            infections or secondary to viral infections.

| 58 | Genus *Neisseria* |

I. *NEISSERIA* SPECIES

    A. Pathogens

Species	Hosts	Specific Diseases	Nonspecific Diseases
N. gonorrhoeae	Man	Gonorrhea	
N. meningitidis	Man	Meningitis	
Other species	Domestic animals		opportunistic

II. HABITAT AND ECOLOGY
    A. Most *Neisseria* species are part of the mucous membrane flora of
        domestic animals and man.

III. CELLULAR, CULTURAL, AND BIOCHEMICAL CHARACTERISTICS
    A. Cellular characteristics
        1. Gram-negative cocci
            a. The cells are often arranged in pairs with their adjacent
                sides flattened. The cells also may occur singly and in
                tetrads.
        2. Nonmotile
    B. Cultural characteristics
        1. Obligate aerobic
        2. Fastidious growth requirements
            a. All *Neisseria* species (other than *N. gonorrhoeae* and *N.
                meningitidis*, which have fastidious nutritional
                requirements) will grow on blood agar, but many species
                require 3 to 8 percent carbon dioxide for growth. The

colony morphology and ability to produce hemolysis varies with the species.
   (1) Chocolate agar, which is a rich source of iron, is commonly used to culture *N. gonorrhoeae* and *N. meningitidis*.
   b. The growth of neisseriae on MacConkey agar is absent or very sparse.
   c. Presumptive identification of these species is based on Gram reaction, cellular morphology, cellular arrangement, and oxidase reactivity. The definitive identification of the *Neisseria* species is largely based on their ability to reduce nitrate and to utilize various monosaccharides and disaccharides.
C. Biochemical characteristics
   1. Oxidase-positive
   2. Respiratory metabolism
      a. Some *Neisseria* species are saccharolytic and utilize glucose oxidatively, but other species are asaccharolytic.

IV. DISEASE OVERVIEW
   A. Infections in domestic animals
      1. Although *Neisseria* species are potential pathogens of domestic animals, they rarely play a significant role in disease.

59	Genus *Pasteurella*

I. *PASTEURELLA* SPECIES
    A. Pathogens

Species	Hosts	Specific Diseases	Nonspecific Diseases
P. haemolytica	Bovine	Respiratory disease complex	pneumonia
	Ovine	Pneumonia, Septicemia	
	Porcine		pneumonia
P. multocida	Bovine	Respiratory disease complex	pneumonia
		Epizootic hemorrhagic septicemia	
	Ovine		pneumonia
	Porcine		pneumonia
			opportunistic
	Canine, feline		bite wounds
Other species	Domestic animals		opportunistic

B. Characteristics of *P. haemolytica* and *P. multocida*
    1. They are heterologous species.
        a. Each species is composed of strains (biovars, capsular types or serovars) with considerable differences in host predilection, pathogenicity, colonial morphology, and antigenic nature.
    2. *P. haemolytica* has two biovars (A and T), based on carbohydrate fermentation reactions. Each biovar has multiple capsular and somatic antigens.
        a. The biovars and their serovars often have a host and/or organ predilection.
            (1) *P. haemolytica* biovar A serovar 1 is frequently isolated from bovine pneumonias.
    3. *P. multocida* has four capsular types (A, B, D, and E) as well as nonencapsulated strains.
        a. Capsular types A and D are found in domestic animals and fowl in the United States. Type A is the most common.
        b. Capsular types B and E are rarely, if ever, found in the United States.
        c. Nonencapsulated strains are commonly isolated from dogs and cats.

II. HABITAT AND ECOLOGY
    A. *Pasteurella* species
        1. The pasteurellae are normal inhabitants of the upper respiratory tract of domestic animals.

a. *P. haemolytica* is a commensal of the upper respiratory tract of healthy cattle and sheep.
   (1) Only biovar A and mainly serovars 1 and 2 have been isolated from cattle. Both biovars A and T and all recognized serovars have been isolated from sheep.
b. *P. multocida* has been recovered from over 40 species of domestic and wild mammals and more than 60 species of birds.
   (1) Capsular types A and D are considered normal respiratory tract flora of domestic animals, but types B and E are not commensals.
   (2) *P. multocida* is normal oral flora of the dog and cat.

III. CELLULAR, CULTURAL, AND BIOCHEMICAL CHARACTERISTICS
A. Cellular characteristics
   1. Gram-negative rods
      a. Cells of *P. multocida* often show bipolar staining.
   2. Nonmotile
   3. Most virulent strains of *P. haemolytica* and *P. multocida* produce capsules of varying size.
      a. Canine and feline strains of *P. multocida* often lack a capsule.
B. Cultural characteristics
   1. Facultative anaerobic
   2. Growth on blood agar and/or MacConkey agar at 37°C
      a. Pasteurellae colonies are round and grayish. *P. haemolytica* produces a zone of beta hemolysis and will grow sparsely on MacConkey agar. *P. multocida* is nonhemolytic, and encapsulated strains produce mucoid colonies that tend to coalesce. *P. multocida* does not grow on MacConkey agar.
C. Biochemical characteristics
   1. Oxidase-positive
   2. Fermentative metabolism
      a. Pasteurellae produce acid, but no gas, from a number of carbohydrates.

IV. DISEASE OVERVIEW
A. *P. haemolytica* and *P. multocida* infections
   1. Bovine respiratory disease complex (BRDC)
      a. BRDC is caused by the interaction of stress and multiple etiologic agents, including numerous viruses and bacterial species.
      b. The pneumonic lesions are characterized as an acute, bilaterial, fibrinonecrotic bronchopneumonia with pleuritis.
      c. Of the bacterial species, *P. haemolytica* biovar A and *P. multocida* capsular types A and D are the most frequently isolated from the lung lesions. Other bacteria,

occasionally isolated include *Actinomyces pyogenes*, *Haemophilus somnus*, *Mycoplasma* species, and *Streptococcus* species.

    (1) These bacteria are frequently present on the oral, nasal, and pharyngeal mucosa of healthy cattle. Thus the bovine lower respiratory tract is constantly exposed to bacteria inhaled on dust particles or aerosolized from the oral and nasal pharyngeal mucosa in droplet nuclei.

  d. Of the viruses, parainfluenza-3 virus is the most commonly isolated from the pneumonic lesions. Other viral agents that have been implicated in BRDC include adenoviruses, bovine virus diarrhea virus, enteroviruses, infectious bovine rhinotracheitis virus, reoviruses, respiratory syncytial viruses, and rhinoviruses.

  2. Bovine and ovine pneumonia

    a. *P. haemolytica* and *P. multocida* are commonly isolated from primary bacterial pneumonias of cattle and sheep.

      (1) Occasionally *P. haemolytica* will produce a fatal septicemia in lambs.

B. *P. multocida* infections

  1. Bovine epizootic hemorrhagic septicemia

    a. Types B and E of *P. multocida* cause the classic hemorrhagic septicemia syndrome. The disease has been characterized as an acute septicemia often resulting in death. It is very rare in the United States but commonly occurs in cattle and water buffalo of South Asia.

  2. Canine and feline infections

    a. Noncapsulated strains of *P. multocida* has been isolated from a wide variety of bacterial infections, often in mixed culture.

      (1) Bite wounds from dogs and cats are often contaminated with *P. multocida*.

      (2) *P. multocida* can induce severe abscesses in cats.

  3. Porcine infections

    a. *P. multocida* is a very common secondary infection of the various respiratory conditions of swine.

      (1) The lesions are a purulent bronchopneumonia.

    b. *P. multocida* type D has been incriminated as a primary etiologic agent of atrophic rhinitis.

60	Genus *Pseudomonas*

I. *PSEUDOMONAS* SPECIES
   A. Pathogens

Species	Hosts	Specific Diseases	Nonspecific Diseases
P. aeruginosa	Domestic animals		opportunistic
P. mallei	Equine	Glanders	
P. pseudomallei	Domestic animals	Melioidosis	
Other species	Domestic animals		opportunistic

II. HABITAT AND ECOLOGY
   A. The pseudomonads are found as free-living saprophytes in soil, water, and many other natural materials, or in association with plants or animals as agents of disease.

III. CELLULAR, CULTURAL, AND BIOCHEMICAL CHARACTERISTICS
   A. Cellular characteristics
       1. Gram-negative rods
       2. All *Pseudomonas* species are motile by polar flagella except *P. mallei*, which is nonmotile. *P. aeruginosa* has a single flagellum, but *P. pseudomallei* is multitrichous.
   B. Cultural characteristics
       1. Obligate aerobic
           a. *P. aeruginosa* can use nitrate instead of molecular oxygen as a terminal electron acceptor and can grow under anaerobic conditions. Thus *P. aeruginosa* and other nitrate-reducing bacteria are functionally facultative anaerobes because they do not require molecular oxygen for growth. This type of metabolism is called anaerobic respiration.
       2. Growth on blood agar and/or MacConkey agar at 37°C
           a. Many *Pseudomonas* species grow better at 20°C than at 37°C.
           b. On blood agar, colonies of *P. aeruginosa* are large, gray, and produce a zone of beta hemolysis. The bacterium also will grow on MacConkey agar.
   C. Biochemical characteristics
       1. Oxidase-positive except for *P. mallei*, which is oxidase-negative.
       2. Respiratory metabolism
           a. *P. aeruginosa*, *P. mallei*, and *P. pseudomallei* utilize glucose oxidatively.

IV. DISEASE OVERVIEW
  A. *P. aeruginosa* infections
    1. Infections in domestic animals
      a. *P. aeruginosa* produces a wide variety of suppurative
          infections that are often due to gross impairment of one or
          more host defense mechanisms. It is often isolated from
          mixed infections.
        (1) The purulent material from *P. aeruginosa*-infected
            lesions may be green.
  B. *P. mallei* infections
    1. Equine glanders
      a. Glanders is primarily a disease of horses.
      b. Forms of the disease include pulmonary glanders, nasal
          glanders, cutaneous glanders or farcy, and ulcerative
          lymphangitis. There also is an acute septicemic form that
          kills the animal before abscesses develop.
      c. Infections are characterized by the formation of
          encapsulated nodules that contain yellow caseous purulent
          material.
      d. Glanders has been eradicated from the United States.
  C. *P. pseudomallei* infections
    1. Infections in domestic animals
      a. Melioidosis (pseudoglanders) can affect all domestic
          animals.
      b. The lesions resemble those of glanders. In the chronic
          form, nodules and abscesses occur in the lungs, liver,
          spleen, lymph nodes, and subcutis.

PART **12**	Commonly Isolated Extracellular Bacteria

61	Culture Requirements of Commonly Isolated Extracellular Bacteria

I. ATMOSPHERIC AND NUTRITIONAL GROWTH REQUIREMENTS
   FOR BACTERIAL PATHOGENS
   A. The culture requirements of extracellular and facultative
      intracellular bacteria commonly isolated from bovines, ovines,
      porcines, equines, canines, and felines are listed (Tables 61.1 to
      61.6).

Table 61.1. Extracellular bacteria commonly isolated from bovines and their culture requirements

Body System / Organisms	Nonfastidious Organisms[a]	Aerobic	Anaerobic	Other[b]	Blood agar	Other
		(Atmospheric Requirements)			*(Nutritional Requirements)*	
Gastrointestinal						
Clostridium perfringens	+					
Escherichia coli					+	
Mycobacterium paratuberculosis						+
Salmonella serovars	+					
Integument and subcutis						
Epidermis						
Dermatophilus congolensis	+					
Abscesses						
Actinobacillus lignieresii	+					
Corynebacterium bovis	+					
Escherichia coli, other coliforms	+					
Musculoskeletal						
Muscle						
Clostridium chauvoei			+			
C. septicum			+		+	
Joints						
Actinomyces pyogenes		+		+		
Haemophilus somnus		+				+
Mycoplasma species		+				+
Staphylococcus aureus	+					
Streptococcus species	+					
Foot						
Bacteroides melaninogenicus and			+	+		
Fusobacterium necrophorum			+		+	+
Nervous						
Brain						
Haemophilus somnus		+				+
Listeria monocytogenes	+					
Ocular						
Moraxella bovis	+					
Respiratory						
Actinomyces pyogenes	+					
Bordetella bronchiseptica	+					
Haemophilus somnus		+				+
Mycoplasma species		+				+
Pasteurella haemolytica	+					
P. multocida	+					

Table 61.1. (continued)

| Body System | Organisms | Nonfastidious Organisms[a] | Fastidious Organisms | | | | | |
| | | | Atmospheric Requirements | | | Nutritional Requirements | | |
			Aerobic	Anaerobic	Other[b]	Blood agar	Other	
Reproductive								
Genital, abortion	*Actinomyces pyogenes*	+						
	Brucella abortus		+				+	
	Campylobacter fetus ss *venerealis*				+	+		
	C. fetus ss *fetus*				+	+		
	Mycoplasma bovigenitalium		+				+	
Mastitis	*Actinomyces pyogenes*	+						
	Brucella abortus				+		+	
	Escherichia coli, other coliforms	+						
	Mycoplasma species		+				+	
	Nocardia asteroides	+						
	Pseudomonas aeruginosa	+						
	Staphylococcus aureus	+						
	Streptococcus agalactiae	+						
	Streptococcus species	+						
Urinary	*Corynebacterium renale*	+						

[a] Growth on blood agar and/or MacConkey agar incubated aerobically at 37°C.
[b] Usually microaerophilic and/or capnophilic.

Table 61.2. Extracellular bacteria commonly isolated from ovines and their culture requirements

Body System	Organisms	Nonfastidious Organisms[a]	Fastidious Organisms				
			Atmospheric Requirements			Nutritional Requirements	
			Aerobic	Anaerobic	Other[b]	Blood agar	Other
Gastrointestinal							
	Clostridium perfringens			+		+	
	Mycobacterium paratuberculosis						+
	Salmonella serovars	+					
Integument and subcutis							
Epidermis	Dermatophilus congolensis	+					
Abscesses	Corynebacterium pseudotuberculosis	+					
Musculoskeletal							
Muscle	Clostridium chauvoei			+		+	
	C. septicum			+		+	
Joints	Actinomyces pyogenes	+					
	Erysipelothrix rhusiopathiae	+					
	Escherichia coli, other coliforms	+					
	Haemophilus agni		+				+
	Mycoplasma species		+				+
	Streptococcus species	+					
Foot	Bacteroides nodosus and			+			+
	Fusobacterium necrophorum			+			+
Nervous							
Brain	Listeria monocytogenes	+					
Respiratory							
	Actinomyces pyogenes	+					
	Mycoplasma species	+					
	Pasteurella haemolytica	+					
	P. multocida	+					
Reproductive							
Genital, abortion	Campylobacter fetus ss fetus				+	+	
	Corynebacterium pseudotuberculosis	+					
	Listeria monocytogenes	+					
Epididymitis	Actinobacillus seminis	+					
	Brucella ovis				+	+	
Mastitis	Actinomyces pyogenes	+					
	Corynebacterium pseudotuberculosis	+					
	Mycoplasma species		+				+
	Staphylococcus aureus	+					
	Streptococcus agalactiae	+					
	Streptococcus species	+					
	Pasteurella haemolytica	+					
	P. multocida	+					

[a] Growth on blood agar and/or MacConkey agar incubated aerobically at 37°C.
[b] Usually microaerophilic and/or capnophilic.

Table 61.3. Extracellular bacteria commonly isolated from porcines and their culture requirements

Body System	Organisms	Nonfastidious Organisms[a]	Fastidious Organisms				
			Atmospheric Requirements			Nutritional Requirements	
			Aerobic	Anaerobic	Other[b]	Blood agar	Other
Gastrointestinal	*Clostridium perfringens*			+		+	
	Escherichia coli	+					
	Salmonella serovars	+					
	Treponema hyodysenteriae			+		+	
Integument and subcutis Jowl abscesses	*Actinomyces pyogenes*	+					
	Streptococcus suis	+					
	Actinobacillus suis	+					
Musculoskeletal Joints	*Actinomyces pyogenes*	+					
	Erysipelothrix rhusiopathiae	+					
	Escherichia coli, other coliforms	+					
	Haemophilus parasuis		+				+
	Mycoplasma hyorhinis		+				+
	Staphylococcus aureus	+					
	Streptococcus species	+					
Nervous Brain	*Listeria monocytogenes*	+					
	Pasteurella multocida	+					
	Streptococcus suis	+					
Respiratory	*Actinobacillus suis*	+					
	A. pleuropneumoniae		+				+
	Actinomyces pyogenes	+					
	Haemophilus parasuis		+				+
	Mycoplasma hyopneumoniae		+				+
	M. hyorhinis		+				
	Pasteurella haemolytica	+					
	P. multocida	+					

Table 61.3. *(continued)*

| Body System | Organisms | Nonfastidious Organisms[a] | Fastidious Organisms | | | | |
| | | | Atmospheric Requirements | | | Nutritional Requirements | |
			Aerobic	Anaerobic	Other[b]	Blood agar	Other
Reproductive							
Genital, abortion	*Actinomyces pyogenes*	+					
	Brucella suis				+	+	
	Mycobacterium species		+				+
	Pasteurella multocida	+					
	Pseudomonas aeruginosa	+					
	Streptococcus species	+					
	Actinobacillus lignieresii	+					
Mastitis	*Actinomyces pyogenes*	+					
	Escherichia coli, other coliforms	+					
	Fusobacterium necrophorum			+			+
	Mycobacterium species		+				+
	Staphylococcus aureus	+					
	Streptococcus species	+					
Urinary	*Eubacterium suis*			+		+	

[a]Growth on blood agar and/or MacConkey agar incubated aerobically at 37°C.
[b]Usually microaerophilic and/or capnophilic.

Table 61.4. Extracellular bacteria commonly isolated from equines and their culture requirements

Body System	Organisms	Nonfastidious Organisms[a]	Fastidious Organisms				
			Atmospheric Requirements			Nutritional Requirements	
			Aerobic	Anaerobic	Other[b]	Blood agar	Other
Gastrointestinal	*Actinobacillus equuli*	+					
	Clostridium perfringens			+		+	
	Escherichia coli	+					
	Rhodococcus equi	+					
	Salmonella serovars	+					
Integument and subcutis Abscesses	*Corynebacterium pseudotuberculosis*	+					
Musculoskeletal Joints	*Actinobacillus equuli*	+					
	Escherichia coli, other coliforms	+					
	Rhodococcus equi	+					
	Staphylococcus aureus	+					
	Streptococcus species	+					
Nervous	*Staphylococcus aureus*	+					
	Streptococcus species	+					
Respiratory	*Actinobacillus equuli*	+					
	Bordetella bronchiseptica	+					
	Klebsiella pneumoniae	+					
	Pasteurella multocida	+					
	Rhodococcus equi	+					
	Streptococcus equi	+					
	S. equisimilis	+					
	S. zooepidemicus	+					
Reproductive Genital, abortion	*Actinobacillus equuli*	+					
	Escherichia coli, other coliforms	+					
	Klebsiella pneumoniae	+					
	Pseudomonas aeruginosa	+					
	Rhodococcus equi	+					
	Salmonella serovars	+					
	Staphylococcus aureus	+					
	Streptococcus zooepidemicus	+					
	Streptococcus species	+					
	Taylorella equigenitalis				+		+
Mastitis	*Staphylococcus aureus*	+					
	Streptococcus species	+					

[a] Growth on blood agar and/or MacConkey agar incubated aerobically at 37°C.
[b] Usually microaerophilic and/or capnophilic.

Table 61.5. Extracellular bacteria commonly isolated from canines and their culture requirements

| Body System | Bacteria | Nonfastidious Organisms[a] | Fastidious Organisms | | | | |
| | | | Atmospheric Requirements | | | Nutritional Requirements | |
			Aerobic	Anaerobic	Other	Blood agar[b]	Other
Gastrointestinal	*Campylobacter jejuni*				+	+	
	Escherichia coli	+					
	Salmonella serovars	+					
Integument and subcutis							
Pyoderma, otitis	*Proteus* species	+					
Externa	*Pseudomonas aeruginosa*	+					
	Staphylococcus aureus	+					
	S. intermedius	+					
Abscesses	*Streptococcus* species	+					
	Polymicrobial infections[c]						
Respiratory							
Tracheobronchitis	*Bordetella bronchiseptica*	+					
Pneumonia	*Actinomyces viscosus*				+	+	
	Bacteroides species				+/-[c]	+/-[c]	
	Bordetella bronchiseptica	+					
	Escherichia coli	+					
	Fusobacterium species			+		+/-[c]	+/-[c]
	Klebsiella pneumoniae	+					
	Nocardia asteroides	+					
	Pasteurella multocida	+					
	Pseudomonas aeruginosa	+					
	Staphylococcus aureus	+					
	Streptococcus species	+					
Reproductive							
Genital, abortion	*Brucella canis*				+	+	
	Escherichia coli, other coliforms	+					
	Pseudomonas aeruginosa	+					
Mastitis	*Staphylococcus* species	+					
	Streptococcus species	+					

[a] Growth on blood agar and/or MacConkey agar incubated aerobically at 37°C.
[b] Usually microaerophilic and/or capnophilic.
[c] Growth requirements are species-dependent.

Table 61.6. Extracellular bacteria commonly isolated from felines and their culture requirements

Body System	Bacteria	Nonfastidious Organisms[a]	Fastidious Organisms				
			Atmospheric Requirements			Nutritional Requirements	
			Aerobic	Anaerobic	Other	Blood agar	Other
Gastrointestinal	*Salmonella* serovars	+					
Integument and subcutis	*Nocardia asteroides*	+					
	Pasteurella multocida	+					
Ocular	*Mycoplasma felis*		+				+
Respiratory	*Bordetella bronchiseptica*	+					
	Nocardia asteroides	+					
	Pasteurella multocida	+					
Reproductive Mastitis	*Staphylococcus aureus*	+					
	Streptococcus species	+					

[a]Growth on blood agar and/or MacConkey agar incubated aerobically at 37°C.

<table>
<tr><td>PART 13</td><td># Hosts of Extracellular Bacteria</td></tr>
</table>

<table>
<tr><td>62</td><td>## Host Range of Selected Bacteria</td></tr>
</table>

I. MAMMALIAN HOSTS OF SELECTED BACTERIA

A. The bacteria are grouped based on oxygen requirements, Gram reaction, and cellular characteristics (Tables 62.1 to 62.11).

1. A subjective scoring schema is used to delineate the host range and relative public health significance of selected extracellular and facultative intracellular bacteria as follows: − = not infected; ± = may be infected but no clinical disease is produced; + = rarely infected with clinical disease; ++ = commonly infected with clinical disease; +++ = primary host(s) of a pathogen; ND = not determined or not common. Other mammalian or avian hosts are listed if they are a primary or reservoir host.

Table 62.1. Aerobic gram-positive cocci

Genus	Species	Bovine	Canine	Equine	Feline	Ovine	Porcine	Man	Other
Micrococcus	*Micrococcus* species	−	−	−	−	−	−	−	−
Staphylococcus	*S. aureus*	++	++	++	++	++	++	++	++
	S. hyicus	ND	ND	ND	ND	ND	+++	ND	ND
	S. intermedius	ND	++	ND	ND	ND	ND	ND	ND
Streptococcus	*S. agalactiae*	+++	−	−	−	−	−	−	−
	S. equi	±	±	+++	±	±	±	±	±
	S. equisimilis	+	+	++	+	+	++	+	+
	S. pneumoniae	−	−	−	−	−	−	+++	+++
	S. pyogenes	++	++	++	++	++	++	++	++
	S. zooepidemicus	+	+	++	+	+	+	+	+

Table 62.2. Family Enterobacteriaceae, aerobic gram-negative rods

Genus	Species/Serovar	Host Range						
		Bovine	Canine	Equine	Feline	Ovine	Porcine	Man
Escherichia	*E. coli*	++	++	++	++	++	++	++
Klebsiella	*K. pneumoniae*	+	+	++	+	+	+	+
Salmonella	*S. choleraesuis*	-	-	-	-	-	+++	-
	S. paratyphi	-	-	-	-	-	-	++
	S. typhi	-	-	-	-	-	-	+++
	S. typhimurium	++	+	++	+	++	++	++
	S. typhisuis	-	-	-	-	-	+++	-
Shigella	*Shigella* species	-	-	-	-	-	-	+++
Yersinia	*Y. pestis*	-	-	-	-	-	-	++

Table 62.3. Aerobic gram-positive rods

us	Species	Host Range							Other
		Bovine	Canine	Equine	Feline	Ovine	Porcine	Man	
inomyces	*A. pyogenes*	++	++	++	++	++	++	++	
ynebacterium	*C. diphtheriae*	-	-	-	-	-	-	+++	
	C. pseudotuberculosis	±	±	+	-	++	±	±	
	C. renale	+++	-	-	-	-	-	-	
matophilus	*D. congolensis*	++	+	+	+	++	+	+	
sipelothrix	*E. rhusiopathiae*	-	-	-	-	+	++	+	
teria	*L. monocytogenes*	++	+	+	+	++	++	+	
obacterium	*M. avium*	±	±	±	±	±	++	+	Poultry
	M. bovis	+++	+	±	+	+	+	++	
	M. leprae	-	-	-	-	-	-	+++	
	M. paratuberculosis	+++	-	-	-	++	-	-	
	M. tuberculosis	++	+	±	±	+	+	+++	
ardia	*N. asteroides*	++	++	+	++	+	+	+	
dococcus	*R. equi*	-	-	++	-	-	+	-	

Table 62.4. Aerobic and anaerobic gram-positive sporeforming rods

Genus	Species	Host Range						
		Bovine	Canine	Equine	Feline	Ovine	Porcine	Man
Bacillus	*B. anthracis*	++	+	+	±	++	+	+
Clostridium	*C. botulinum*	+	-	+	-	+	-	++
	C. chauvoei	++	-	-	-	++	-	-
	C. haemolyticum	++	-	-	-	++	-	-
	C. novyi	++	-	-	-	++	-	-
	C. perfringens	++	+	++	±	++	+	+
	C. septicum	++	-	-	+	++	+	+
	C. tetani	+	+	++	+	+	+	+

Table 62.5. Anaerobic gram-positive and gram-negative cocci

Genus	Species	Bovine	Canine	Equine	Feline	Ovine	Porcine	Man
					Host Range			
Peptococcus	*Peptococcus* species	+	++	+	+	+	+	++
Peptostreptococcus	*Peptostreptococcus* species	+	++	+	+	+	+	++
Veillonella	*Veillonella* species	+	+	+	+	+	+	+

Table 62.6. Anaerobic gram-positive rods

Genus	Species	Bovine	Canine	Equine	Feline	Ovine	Porcine	Man
					Host Range			
Actinomyces	*A. bovis*	++	-	++	-	-	-	+
	A. israelii	-	-	-	-	-	-	++
	A. viscosus	-	++	-	+	-	-	-
Eubacterium	*E. suis*	±	±	±	±	±	++	±

Table 62.7. Anaerobic gram-negative rods

Genus	Species	Bovine	Canine	Equine	Feline	Ovine	Porcine	Man
					Host Range			
Bacteroides	*B. melaninogenicus*	++	+	±	±	+	+	+
	B. nodosus	+	-	-	-	+++	-	-
Fusobacterium	*F. necrophorum*	++	++	+	+	++	++	++

Table 62.8. Aerobic and anaerobic spirochetes

Genus	Species/Serovars	Bovine	Canine	Equine	Feline	Ovine	Porcine	Man	Other[a]
					Host Range				
Borrelia	*B. burgdorferi*	-	++	-	-	-	-	++	
	B. recurrentis	-	-	-	-	-	-	++	
	B. theileri	++	-	++	-	-	-	-	
Leptospira	*L. canicola*	+	+++	+	-	-	-	++	
	L. grippotyphosa	+	++	++	-	-	++	+	Wild anima
	L. hardjo	+++	-	-	-	-	-	-	
	L. icterohaemorrhagiae	+	++	++	-	-	++	++	
	L. pomona	+++	-	-	-	++	++	-	Wild anima
	L. szwajizak	+++	-	-	-	++	-	-	
Treponema	*T. hyodysenteriae*	-	-	-	-	-	++	-	
	T. pallidum	-	-	-	-	-	-	+++	

[a]Reservoir hosts.

Table 62.9. Aerobic gram-negative helical rods

		Host Range						
Genus	Species	Bovine	Canine	Equine	Feline	Ovine	Porcine	Man
Campylobacter	*C. fetus* ss *fetus*	+	−	−	−	++	−	−
	C. fetus ss *venerealis*	+++	−	−	−	−	−	−
	C. jejuni	ND	+	ND	ND	ND	+	++
	C. sputorum ss *mucosalis*	−	−	−	−	−	++	−
Vibrio	*V. cholerae*	−	−	−	−	−	−	+++

Table 62.10. Family Mycoplasmataceae, aerobic pleomorphic cells

		Host Range						
Genus	Species	Bovine	Canine	Equine	Feline	Ovine	Porcine	Man
Mycoplasma	*M. agalactiae*	−	−	−	−	+++	−	−
	M. hyopneumoniae	−	−	−	−	−	+++	−
	M. mycoides ss *mycoides*	+++	−	−	−	−	−	−
	M. ovipneumoniae	−	−	−	−	+++	−	−
	M. pneumoniae	−	−	−	−	−	−	+++

Table 62.11. Aerobic gram-negative cocci and rods

		Host Range						
Genus	Species	Bovine	Canine	Equine	Feline	Ovine	Porcine	Man
Actinobacillus	*A. equuli*	−	−	++	−	−	+	−
	A. lignieresii	++	−	−	−	−	−	−
	A. pleuropneumoniae	−	−	−	−	−	+++	−
	A. seminis	−	−	−	−	++	−	−
	A. suis	−	−	−	−	−	++	−
Bordetella	*B. bronchiseptica*	++	++	++	+	+	++	++
	B. pertussis	−	−	−	−	−	−	+++
Brucella	*B. abortus*	+++	+	+	+	++	+	++
	B. melitensis	++	+	+	−	+++	+	++
	B. suis	++	+	−	−	−	+++	++
	B. canis	−	+++	−	−	−	−	+
	B. ovis	−	±	−	−	+++	−	ND
Francisella	*F. tularensis*	−	−	−	−	−	−	++
Haemophilus	*H. influenzae*	−	−	−	−	−	−	+++
	H. parasuis	−	−	−	−	−	+++	−
	H. somnus	+++	−	−	−	ND	−	−
Taylorella	*T. equigenitalis*	−	−	+++	−	−	−	−
Legionella	*Legionella* species	−	−	−	−	−	−	+++
Moraxella	*M. bovis*	+++	+	+	+	+	+	+
Neisseria	*N. gonorrhoeae*	−	−	−	−	−	−	+++
	N. meningitidis	−	−	−	−	−	−	+++
Pasteurella	*P. haemolytica*	++	++	++	++	++	++	++
	P. multocida	++	++	++	++	++	++	++
Pseudomonas	*P. aeruginosa*	++	++	++	++	++	++	++
	P. mallei	−	−	+++	−	−	−	−

SECTION IV

Obligate Intracellular and Cell-associated Bacteria

PART **1**	# Classification and Characteristics

63	# Orders Chlamydiales and Rickettsiales

I. OBLIGATE INTRACELLULAR AND CELL-ASSOCIATED BACTERIA
A. Classification of pathogens (Table 63.1)

Table 63.1. Pathogens, orders Chlamydiales and Rickettsiales

Orders	Families	Genera[a]
Chlamydiales	Chlamydiaceae	*Chlamydia*
Rickettsiales	Anaplasmataceae	*Anaplasma*
		Eperythrozoon
		Haemobartonella
	Rickettsiaceae	*Cowdria*
		Coxiella
		Ehrlichia
		Neorickettsia
		Rickettsia

[a]Only genera that have species pathogenic for domestic animals are listed.

1. Two characteristics are commonly used to distinguish the orders Chlamydiales and Rickettsiales.
   a. Bacterial species in the order Chlamydiales are metabolically deficient and cannot synthesize ATP, relying on host cells for this substrate, whereas bacterial species in the order Rickettsiales synthesize their own ATP.
   b. Bacterial species in the order Chlamydiales have a unique developmental cycle with two morphologically distinct cell types called elementary bodies and reticulate bodies, whereas bacterial species in the order Rickettsiales have only one morphologic cell type.

B. Characteristics of families (Table 63.2)

Table 63.2. Differential characteristics of families Chlamydiaceae, Rickettsiaceae, and Anaplasmataceae

Characteristic	Chlamydiaceae	Rickettsiaceae	Anaplasmataceae
Gram reaction	-	-	-
Cellular morphology	Pleomorphic	Pleomorphic	Pleomorphic
Motility	-	-	-
Growth in cell-free media	-	-	-
Multiplication in host cells			
Nucleated cells	+[a]	+[b]	-
Erythrocytes	-	-	+[c]

[a]Chlamydiaceae infect a variety of nucleated cell types.
[b]The parasitic species are associated with reticuloendothelial and/or vascular endothelial cells.
[c]The parasitic species are found within erythrocytes, on the surface of erythrocytes, or free in the blood plasma.

1. The aerobic, nonmotile, gram-negative bacteria in the families Chlamydiaceae, Rickettsiaceae, and Anaplasmataceae have marked differences in the structure and composition of their cell walls.
   a. The Chlamydiaceae and Rickettsiaceae have trilaminar cell walls, but the Anaplasmataceae do not.
   b. The Rickettsiaceae have muramic acid in their cell walls, whereas the Chlamydiaceae contain little, if any, muramic acid.
2. Although these obligate intracellular and cell-associated bacteria are classified as gram-negative, they stain poorly with the Gram stain method.
   a. Three stain methods commonly used are Giemsa, Gimenez, and Macchiavello techniques.
C. Pathogenic species (Table 63.3)
   1. The host range of the obligate intracellular and cell-associated bacteria is often determined by their modes of transmission.
      a. *C. psittaci* is generally transmitted by the ingestion or inhalation of the extracellular elementary bodies, which are highly resistant to environmental conditions.
         (1) *C. psittaci* has a wide host range and can induce clinical disease in numerous avian and mammalian species as well as man.
         (2) *C. psittaci* has been isolated from numerous arthropods; however, infected insects play little, if any, role in its natural transmission.
      b. Pathogenic species in the family Rickettsiaceae require biologic vectors for transmission and have a limited host range, except *Coxiella burnetii*, which can be transmitted by ingestion or inhalation of bacteria in the environment.
         (1) *C. burnetii*, like *C. psittaci*, has a broad host range and can infect numerous mammalian species as well as man.
         (2) The geographic distribution of *C. ruminantium*,

Table 63.3. Hosts, vectors, and tissue tropism of obligate intracellular and cell-associated pathogens

Families	Species	Hosts[a]							Vectors		Tissue Tropism	
		Bovine	Canine	Equine	Feline	Ovine	Porcine	Man	Arthropod	Trematode	Nucleated Cells	Erythrocytes
Chlamydiaceae	*Chlamydia psittaci*	++	+	++	++	++	++	++	+[b]	-	Variety of cell types	-
Rickettsiaceae	*Cowdria ruminantium*	++	-	-	-	++	-	-	Tick	-	Vascular endothelial cells	-
	Coxiella burnetii	+	-	-	-	+	-	++	Tick	-	Vascular endothelial cells	-
	Ehrlichia canis	-	++	-	-	-	-	-	Tick	-	Leukocytes	-
	E. equi	-	-	++	-	-	-	-	ND	-	Leukocytes	-
	E. phagocytophila	++	-	-	-	++	-	-	Tick	-	Leukocytes	-
	E. risticii	-	-	+	-	-	-	-	ND	-	Leukocytes	-
	Neorickettsia helminthoeca	-	++	-	-	-	-	-	-	+	Reticular cells of lymphoid tissue	-
	Rickettsia rickettsii	-	++	-	-	-	-	++	Tick	-	Vascular endothelial cells	-
Anaplasmataceae	*Anaplasma caudatum*	++	-	-	-	-	-	-	Tick	-	-	+
	A. centrale	++	-	-	-	-	-	-	Tick	-	-	++
	A. marginale	++	-	-	-	-	-	-	Tick	-	-	++
	A. ovis	+	-	-	-	++	-	-	Tick	-	-	++
	Eperythrozoon ovis	-	-	-	-	++	-	-	+[b]	-	-	++
	E. parvum	-	-	-	-	-	+	-	Louse	-	-	++
	E. suis	-	-	-	-	-	++	-	ND	-	-	++
	E. wenyonii	++	-	-	-	-	-	-	ND	-	-	++
	Haemobartonella canis	-	+	-	-	-	-	-	-	-	-	++
	H. felis	-	-	-	++	-	-	-	-	-	-	+

a = no infection occurs; + = infection occurs without clinical disease; ++ = infection occurs with clinical disease.
b Numerous arthropods have been incriminated as vectors.
ND = not determined.

Ehrlichia species, *Neorickettsia helminthoeca*, and
Rickettsia rickettsii is restricted to the location of
their biologic arthropod and tremode vectors.

c. Pathogenic species in the family Anaplasmataceae tend to be
highly host-adapted.

   (1) Numerous arthropods have been incriminated as biologic
vectors, mechanical vectors, or both. However, the
natural modes of transmission for many of these
pathogens has not been delineated.

2. The cell type infected often determines the clinical syndrome
produced.

a. Chlamydiaceae

   (1) *Chlamydia* species are capable of infecting a variety
of nucleated cell types, where they proliferate in
cytoplasmic vacuoles producting intracytoplasmic
inclusions.

      (a) The host and cell type infected may be determined
by the bacterial serotype.

b. Rickettsiaceae

   (1) Pathogenic species only infect nucleated cells, where
they proliferate within the cytoplasm except *R.
rickettsii*, which can proliferate both in the
cytoplasm and nucleus of infected cells.

c. Anaplasmataceae

   (1) Infections induced by members of family
Anaplasmataceae are associated with erythrocytes
within the various hosts.

      (a) *Anaplasma* species are found predominantly within
erythrocytes and seldom in the plasma.

      (b) *Eperythrozoon* species are found loosely adhered
to the surface of erythrocytes or free in the
plasma in about equal frequency.

      (c) *Haemobartonella* species are tightly adhered to
the surface of erythrocytes, and a few can be
observed free in the plasma.

PART 2

Family Chlamydiaceae

64 | Genus *Chlamydia*

I. *CHLAMYDIA* SPECIES
  A. Pathogens of domestic animals

Species	Hosts	Clinical Infections
C. psittaci	Bovine	Chlamydial abortion, Orchitis, Sporadic encephalomyelitis
	Equine	Abortion, Diarrhea
	Feline	PNEUMONITIS
	Ovine	ENZOOTIC ABORTION, Diarrhea, Pneumonia
	Porcine	Diarrhea, Pneumonia

  B. Pathogens of man

Species	Clinical Infections
C. psittaci	Psittacosis
C. trachomatis biovar *trachoma*	Trachoma
C. trachomatis biovar *lymphogranuloma venereum*	Lymphogranuloma venereum

    1. There are two species in the genus.
  C. Antigens
    1. The chlamydiae possess group (genus)-specific cell wall antigens, which are part of the lipopolysaccharide complex. These heat-stable antigens are shared by both *C. psittaci* and *C. trachomatis.*
    2. *C. psittaci* and *C. trachomatis* also possess species-specific and serotype-specific antigens. These antigens are mostly heat-labile proteins.
      a. Some chlamydiae strains that induce specific disease

syndromes in domestic animals and man have identifiable
antigens associated with them.

D.   Developmental cycle
   1.   Chlamydiae multiply only within the cytoplasm of nucleated
        eucaryotic cells by a developmental cycle that is unique among
        bacteria. In the developmental cycle, chlamydiae occur in two
        distinct morphologic forms, elementary bodies and reticulate
        bodies (Table 64.1).

Table 64.1. Characteristics of the two cell types of *Chlamydia* species

Characteristic	Elementary Bodies	Reticulate Bodies
Infectivity for host cells	+	-
Intracellular multiplication	-	+[a]
Diameter	0.2-0.4 μm	0.5-1.5 μm

[a]Reticulate bodies develop in cytoplasmic vacuoles and divide by
a process analogous to binary fission.

   2.   There are three phases of the chlamydial developmental cycle.
        a.   The extracellular elementary bodies attach to susceptible
             host cells by specific receptors and are ingested by the
             host cells, in a process analogous to phagocytosis.
             (1) The ingested elementary bodies enter host cells inside
                  phagosomes; however, there is no fusion of the
                  lysosomes and phagosomes.
             (2) Within the phagosomes, the elementary bodies rearrange
                  into reticulate bodies.
        b.   Multiplication of the reticulate bodies occurs by binary
             fission, forming cytoplasmic inclusions composed of
             bacterial microcolonies.
             (1) The cytoplasmic inclusions generally contain from 10
                  to 100 bacteria and are first observed 12 to 15 hours
                  after infection.
        c.   Reticulate bodies convert to elementary bodies and are
             released into the extracellular environment when the host
             cells are lysed.
             (1) Chlamydiae have been demonstrated to inhibit protein
                  and nucleic acid synthesis in infected cells.
             (2) The development cycle (from infection of the host cell
                  until its lysis) is usually completed in 48 to 72
                  hours.

II. VECTORS AND HOST RANGE
   A.   Vectors
       1.   Arthopods may harbor *C. psittaci*, but their role as vectors has
            not been proven.
   B.   Host range
       1.   *C. psittaci* has a broad host range and has been isolated from a
            large number of avian and mammalian species.

a. Some avian strains are highly infectious and produce human psittacosis but are not generally considered to be infectious for domestic animals.

b. Mammalian strains do not readily infect man and generally have a limited host range in domestic animals.

III. CELLULAR, CELL-ASSOCIATION, AND CULTURAL CHARACTERISTICS
A. Cellular characteristics
1. Gram-negative pleomorphic cells
B. Cell-association characteristics
1. Chlamydiae are parasites of a variety of eukaryotic cells. For these bacteria to proliferate, they need precursor substances and energy from the host cell.
   a. Chlamydiae are metabolically deficient bacteria that are unable to produce or store ATP, which is an essential growth requirement. These bacteria, however, are capable of synthesizing their own lipids, proteins, and nucleic acids.
   (1) The energy dependence of the chlamydiae has been postulated to be the factor responsible for their inability to multiply extracellulary.
C. Cultural characteristics
1. Chlamydiae do not grow in cell-free media.
2. The laboratory isolation of chlamydiae requires living eucaryotic cells in which the chlamydiae form intracytoplasmic inclusions.
   a. Shortly after being internalized in the host cells, the elementary bodies develop in cytoplasmic inclusions into the larger reticulate bodies.
3. Characteristics used to differentiate *C. psittaci* and *C. trachomatis*
   a. The intracytoplasmic inclusions of *C. trachomatis* contain more glycogen than those of *C. psittaci*. Therefore inclusions of *C. trachomatis*, but not those of *C. psittaci*, stain brown with iodine.
   b. The relative difference in susceptibility to D-cycloserine and sulfonamides differentiates the two species of *Chlamydia*. *C. trachomatis* is resistant to D-cycloserine but sensitive to sulfadiazine, whereas *C. psittaci* is sensitive to D-cycloserine but resistant to sulfadiazine.

IV. DISEASE OVERVIEW
A. *C. psittaci*
1. Infections in domestic animals
   a. Ingestion and inhalation of elementary bodies, the infectious form of chlamydiae that survive under adverse conditions outside an animal host, are the primary modes of transmission.
   (1) Animals with subclinical chronic infections often

continuously excrete chlamydiae into the environment of susceptible animal groups.

    (a)   In cattle and sheep, fecal shedding from asymptomatic carriers is important in the spread and maintenance of the infection within the herds and flocks.

b.   *C. psittaci* induces a wide range of clinical manifestations, including respiratory and intestinal infections, conjunctivitis, polyarthritis, fetal death and abortion, and genital disease. All chlamydial infections tend to persist in chronic or clinically inapparent forms.

c.   Clinical intestinal infections with diarrhea are usually limited to the newborn and may be accompanied by polyarthritis and polyserositis.

d.   Chlamydial pneumonia is a mild disease and seldom recognized as a clinical entity.

2.   Bovine infections

a.   *C. psittaci* has the ability to establish placental and fetal infections, resulting in abortions, stillbirths, or the birth of weak calves. Most abortions occur in the seventh to ninth month of gestation. Retained placentas are common.

b.   *C. psittaci* has been reported as a cause of seminal vesiculitis in young bulls.

c.   Milk production often decreases in *C. psittaci*-infected dairy cows.

d.   Sporadic bovine encephalomyelitis often follows systemic *C. psittaci* infection. The mortality rate of affected animals is about 50 percent.

    (1)   Calves less than 6 months of age are the most susceptible to this neurological disease.

3.   Equine infections

a.   Horses are susceptible to *C. psittaci* infection and have a disease spectrum similar to that seen in cattle and sheep.

    (1)   *C. psittaci* has been reported as a cause of naturally occurring abortion in mares.

4.   Feline pneumonitis (see Chap. 117)

a.   *C. psittaci* is a major cause of conjunctivitis and pneumonitis in neonatal kittens, which are more susceptible than adults. Infections in adult cats are often mild or subclinical.

b.   Feline pneumonitis is highly contagious, transmitted by inhalation of infected droplets expelled by sneezing or by contaminated ocular discharges. The clinical syndrome is characterized by absence of significant fever, droolings of saliva, depression, anorexia, and serous discharges from the eyes and nose, which often become mucopurulent due to secondary bacterial infection. The disease is debilitating; it may linger for weeks without change in the symptomology and then is followed by a slow recovery.

5. Ovine enzootic abortion (see Chap. 94)
    a. *C. psittaci* persists as a latent infection in pregnant ewes until the fourth month of gestation when the bacterium invades the placenta, causing a placentitis that results in abortions, stillbirths, and premature lambing (the only clinical manifestations of the infection).
6. Porcine infections
    a. *C. psittaci* has been reported as a cause of abortion, conjunctivitis, pneumonia, and polyarthritis in swine.

B. Avian-associated human chlamydiosis
1. *C. psittaci* infections are called psittacosis in psittacine birds and ornithosis in other avian species. More than a hundred species of birds have been known to be infected with *C. psittaci* and are potential reservoirs of human psittacosis.
    a. Man usually acquires psittacosis after the inhalation of infected avian fecal material. The disease may appear clinically as one of two distinct syndromes: the more common atypical pneumonia form and the less common septicemic form in which pneumonia may be absent.
    b. The majority of the human psittacoses occurs in poultry workers, who contract the infections from infected nonpsittacine domestic birds. Turkeys are the major reservoir for transmitting *C. psittaci* to man in the United States.
    c. Owners of infected psittacine birds, which may be either clinically affected or carriers, are occasionally affected.
        (1) In their natural state, psittacine birds have a low level of infection, and most infections are either subclinical or latent. During the capture and transport of psittacine birds, the resulting stress may increase the incidence of the disease and lead to exposure outbreaks in both avian species and man. In response to this problem, all psittacine birds imported into the United States are required to undergo a chlortetracycline prophylactic regimen. This procedure does not eradicate the organism in every imported bird, however, and some birds remain carriers of *C. psittaci*.

PART **3**	# Family Rickettsiaceae

65	Genus *Cowdria*

I. *COWDRIA* SPECIES
   A. Pathogens of domestic animals

Species	Hosts	Clinical Infection
C. ruminantium	Bovine	Heartwater
	Ovine	Heartwater

      1. It is the only species in the genus.

II. ARTHROPOD VECTORS AND HOST RANGE
   A. Arthropod vectors
      1. *C. ruminantium* is transmitted by the bont tick, *Amblyomma hebraeum*. The tick has a transstadial transmission.
   B. Host range
      1. *C. ruminantium* is an obligate parasite of ruminants.

III. CELLULAR, CELL-ASSOCIATION, AND CULTURAL CHARACTERISTICS
   A. Cellular characteristics
      1. Gram-negative pleomorphic cells
   B. Cell-association characteristics
      1. The bacterium is a parasite of vascular endothelial cells.
   C. Cultural characteristics
      1. The bacterium has not been cultivated in cell-free media.

IV. DISEASE OVERVIEW
   A. Bovine and ovine heartwater
      1. Susceptible cattle and sheep are infected when infested with ticks that are biological vectors of *C. ruminantium*.
         a. Heartwater is geographically restricted to areas where the

ticks occur. The disease is endemic in many areas of
Africa but is not present in the United States.
2. In the ruminant, the bacteria initially infect the cells of the
reticuloendothelial system and later the vascular endothelial
cells. After an incubation period of 1 to 2 weeks, the acute
disease phase, which generally lasts 2 to 7 days, is
characterized by fever and gastroenteritis and frequently
terminates in convulsions and death. The case fatality rate is
50 to 100 percent. Animals that recover from acute disease
often remain carriers of *C. ruminantium* for a few weeks to
several months.
3. Heartwater is characterized by hydropericardium, resulting from
serous effusions into the pericardial sac. There also are
serous effusions into the peritoneal and pericardial cavities.

66	Genus *Coxiella*

I. *COXIELLA* SPECIES
  A. Pathogens

Species	Hosts	Nonclinical Infections	Clinical Infection
C. burnetii	Bovine, Ovine	+	
	Man		Q fever

    1. It is the only species in the genus.

II. ARTHROPOD VECTORS AND HOST RANGE
  A. Arthropod vectors
    1. Several genera of ticks are commonly infected with *C. burnetii*
and serve as carriers of the infection: *Amblyomma, Dermacentor,
Haemaphysalis, Myalomma, Ixodes, Ornithodorus,* and
Rhipicephalus.
      a. Infected ticks shed *C. burnetii* in their feces and transmit
the infection by biting susceptible animals.
      b. The transmission of *C. burnetii* in domestic animals and man
is not dependent on arthropods.

B.   Host range
  1.   *C. burnetii* can infect numerous wild and domesticated animals, including dogs, cattle, horses, pigs, and sheep. Domestic animals rarely exhibit clinical signs.
     a.   Cattle and sheep can serve as sources of infection for man.
  2.   Man is very susceptible to infection.
     a.   The infections are usually acquired by the aerosol route but can also be transmitted by drinking unpasteurized milk from infected cows.

III. CELLULAR, CELL-ASSOCIATION, AND CULTURAL CHARACTERISTICS
A.   Cellular characteristics
  1.   Gram-negative pleomorphic cells
     a.   Some have reported the microorganism as gram-positive.
  2.   Endosporelike structures provide *C. burnetii* with a high degree of resistance to physical and chemical agents, comparable to sporogenic bacteria in the genera *Bacillus* and *Clostridium*.
B.   Cell-association characteristics
  1.   The bacterium is a parasite of the vascular endothelial cells and multiplies within the phagolysosome of the infected host cell.
C.   Cultural characteristics
  1.   The bacterium has not been cultivated in cell-free media.

IV. DISEASE OVERVIEW
A.   Bovine and ovine infections
  1.   *C. burnetii* infections are asymptomatic in cattle and sheep; however, the organism grows to high levels in their placentas and is commonly found in their milk.
B.   Infections in man
  1.   Q fever in man is characterized by fever and interstitial pneumonia.
  2.   Most infections are acquired by inhalation, but a few are acquired by ingesting contaminated milk.
  3.   Sources of infection from domestic animals
     a.   Infected dried placentas of cattle and sheep contain billions of organisms, which remain viable for extended periods of time and contaminate the surrounding area.
     b.   Dust from tick feces are deposited on the hides of animals.
     c.   Many dairy herds are infected with *C. burnetii*, and lactating cows shed these organisms in their milk. It is noteworthy that the low temperature-long holding pasteurization method was increased to $62.7^{\circ}C$ for 30 minutes in order to inactivate the bacterium.

67 | Genus *Ehrlichia*

I. *EHRLICHIA* SPECIES
   A. Pathogens of domestic animals

Species	Hosts	Clinical Infections
E. canis	Canine	EHRLICHIOSIS
E. equi	Equine	Ehrlichiosis
E. phagocytophila	Bovine	Ehrlichiosis
	Ovine	Ehrlichiosis
E. risticii	Equine	Potomac horse fever

      1. Four of the five species in the genus infect domestic animals.
   B. Pathogens of man
      1. *E. sennetsu*

II. ARTHROPOD VECTORS AND HOST RANGE
   A. Transmission by tick vectors has been established for *E. canis* and *E. phagocytophila.*
      1. *Rhipicephalus sanguineus*, the brown dog tick, has been demonstrated to transmit *E. canis.*
      2. *Ixodes* species can transmit *E. phagocytophila.*
      3. The vectors and reservoir hosts of *E. risticii* are not known at this time.
   B. Host range
      1. *Ehrlichia* species are obligate parasites.
         a. Infections are usually restricted to one animal species or to a few closely related host species.

III. CELLULAR, CELL-ASSOCIATION, AND CULTURAL CHARACTERISTICS
   A. Cellular characteristics
      1. Gram-negative pleomorphic cells
   B. Cell-association characteristics
      1. They are parasites of reticuloendothelial cells and leukocytes and are located in the cytoplasm of parasitized cells (Table 67.1).
         a. In blood smears stained by Romanowsky's methods, ehrlichiae stain bluish purple.
   C. Cultural characteristics
      1. Ehrlichiae have not been cultivated in cell-free media.

Table 67.1. Types of leukocytes infected with *Ehrlichia* species

Species	Cell Type
E. canis	Monocytes, lymphocytes, and neutrophils[a]
E. equi	Granulocytes
E. phagocytophila	Granulocytes
E. risticii	Monocytes

[a]Neutrophils are rarely infected.

IV. DISEASE OVERVIEW

A. Canine ehrlichiosis (see Chap. 111)

1. *E. canis* is the causative agent of canine ehrlichiosis, a febrile disease characterized by pancytopenia, anorexia, emaciation, hemorrhage, and death.

B. Equine ehrlichiosis and Potomac horse fever

1. *E. equi* is the causative agent of equine ehrlichiosis, a febrile disease characterized by edema, lymphadenopathy, and thrombocytopenia.

2. *E. risticii* is the causative agent of Potomac horse fever. Clinical symptoms vary markedly and include one or all of the following: fever, depression, anorexia, leukopenia, distal edema of the limbs, laminitis, mild to severe diarrhea, and colic.

C. Bovine and ovine ehrlichiosis

1. *E. phagocytophila* is the cause of ehrlichiosis in cattle and sheep. Affected animals are generally asymptomatic.

68	Genus *Neorickettsia*

I. *NEORICKETTSIA* SPECIES
  A. Pathogens of domestic animals

Species	Hosts	Clinical Infection
N. helminthoeca	Canine	SALMON POISONING

  1. It is the only species in the genus.

II. TREMATODE VECTORS AND HOST RANGE
  A. Trematode vectors
      1. *N. helminthoeca* is found in all stages (eggs, cercariae, and
         adults) of the fluke *Nanophyetus salmincola*. This fluke is
         found in salmon and trout on the West Coast of the United
         States.
         a. Dogs acquire the infection by ingesting infected salmon and
            trout.
  B. Host range
      1. Dogs are the only domestic animal infected.

III. CELLULAR, CELL-ASSOCIATION, AND CULTURAL CHARACTERISTICS
  A. Cellular characteristics
      1. Gram-negative pleomorphic cells
  B. Cell-association characteristics
      1. They are parasites of nucleated cells.
      2. The organisms are located in the cytoplasm of reticular cells of
         lymphoid tissues.
         a. In histopathologic sections, the coccoid forms are most
            common, but short rods and rings also occur. The cocci are
            0.3 to 0.4 um in diameter.
  C. Cultural characteristics
      1. The bacterium has not been grown in cell-free media.

IV. DISEASE OVERVIEW
  A. Canine salmon poisoning (see Chap. 114)
      1. *N. helminthoeca* causes an acute, often fatal disease in dogs
         that is characterized by a hemorrhagic enteritis and
         lymphadenopathy.
         a. Clinically salmon poisoning is diagnosed by clinical signs
            and the presence of fluke eggs in the dog's feces.

69	Genus *Rickettsia*

I. *RICKETTSIA* SPECIES
   A. Pathogens of domestic animals

Species	Host	Vector	Clinical Infection
R. rickettsii	Canine	Tick	ROCKY MOUNTAIN SPOTTED FEVER

   1. There are 12 species in the genus, but only *R. rickettsii* causes clinical disease in domestic animals.
   B. Pathogens of man

Disease Groups	Species	Vectors
Scrub typhus	*R. tsutsugamushi*	Mite
Spotted fever	*R. akari*	Mite
	R. australis	Tick
	R. conorii	Tick
	R. montana	Tick
	R. parkeri	Tick
	R. rhipicephali	Tick
	R. rickettsii	Tick
	R. sibirica	Tick
Typhus	*R. canada*	Tick
	R. prowazekii	Louse
	R. typhi	Flea

II. ARTHROPOD VECTORS AND HOST RANGE
   A. Arthropod vectors
      1. Selected genera and species of fleas, lice, mites, and ticks can serve as biological vectors for the *Rickettsia* species.
      2. The primary tick vectors of canine Rocky Mountain spotted fever are the dog tick, *Dermacentor variabilis*, in the eastern United States and the wood tick, *D. andersoni*, in the western United States.
         a. Numerous other tick species have been found naturally infected with *R. rickettsii* and are potential vectors of the disease.
   B. Host range
      1. *R. rickettsii* causes clinical disease in both dogs and man.
         a. The distribution of infections in dogs is limited to the geographic distribution of the tick vectors. In the United States, the disease occurs in the middle Atlantic states and the Rocky Mountain states.

III. CELLULAR, CELL-ASSOCIATION, AND CULTURAL CHARACTERISTICS
A. Cellular characteristics
  1. Gram-negative pleomorphic rods
     a. Rickettsiae are gram-negative but stain poorly by the Gram technique.
     b. Rickettsiae stain purple by the Giemsa stain and red by the Gimenez and Macchiavello techniques.
B. Cell-association characteristics
  1. They are parasites of nucleated cells.
     a. *R. rickettsii* are located both in the cytoplasm and nucleus of vascular endothelial cells.
        (1) In histopathologic sections, the bacteria are 0.3 to 0.5 um in diameter and 0.8 to 2.0 um in length.
C. Cultural characteristics
  1. They have not been grown in cell-free media.
     a. The rickettsiae can be grown in the yolk sac of embryonated hen eggs.

IV. DISEASE OVERVIEW
A. Canine Rocky Mountain spotted fever (see Chap. 113)
  1. Rocky Mountain spotted fever is an acute, often fatal disease of dogs.
     a. *R. rickettsia* has a predilection for the vascular endothelium and stimulates the cells lining the small vessels to swell and proliferate.
     b. The clinical manifestations of Rocky Mountain spotted fever result largely from the hyperplasia of the endothelial cells, localized thrombus formation, and the accumulation of erythrocytes in the extravascular tissues.

PART 4	Family Anaplasmataceae

70	Genus *Anaplasma*

I. *ANAPLASMA* SPECIES
   A. Pathogens of domestic animals

Species	Hosts	Nonclinical infection	Clinical Infection
A. caudatum	Bovine		Anaplasmosis
A. centrale	Bovine		Anaplasmosis
	Ovine		Anaplasmosis
A. marginale	Bovine		ANAPLASMOSIS
A. ovis	Ovine		Anaplasmosis
	Bovine	+	

   1. There are four species in the genus.

II. ARTHROPOD VECTORS AND HOST RANGE
   A. Arthropod vectors
      1. *Anaplasma* species are transmitted by numerous bloodsucking arthropods, including ticks, which can act as biological vectors. Other biting arthropods can serve as mechanical vectors.
         a. *Dermacentor andersoni* has shown transstadial transmission of *A. marginale*.
   B. Host range
      1. Infections with *Anaplasma* species are limited to ruminants.

III. CELLULAR, CELL-ASSOCIATION, AND CULTURAL CHARACTERISTICS
   A. Cellular characteristics
      1. Gram-negative cocci, often with appendages
   B. Cell-association characteristics
      1. *Anaplasma* species parasitize erythrocytes (Table 70.1).
         a. In blood smears stained by Romanowsky-type stains, the organisms appear within the erythrocytes as round bluish

Table 70.1. Location of *Anaplasma* species in parasitized erythrocytes

Species	Location in Erythrocyte
A. *caudatum*	Marginal
A. *centrale*	Central
A. *marginale*	Marginal
A. *ovis*	Marginal

purple inclusions 0.3 to 1.0 um in diameter. The predominant location of the inclusion bodies within the erythrocyte is a diagnostic aid.

C. Cultural characteristics
   1. They have not been cultivated in cell-free media.

IV. DISEASE OVERVIEW
   A. Bovine and ovine *Anaplasma* species infections (Table 70.2)
      1. Anaplasmosis is characterized by anemia and icterus. Severe disease can be fatal.

Table 70.2. Occurrence of infection by *Anaplasma* species

Species	Bovine	Ovine
A. *caudatum*	++	−
A. *centrale*	++	++
A. *marginale*	+++	−
A. *ovis*	+	+

Note: − = no infection occurs; + = infection occurs without disease; ++ = infection causes mild to severe disease; +++ = infection causes severe disease.

   B. Bovine *A. marginale* infections (see Chap. 75)
      1. Cattle of all ages may become infected with *A. marginale*. The age of the animal when infected largely determines the outcome.
         a. Calves less than 6 months of age are susceptible to infection but seldom exhibit signs of anaplasmosis. The infection endows the affected animals with a state of preimmunity for the duration of the infection, which may persist for life.
         b. The severity and mortality of anaplasmosis is markedly increased in cattle over 6 months of age. Cattle over 3 years of age with clinical anaplasmosis frequently have a mortality rate from 25 to 50 percent.
      2. Outbreaks of clinical anaplasmosis under natural conditions often follows the seasons, determined by the prevalence of biological and mechanical insect vectors. The incubation period from infection until clinical signs are exhibited is usually 1 to 3 months or longer. Cattle with an acute anaplasmosis episode will exhibit an intermittent fever, anemia, and icterus. Animals that die during an acute phase of the infection do not

exhibit any pathognomonic gross lesions on necropsy. The acute episodes may occur at various time intervals either until the animal succumbs to the infection or develops immunity and establishes a carrier state.

3. Most diagnoses are based on history, clinical signs, and the presence of anaplasma bodies in Giemsa-stained blood smears. The anaplasmosis card test and complement-fixation test are used to detect antibodies to parasitized erythrocytes.

71	Genus *Eperythrozoon*

I. *EPERYTHROZOON* SPECIES
  A. Pathogens of domestic animals

Species	Hosts	Nonclinical Infections	Clinical Infection
E. ovis	Ovine		Eperythrozoonosis
E. parvum	Porcine	+	
E. suis	Porcine		EPERYTHRO-ZOONOSIS
E. wenyonii	Bovine		Eperythrozoonosis

  1. Four of the five species in the genus infect domestic animals.

II. ARTHROPOD VECTORS AND HOST RANGE
  A. Arthropod vectors
    1. Some species have been shown to be transmitted by vectors.
      a. *E. ovis* can be transmitted by horse flies, as well as by other arthropods.
      b. *E. parvum* can be transmitted by the pig louse, *Haematopinus suis.*
  B. Host range
    1. *Eperythrozoon* species are obligate parasites.
      a. Most species are host-specific.

III. CELLULAR, CELL-ASSOCIATION, AND CULTURAL CHARACTERISTICS
  A. Cellular characteristics
    1. Gram-negative pleomorphic cells

B. Cell-association characteristics
   1. They are parasites of erythrocytes. The organisms occur on erythrocytes or free in plasma with about equal frequency.
      a. In blood smears stained by Giemsa and Romanowsky-type stains, the organisms appear as bluish or pinkish violet rings or cocci 0.4 to 1.5 um in diameter.
C. Cultural characteristics
   1. They have not been cultivated in cell-free media.

IV. DISEASE OVERVIEW
A. Bovine eperythrozoonosis
   1. *E. wenyonii* cause a mild anemia and parasitemia, but no other clinical signs occur. Latent infections are common.
B. Ovine eperythrozoonosis
   1. *E. ovis* can cause anemia and failure to gain weight in young lambs. Symptoms are mild in adult sheep.
C. Porcine eperythrozoonosis (see Chap. 101)
   1. *E. suis* infections are characterized by fever and anemia. Icterus occurs in the most severe cases.
      a. Pigs less than 1 week old are the most likely group in a herd to exhibit clinical signs. The infections in neonatal pigs are often fatal.
      b. The morbidity of porcine eperythrozoonosis is low; however, pigs that acquire the infection often remain carriers of the bacterium.
      c. At postmortem, there are icterus, watery blood, serous effusions, and splenomegaly.
   2. *E. parvum* is nonpathogenic for domestic pigs.

72 | Genus *Haemobartonella*

I. *HAEMOBARTONELLA* SPECIES
   A. Pathogens of domestic animals

Species	Hosts	Nonclinical Infections	Clinical Infection
H. canis	Canine	+	
H. felis	Feline		HAEMOBARTO-NELLOSIS

   1. Two of the three species in the genus infect domestic animals.

II. ARTHROPOD VECTORS AND HOST RANGE
   A. Arthropod vectors
      1. Biological transmission by arthropod vectors has not been established for either *H. canis* or *H. felis*.
   B. Host range
      1. *Haembartonella* species are obligate parasites.
         a. Infections are restricted to one animal species or to a few closely related host species.

III. CELLULAR, CELL-ASSOCIATION, AND CULTURAL CHARACTERISTICS
   A. Cellular characteristics
      1. Gram-negative pleomorphic cells
   B. Cell-association characteristics
      1. They are parasites of erythrocytes, and the organisms are located on or within erythrocytes.
         a. In blood smears stained by Giemsa- and Romanowsky-type stains, the organisms appear as bluish or pinkish violet cocci or rods. The cocci are 0.1 to 0.8 um in diameter, and the rods are 0.2 to 0.5 by 1.0 to 1.5 um.
   C. Cultural characteristics
      1. They have not been cultivated in cell-free media.

IV. DISEASE OVERVIEW
   A. Canine haemobartonellosis
      1. *H. canis* does not produce clinical disease in dogs.
   B. Feline haemobartonellosis (see Chap. 116)
      1. *H. felis* produces a severe, sometimes fatal hemolytic anemia in cats. A patent parasitemia and a nonclinical carrier state are common manifestations of the infections.
         a. The infection can be transmitted by the oral, intravenous,

           intraperitoneal, and intrauterine routes. *H. felis* also can be transmitted during cat fights.

b. The most common clinical signs are depression, anorexia, weight loss, splenomegaly, and anemia.

c. Postmortem appearance is dominated by pallor with or without icterus, splenomegaly, and enlargement of the mesenteric lymph nodes.

SECTION V

Bacterial Diseases of Domestic Animals

PART **1**	Bovine Diseases

73	Actinobacillosis

I. ETIOLOGY
   A. *Actinobacillus lignieresii* is a facultative anaerobic, gram-negative bacillus.
      1. Virulence factors of the bacterium are poorly understood.

II. TRANSMISSION
   A. The bacterium is implanted into the tongue and soft tissues of the head and neck from endogenous oral flora.
      1. *A. lignieresii* is a common inhabitant of the bovine oral and rumen flora.

III. CLINICAL FEATURES
   A. The disease is sporadic in nature.
   B. The classical picture of wooden tongue, in which the lesions are located in the lingual musculature, are enlargement and protrusion of the tongue with eventual interference with feeding. Affected animals exhibit a gradual weight loss.

IV. PATHOGENESIS
   A. After *A. lignieresii* is implanted into the soft tissues of the head and neck, the suppurative lesions gradually enlarge and are first grossly visible about 10 days after infection.
      1. The lesions become encapsulated and form abscesses, but many lesions will rupture and drain through the skin.
      2. The infection is a lymphangitis and spreads by lymphogenous extension. The regional lymph nodes are frequently involved.

V. PATHOLOGY
   A. Pyogranulomatous lesions can be present in the tongue, cheeks, gums, and lymph nodes draining the head and neck.

VI. DIAGNOSIS
  A. Clinical signs
    1. Infection of the tongue (wooden tongue) is a characteristic lesion.
  B. Pathology
    1. Abscesses are present in the soft tissues of head and neck regions with sulfur granules in the exudate.
  C. Direct smears
    1. Gram-stained sulfur granules are pathognomonic for actinobacillosis. The granules have a central mass of gram-negative bacilli.
  D. Culture
    1. Isolation and biochemical identification of *A. lignieresii*

VII. IMMUNIZATION
  A. Commercial vaccines for *A. lignieresii* are not available.

---

74 | Actinomycosis

I. ETIOLOGY
  A. *Actinomyces bovis* is a facultative anaerobic, gram-positive bacillus.
    1. Virulence factors of the bacterium are poorly understood.

II. TRANSMISSION
  A. The bacterium is implanted into the mandible or maxilla from endogenous oral flora.

III. CLINICAL FEATURES
  A. Bovine actinomycosis (lumpy jaw) is a proliferative osteomyelitis of the bones of the jaw.
    1. The infection is usually a chronic process that may last for months or years and is spread by contiguity.
    2. The lesions are painless hard swellings on the mandible or maxilla. If the adjacent soft tissues are involved, granulomatous lesions are formed, often with draining tracts.

B.   The animal is afebrile and may be emaciated through interference with mastication.

IV. PATHOGENESIS
A.   The infection destroys the bone and stimulates new growth.
1.   This proliferative osteomyelitis is characterized by a destructive rarefaction and regenerative proliferation.
B.   When soft tissues are infected, granulomatous lesions with sulfur granules are formed.
C.   Immunity to the infection is poorly understood.

V. PATHOLOGY
A.   Bone lesions are characterized by destructive rarefaction and regenerative proliferation.

VI. DIAGNOSIS
A.   Clinical signs (above)
B.   Direct smears
1.   In gram-stained smears, diffuse gram-positive branching rods and filaments are observed.
2.   Sulfur granules found in the exudate of actinomycotic lesions are yellowish to brownish particles about 3 mm in diameter.
a.   In gram-stained smears, the bacterial colony is gram-positive and the surrounding hyaline matrix stains pink.
C.   Culture
1.   Isolation and biochemical identification of *A. bovis*
a.   Anaerobic bacterial culture procedures are generally used to identify the bacterium, which grows well under anaerobic culture conditions. The bacterium can be identified to generic level by gas chromatographical analysis of volatile and nonvolatile fatty acid products of glucose metabolism.

VII. IMMUNIZATION
A.   Commercial vaccines for *A. bovis* are not available.

75 | Anaplasmosis

I. ETIOLOGY
  A. *Anaplasma caudatum*, *A. centrale*, and *A. marginale* are aerobic, gram-
      negative bacteria.
      1. *A. marginale* is the primary etiologic agent of bovine
          anaplasmosis and causes the most severe disease, whereas *A.
          caudatum* and *A. centrale* are rarely incriminated in severe
          disease.
      2. These bacterial species are found within bovine erythrocytes and
          rarely, if ever, free in the plasma.

II. TRANSMISSION
  A. Biological arthropod vectors
      1. Transstadial transmission of *A. marginale* can occur in several
          species of ticks, which include *Boophilus anulatus*, *B.
          microplus*, *Dermacentor andersoni*, *D. occidentalis*, and *D.
          variabilis*.
          a. In the temperate climates of the United States, ticks must
              harbor *A. marginale* transstadially from one season to the
              next to be successful vectors of the bacterium.
  B. Mechanical arthropod vectors
      1. Bloodsucking arthropods (flies, mosquitoes, and ticks) can serve
          as mechanical vectors of *A. marginale*.
          a. Tabinid flies, stable flies, and mosquitoes are commonly
              incriminated in the natural transmission of bovine
              anaplasmosis.
  C. Fomites
      1. Blood-contaminated needles, syringes, and surgical instruments,
          which are used to bleed, vaccinate, dehorn, and castrate cattle,
          can serve as vehicles for the spread of the disease.

III. CLINICAL FEATURES
  A. Clinical signs
      1. Anemia and intermittent fever with or without icterus are the
          principal clinical manifestations of bovine anaplasmosis.
          a. Acute episodes may occur at various time intervals until
              the animal succumbs to the infection or develops immunity
              and establishes a carrier state.
  B. Age susceptibility
      1. Cattle of all ages may become infected with *A. marginale*;
          however, the age of the animal when infected largely determines
          the outcome.

     a. Calves less than 6 months of age seldom exhibit signs of anaplasmosis, and the asymptomatic infection endows the affected animal with a state of preimmunity for the duration of the infection, which may persist for life.

     b. In cattle over 6 months of age, the severity and mortality of anaplasmosis are markedly increased.

        (1) Cattle over 3 years of age often have a mortality rate of 25 to 50 percent.

C. Geographic distribution and seasonal incidence

   1. The geographic distribution and seasonal incidence of bovine anaplasmosis is largely determined by the geographic distribution of the biological tick vectors, while the seasonal incidence is determined by both biological and mechanical vectors of *A. marginale*.

     a. Under natural conditions, outbreaks of clinical anaplasmosis often follow the seasons, determined by the prevalence of bloodsucking vectors.

IV. PATHOGENESIS

A. Cattle can acquire the infection from biological insect vectors, mechanical insect vectors, or from blood-contaminated bleeding and surgical instruments.

   1. The incubation period (time from infection until clinical signs are first observed) is 1 to 3 months or longer.

     a. The bacteria are taken up by the erythrocytes by a phagocytic-type process, form vacuoles within the cytoplasm, proliferate by binary fission, and form microcolonies (inclusions).

     b. Large numbers of infected erythrocytes are observed in the peripheral blood 5 to 10 days prior to a hemolytic crisis.

     c. The level of serum opsonins to parasitized erythrocytes is markedly increased prior to the hemolytic crisis, when large numbers of infected erythrocytes are removed by the monocyte-macrophage system, particularly in the spleen. The removal and destruction of infected erythrocytes results in anemia and icterus.

        (1) The infected erythrocytes may be removed over a period of a few days, and the volume of circulating erythrocytes may decrease by 50 to 75 percent. During this period the animal has an elevated body temperature and is often anorexic and depressed.

        (2) In a hemolytic crisis in which the erythrocytes are being destroyed in the spleen by the reticulo-endothelial system, bilirubin accumulates in the plasma and tissues due to the inability to excrete it as rapidly as it is produced.

   2. Various stress factors, particularly splenectomy, can cause a recrudescence of asymptomatic infections, resulting in clinical disease.

B. The immunity to bovine anaplasmosis is poorly understood.

V. PATHOLOGY
  A. Clinical pathology
    1. The number of infected erythrocytes is greatest just prior to
        the hemolytic crisis, and within 4 to 7 days after the hemolytic
        crisis, the anaplasma bodies may be too few to permit a
        diagnosis based on blood smear examination.
  B. Gross pathology
    1. Characteristic postmortem findings are anemia with thin watery
        blood, icterus, splenomegaly, and hepatomegaly, in which the
        liver has an orange color.
      a. Cattle that die during the acute phase of the infection
          often do not exhibit any pathognomonic lesions.

VI. DIAGNOSIS
  A. Clinical signs and history (above)
  B. Clinical pathology
    1. In Giemsa-stained blood smears, *Anaplasma* species are identified
        based on their location within erythrocytes. *A. caudatum* and *A.
        marginale* are located near the periphery of the erythrocytes,
        whereas *A. centrale* is located in the center of the erythro-
        cytes.
  C. Gross pathology (above)
  D. Serology
    1. The anaplasmosis card and complement-fixation tests are used to
        determine carrier animals in a herd, which have detectable
        levels of antibodies but may not exhibit a detectable bacteremia
        on stained blood smears.
      a. Serologic reactions are often negative or negligible during
          the incubation stage of infection.

VII. IMMUNIZATION
  A. A commercial *A. marginale* vaccine is available.
    1. The vaccine aids in the prevention of clinical disease but does
        not prevent infection.

76	Anthrax

I. ETIOLOGY
  A. *Bacillus anthracis* is a facultative anaerobic, gram-positive, sporeforming bacillus.

II. TRANSMISSION
  A. Ingestion
    1. Cattle infections usually result from the ingestion of contaminated feed or soil.
       a. Spores of *B. anthracis* are found in soil and pasture contaminated with vegetative cells from dead and dying animals. The spores can remain viable for years in contaminated soil.
       b. *B. anthracis* is associated with alkaline or calcareous soils.
       c. Epidemic outbreaks of anthrax are often associated with extreme changes in the general climatic conditions. These changes are believed responsible for germination of spores and proliferation of the bacterium.
       d. Anthrax is endemic in parts of the southwestern and western United States.
  B. Disposal of dead animals
    1. To reduce the level of environmental contamination, dead animals are disposed of by burning or by burying in quicklime.

III. CLINICAL FEATURES
  A. Age and sex susceptibility
    1. Calves are seldom affected.
    2. Bulls appear to be much more susceptible to infection than are cows.
  B. Morbidity and mortality
    1. The number of animals in a herd that contract anthrax during an epidemic is highly variable; however, the case fatality ratio of cattle with clinical anthrax is greater than 90 percent.
  C. Clinical signs
    1. There are three clinical courses of bovine anthrax.
       a. Peracute septicemia
          (1) Peracute septicemia is the most common form of bovine anthrax.
          (2) Death usually occurs within 2 hours after the first clinical signs are observed. Sudden death in cattle that appeared normal a few hours earlier is common.

      b. Acute septicemia
         (1) Death usually occurs within 48 to 96 hours after clinical signs are first observed. Occasionally an animal survives this form of the disease without treatment, but this is a rare occurrence.
         (2) Clinical signs include fever, anorexia, ruminal statis, hematuria, and blood-tinged diarrhea. Pregnant animals may abort, and milk production often abruptly decreases. Terminal signs include severe depression, respiratory distress, and convulsions.
      c. Chronic infections
         (1) Chronic anthrax infections, in which clinical signs are manifested for more than 6 days, are rare.

IV. PATHOGENESIS

  A. Infections
    1. Ingestion of contaminated forages is the primary mode of infection, and the intestinal tract, the primary portal of entry.
    2. The virulence of *B. anthracis* is dependent on both the D-glutamic acid polypeptide capsule and the exotoxin complex.
      a. The capsule is antiphagocytic and is important in the establishment of the infection.
      b. The exotoxin complex is responsible for the clinical signs seen in the toxemia stage of the infection. The level of lethal toxin increases rapidly late in the course of the disease.
  B. Immunity
    1. Antibodies to the capsular polypeptide act as opsonins and prevent the establishment of the infection.
    2. Antibodies to factor II of the exotoxin complex prevents the expression of factors I (edema factor) and III (lethal factor).

V. PATHOLOGY

  A. Gross pathology
    1. The carcasses of animals that have died of anthrax putrefy rapidly and develop incomplete rigor mortis.
      a. The blood is dark, clots poorly, and may exude from the nose, mouth, and anus.
      b. The spleen is greatly enlarged, dark, and friable.
      c. The lymph nodes, particularly in the region of the initial infection site, will be hemorrhagic and edematous.
      d. Ecchymotic hemorrhages on the serosal surfaces of the abdomen, thorax, epicardium, and endocardium are common.
      e. Subcutaneous edematous swellings are often present on the ventral aspect of the neck.
    2. If anthrax is suspect, complete necropsy of affected animals should be avoided to reduce environmental contamination and

health risks to veterinarians.
    a.   Carcasses are often buried at the site.

VI. DIAGNOSIS
    A.   Endemic areas, clinical signs, and pathology
        1.   Presumptive diagnoses of bovine anthrax are often made based on clinical signs and the gross pathology of animals in endemic areas.
    B.   Direct examination and culture
        1.   Gram-stained blood smears show the vegetative cells of *B. anthracis* as single to short chained bacilli with squared ends.
        2.   Giemsa-stained blood smears will demonstrate the capsule of *B. anthracis*.
        3.   Cultural isolation and biochemical identification of *B. anthracis* is used to confirm the diagnosis.
            a.   On blood agar incubated aerobically, colonies are large, flat, gray, and nonhemolytic. The colony is composed of parallel chains of cells, which give the margin of the colony its "Medusa head" appearance.
                (1) Endospores are easily demonstrated in direct smears prepared from the colonies, but capsules do not form in artificial culture media.

VII. IMMUNIZATION
    A.   The attenuated Stern strain of *B. anthracis* is used to immunize cattle in the United States.
        1.   The vaccine is administered subcutaneously.
            a.   The spores germinate in vivo.
            b.   The vegetative cells are nonencapsulated but produce the exotoxin complex. Since the organisms are not equipped with both antiphagocytic factors (capsule and exotoxin), there is insufficient bacterial proliferation and consequent toxin production to initiate clinical disease. The bacterial proliferation and toxin production are sufficient, however, to satisfactorily induce antibodies to factor II to provide protective immunity to the vaccinates before the nonencapsulated cells are phagocytized and the infection is eliminated.
            c.   The protective humoral antibodies, which are against factor II of the exotoxin complex, develop from 7 to 10 days after vaccination and last about 1 year.
            d.   Localized subcutaneous edema commonly occurs within 24 hours at the injection site and lasts several days.
        2.   Annual vaccination of cattle in areas of endemic anthrax is recommended.

77	Bacillary Hemoglobinuria

I. ETIOLOGY
    A. *Clostridium haemolyticum* is an obligate anaerobic, gram-positive, sporeforming bacillus.

II. TRANSMISSION
    A. *C. haemolyticum* is ingested, passes through the intestinal wall, and lodges in the liver. The spores remain as a latent infection until an anaerobic environment is created by hepatic injury.
        1. The organism grows best in marshy soil that is rich in organic matter and has alkaline water.
        2. The organism is a frequent inhabitant of the intestinal tract.
    B. Predisposing factors
        1. *Fasciola hepatica*, the common liver fluke, is a primary initiating factor of the disease. The adult fluke is found in the liver, bile ducts, and gall bladder.
            a. The migration of the liver fluke in the hepatic parenchyma causes necrosis with an anaerobic environment, which allows the bacterium to proliferate and produce exotoxins.
    C. Life cycle of the fluke
        1. The hermaphrodic adults live in the bile ducts of cattle and sheep.
            a. The fluke eggs are eliminated in the bile and are carried from the bile ducts into the small intestine. The eggs in the feces contaminate the pasture.
            b. The egg hatches, releasing a miracidium, the first larval stage.
            c. The miracidium is actively motile and penetrates the tissues of a snail, an intermediate host for the fluke. In the snail, the miracidium develops into a sporocyst, the second larval stage.
            d. The sporocysts germinate and produce several rediae, the third larval stage.
            e. The rediae leave the sporocyst, and each transforms to the fourth and final larval stage, the cercariae.
            f. The cercariae leave the snail and encyst in the environment to become metacercariae. Encystment occurs on plants or other objects in water.
            g. The metacercariae are ingested by cattle or sheep. Exsheathment occurs in the duodenum, releasing the young adult flukes.

     h.   The young flukes penetrate the intestinal wall, cross the peritoneal cavity, penetrate the capsule of the liver, and migrate through the hepatic parenchyma for a month or more before entering the bile ducts to mature. The acute lesions in the liver caused by the migratory flukes are hemorrhagic foci approximately 2 mm in diameter surrounded by hepatic parenchyma undergoing coagulation necrosis.

III. CLINICAL FEATURES
    A.   Clinical signs
       1.   Bacillary hemoglobinuria (red water disease) is an acute hemolytic anemia.
          a.   Clinical signs include high temperature, anemia, icterus, and hemoglobinuria.
          b.   Cattle usually die within 1 or 2 days after manifesting clinical signs. Death is usually attributed to anoxia.
    B.   Geographic distribution
       1.   The distribution of bacillary hemoglobinuria parallels the distribution of *F. hepatica*, which in turn is determined by the distribution of the snails. The snails serve as intermediate hosts of the flukes.
          a.   In the United States, bacillary hemoglobinuria occurs primary in the northwestern states, southern states, and Wisconsin.

IV. PATHOGENESIS
    A.   Bacillary hemoglobinuria is an intoxication following an infection.
       1.   Primary liver damage by liver flukes or other causes predispose the liver to infection with *C. haemolyticum*, which proliferates and produces a number of exotoxins.
          a.   Phospholipase C, a hemolytic toxin, is the principal toxin involved.
    B.   Clinically affected animals die before protective immunity develops.

V. PATHOLOGY
    A.   The hepatic infarcts, which are the foci of infection for *C. haemolyticum*, are usually single and much larger than the infarcts observed in infectious necrotic hepatitis.
       1.   The migratory hepatic lesions are attributed to *F. hepatica*, if adult flukes are found in the bile ducts. The adult flukes are 2 to 3 cm in length.
    B.   Other pathologic findings are a severe anemia, the kidneys speckled reddish or brown by hemoglobin, and a port wine-colored urine.

VI. DIAGNOSIS
    A.   Clinical signs
       1.   Bacillary hemoglobinuria is characterized by intravascular hemolysis with anemia and hemoglobinuria.

    B. Pathology
        1. Liver infarcts, liver flukes, anemia, and port wine-colored urine are characteristic in animals that have died from the disease.
    C. Culture
        1. Isolation and biochemical identification of *C. haemolyticum*

VII. IMMUNIZATION
    A. Commercial *C. haemolyticum* vaccines provide solid protective immunity.

78	Blackleg

I. ETIOLOGY
    A. *Clostridium chauvoei* is an obligate anaerobic, gram-positive, sporeforming bacillus.

II. TRANSMISSION
    A. It has been postulated that spores found in soil and forages are ingested, after which the organisms penetrate the intestinal tract and eventually lodge in muscle tissues where they reside latently until the infections are activated.

III. CLINICAL FEATURES
    A. Susceptibility factors
        1. Most clinical infections occur in cattle from 6 months to 2 years of age.
           a. Calves less than 6 months of age are apparently resistant to clinical disease, and cattle over 3 years old are seldom involved.
        2. Blackleg occurs chiefly in animals in good body condition that are kept on permanent pasturage.
           a. It is sometimes associated with particular farms or pastures.
    B. Clinical signs
        1. Blackleg is an acute febrile disease with lameness that is almost always associated with a characteristic crepitant

fluctuating swelling in the heavily muscled areas of the body, particularly in the hip, shoulder, back, and neck. Untreated animals usually die within 3 days after symptoms appear.
2. Affected animals are often found dead without clinical signs having been observed.

IV. PATHOGENESIS
   A. Ingestion
      1. The infections are acquired by the ingestion of spores.
         a. The spores are probably transported across the alimentary mucosa in macrophages and then distributed in the muscles as well as other tissues.
      2. The spores reside in the muscle as a latent infection until the muscle is injured by bruising or other injuries that devitalize the tissues.
         a. Germination of the spores and vegetative growth require an alkaline pH and a low oxidation-reduction potential.
      3. Once the vegetative cells become established in the initial focus of infection, the toxins produced by the bacteria provide a suitable and expanding environment for further bacterial growth.
         a. In the devitalized muscle, there is extensive necrosis, edema, and gas formation. This clostridial myonecrosis is due to the numerous exotoxins and enzymes produced by *C. chauvoei*.
         b. There is usually evidence of infection with crepitant fluctuating swelling in the heavy muscle areas within 24 hours of spore germination.
      4. The incubation period is 1 to 5 days, and blackleg is usually fatal 1 to 3 days after symptoms appear.
         a. Death results from a systemic intoxication.

V. PATHOLOGY
   A. Gross lesions
      1. The carcasses of affected animals have crepitant swellings in the musculature, particularly of the extremities, with a stiff characteristic extension of the limbs. Depending on how long the animal has been dead and the environmental temperature, the carcass may be greatly distended with gas.
         a. Affected muscles are dark brown or dark red and streaked with black. Similar lesions are frequently found in the heart and occasionally the tongue.
         b. The subcutaneous tissue in the area of infection has a blood-tinged exudate that contains large deposits of gas bubbles.

VI. DIAGNOSIS
   A. Clinical signs and gross lesions
       1. The crepitant swelling in the affected area, muscle lesions, and
           stiff-limbed posture of a carcass distended with gas are
           characteristic of blackleg.
   B. Culture
       1. Isolation and biochemical identification of *C. chauvoei*
           a. On sheep blood agar incubated anerobically at 37°C, *C.
               chauvoei* produces small colonies with raised centers
               surrounded by a wide zone of hemolysis.

VII. VACCINATION
   A. Commercial *C. chauvoei* bacterins provide productive immunity.
       1. Calves are usually vaccinated about the time they are weaned.

79	Brucellosis

I. ETIOLOGY
   A. *Brucella abortus*, an obligate aerobic, gram-negative bacillus, is a
       facultative intracellular pathogen.

II. TRANSMISSION
   A. Ingestion
       1. Ingestion of infective material is the primary mode of
           transmission.
           a. Reproductive tract exudates, placentas, aborted fetuses,
               and live calves from infected cows are the major sources of
               the organisms.
           b. Brucellae are shed in the milk of approximately 50 percent
               of infected cows.
           c. In brucellae-contaminated feed and water, *B. abortus* can
               survive for up to 6 months if conditions are ideal.
   B. Mucous membranes
       1. *B. abortus* is highly invasive and readily penetrates intact
           mucous membranes.
           a. Infection through the conjunctiva and mucous membranes of

the upper respiratory tract occurs when the concentration of infective cattle is high.
  C. Venereal
    1. Venereal transmission can occur from contaminated semen.
      a. Transmission is rare during natural service with an infected bull but more common during artificial insemination.
  D. Congenital
    1. Congenital transmission is rare but has been reported.
      a. Heifers exposed to brucellae in utero or at parturition will almost always eliminate the infection before they are sexually mature.

III. CLINICAL FEATURES
  A. Age and sex factors
    1. In young cattle prior to sexual maturity, brucellosis has developed a near perfect state of parasitism and is manifested as a mild chronic type of infection, in which the brucellae do not multiply extensively or demonstrate a particular affinity for any tissue.
    2. In sexually mature females, abortion during or after the fifth month of the first gestation is the cardinal clinical feature. Many infected animals never show clinical signs after the first gestation and have healthy calves but frequently shed brucellae after parturition. A retained placenta and metritis are common sequelae.
    3. Orchitis and epididymitis occur occasionally in bulls.
  B. Incidence
    1. In 1934, the United States Department of Agriculture initiated a nationwide cooperative state-federal brucellosis eradication program. Since 1934 there has been a marked reduction in the prevalence of the disease in cattle, from approximately 11 percent to the present level of less than 1 percent.
      a. Today many northern and western states are free of the disease; however, many southeastern and southwestern states still have a relatively high incidence.

IV. PATHOGENESIS
  A. Infection
    1. *B. abortus* is highly invasive and readily penetrates the intact mucous membranes of the oral pharynx and alimentary tract.
    2. The brucellae are phagocytized either by neutrophils, which frequently kill the bacteria, or by macrophages where the bacteria survive and multiply intracellularly.
    3. The brucellae are transported primarily by macrophages to the regional lymph nodes, where cattle can maintain these foci of infection for the duration of their lives.
    4. An intermittent macrophage-associated bacteremia disseminates

the infection to other lymph nodes, spleen, liver, and bone marrow, as well as to the udder and uterus of females and testes of males.

5. The brucellae grow slowly in vivo except in the gravid uterus, where erythritol is produced in the placenta from the fifth to the ninth month of gestation. Erythritol greatly enhances the proliferation of *B. abortus* in the placenta, chorion, and fetal membranes.

B. Anti-*B. abortus* serum antibodies
   1. Predominant immunoglubulin classes
      a. The presence of serum antibodies to *B. abortus* of the IgG class is usually indicative either of infection with virulent field strains of *B. abortus* or of passively acquired colostral antibody from infected cows. Serum antibodies of the IgM classes are generally indicative of vaccination with live attenuated *B. abortus* strain 19, low titers of natural antibodies, or from the non-*Brucella* bacteria that cross react with *B. abortus* antigens.
   2. Naturally infected cattle
      a. In cattle naturally infected with *B. abortus*, IgM is the first immunoglobulin class to appear in the serum and usually attains high titers in acute infections. IgG appears shortly thereafter, becoming the predominant class as the IgM response wanes. IgG usually persists as long as the animal remains infected. Of the two subclasses of IgG in bovine serum (IgG_1 and IgG_2), IgG_1 is the most abundant and is the predominant agglutinin and complement-fixing antibody.
   3. Colostral antibodies
      a. Passively acquired antibodies obtained from the ingestion of colostrum from infected cows progressively decrease, and few, if any, anti-*B. abortus* antibodies remain in the sera of calves by the time they are 1 year of age.
   4. Vaccinal antibodies
      a. *B. abortus* strain 19 is a live attenuated *B. abortus* biovar 1 strain. Strain 19 vaccination was officially approved in 1939 for the USDA brucellosis eradication program. The vaccine may cause persistent serologic reactions, especially when cattle are vaccinated as adults. Currently a reduced-dose vaccine is administered only to heifers between 4 and 12 months of age. In strain 19-vaccinated calves, IgM appears first, followed as early as 10 days by IgG. The IgG anti-*Brucella* antibodies decrease with time, and the occasional persistent agglutinins are attributed to IgM class antibodies.
   5. Natural agglutinins
      a. IgM is the main component of natural *B. abortus* agglutinins. IgG is frequently involved but to a much

lesser extent. Most natural agglutinins are attributed to antigenically cross reactive bacteria, which include certain strains and serotypes of *Yersinia enterocolitica*, *Pasteurella* species, *Campylobacter* species, *Salmonella* serovars, and *Escherichia coli*.

  C. Immunity
    1. Natural resistance
      a. Cattle less than 1 year of age are generally resistant to brucellosis and eliminate the infection before they reach sexual maturity.
    2. Protective immunity
      a. Antibodies to *B. abortus* do not provide protective immunity.
      b. Cell-mediated immunity provides some protective immunity.

V. PATHOLOGY
  A. Aborted fetuses
    1. Fetuses that are aborted from the fifth month of gestation to term are often edematous with excessive subcutaneous fluid but exhibit few other distinctive lesions.
    2. The placental lesions are generally nondescript, but affected cotyledons are often necrotic and covered by a brown exudate.
  B. Cows
    1. The gross appearance of the pregnant uterus and the postparturient uterus is normal. Following abortion, there is often a mild to moderately severe endometritis, which usually returns to normal in 30 to 90 days.

VI. DIAGNOSIS
  A. The definitive diagnosis of brucellosis requires the isolation and identification of the causative bacterium; however, it is not always possible to recover *B. abortus* from live infected animals. Therefore most diagnoses are based on the results of serologic tests.
  B. Culture
    1. *B. abortus* is often present in milk, vaginal specimens, and tissues in very small numbers, but aborted fetuses, infected full-term calves, and fetal membranes usually contain large numbers of brucellae.
      a. *B. abortus* can be isolated from the milk in about 50 percent of the infected cows. Infection of the udder may be confined to one or more quarters. Therefore it is essential that the sample contain milk from all the quarters.
      b. Brucellae can often be recovered from vaginal and uterine specimens taken in the 6-week period following abortion or parturition.
      c. Tissues from which brucellae can most often be isolated are the lymph nodes associated with the digestive tract, udder,

supramammary lymph nodes, and postparturient uterus.

    d.   The best specimens for cultural examination are the stomach contents, liver, and spleen from aborted fetuses and infected full-term calves. The lymph nodes associated with the gastrointestinal tract also are commonly culture-positive for brucellae.

  2. Most field strains of *B. abortus* require the presence of 5 percent serum in the agar medium and 8 to 10 percent carbon dioxide for growth.

    a.   *B. abortus* strain 19 is carbon dioxide-independent.

C. Serology

  1. Standardized serologic tests (Table 79.1)

    a.   Reference antigens, antisera and uniform methods have standardized the agglutination tests commonly used to diagnose bovine brucellosis.

      (1) The whole smooth cell of *B. abortus* USDA reference strain 1119-3 is the antigen.

      (2) The international standard anti-*B. abortus* serum is used as the antisera.

Table 79.1. Serologic tests for bovine brucellosis

Test	Predominant Antibody Classes Detected	Principle of Test
Standard tube	IgM, IgG (combined level)	Agglutination (quantitative)
Card	IgG	Agglutination (qualitative)
Rivanol	IgG	Agglutination (quantitative)
Mercaptoethanol	IgG	Agglutination (quantitative)

    b.   Standard tube agglutination test

      (1) The disadvantages of the standard tube agglutination (STA) test include the detection of nonspecific antibodies as well as specific antibodies arising from natural *B. abortus* infection or strain 19 vaccination. It is often the last test to reach diagnostically significant levels in the incubation stages of the disease and after abortion. In the chronic stages of the disease, the STA test often becomes negative when the results of the supplemental tests are positive.

      (2) Traditionally the infection status of both vaccinated and nonvaccinated cattle has been based on STA titers (Table 79.2).

    c.   Card test

      (1) The card test will usually detect infection earlier than will the standard tube agglutination, rivanol, or mercaptoethanol tests. In naturally infected animals, the card test will usually become positive first,

Table 79.2. Classification of infection status of bovine brucellosis

| Classification | STA Titers | |
	Official vaccinates[a]	All others
Negative	$\leq + 1:50$	$<1:50$
Suspect	$I1:100$ to $\leq I1:200$	$I1:50$ to $\leq I1:100$
Positive	$\geq + 1:200$	$\geq 1:100$

Note: I = incomplete agglutination; + = complete agglutination.
[a]Heifers vaccinated between 4 and 12 months of age with reduced-dose *B. abortus* strain 19 vaccine.

followed by the mercaptoethanol and rivanol tests. In strain 19-vaccinated cattle, as the titer recedes the rivanol test is usually the first to go negative, the mercaptoethanol second, and the card test last. False-positive reactions with the card test are estimated to be between 1 and 3 percent, depending on the level of infection and vaccination history of the herd. False-negative reactions are estimated to range from 1 to 2 percent.

    d.   Rivanol and mercaptoethanol tests

        (1) These supplemental tests are used to differentiate between antibody responses associated with non-*Brucella* antigens, strain 19 vaccination, and infection with field strains of *B. abortus*. Titers indicate the amount, if any, of anti-*Brucella* IgG agglutinin present in the serum. Since IgG is generally associated with the presence of active infection, any positive titer should be regarded as an indication of infection or at least as a suspicion of infection. Low to moderate STA titers in vaccinated cattle are not considered significant when the rivanol and/or mercaptoethanol tests are negative but do indicate the presence of *B. abortus* infection when the rivanol and/or mercaptoethanol tests are positive.

  2. Complement-fixation (CF) tests

    a.   There are a number of different techniques available for the CF test, so the CF results from laboratory to laboratory are often not comparable. The predominant complement-fixing antibody is IgG_1.

    b.   The CF tests rarely exhibit nonspecific reactions and are considered the most reliable tests in differentiating calfhood vaccination serologic responses from those due to infection with field strains of *B. abortus*. After infection with virulent *B. abortus*, CF titers often reach diagnostic levels sooner than STA titers, but unlike STA titers, these do not wane as the disease becomes chronic. The CF test is less sensitive than the card, rivanol, or mercaptoethanol tests.

3. Common problems associated with serologic diagnoses of bovine brucellosis
   a. The long and variable incubation of bovine brucellosis
   b. The variability of an animal's humoral response to infection with both strain 19 vaccine and virulent field strains of *B. abortus*
   c. The relationship of a cow's humoral response to the stage of pregnancy at the time of exposure
   d. The presence of cross-reacting nonspecific antibodies

D. Milk ring test
   1. It is a qualitative agglutination test that is used to screen dairy herds for brucellosis.
      a. Infected diary herds are recognized by detecting antibodies to *B. abortus* in pooled milk samples.
         (1) Udder infection normally follows systemic infection, and there is not a significant level of anti-*B. abortus* antibodies in the milk until the udder is infected.
      b. The milk ring test is very sensitive and uses *B. abortus* antigen stained with hematoxylin (red) or tetrazolium (blue) dyes.
         (1) A concentrated suspension of stained brucellae is added to the milk. In positive tests, the antibodies agglutinate the brucellae, which rise to the surface with the fat globules and form a red or deep blue ring in the cream layer.
      c. If the tested milk gives a positive reaction, the dairy herd is classified as suspect for brucellosis. In suspect herds, individual cows must be blood-tested to determine the infection status of each animal.

VII. IMMUNIZATION
A. Strain 19 vaccination was officially approved by the USDA in 1939 for the brucellosis eradication program.
   1. *B. abortus* strain 19 has all the characteristics of biovar 1 strains except it does not require carbon dioxide for growth and is not stimulated by erythritol.
   2. Only females are vaccinated.
   3. The vaccine will cause orchitis in bulls.
B. Calfhood vaccination
   1. The vaccine should be administered only to heifers between 4 and 12 months of age.
   2. A reduced-dose vaccine that contains 3×10^9 cells of strain 19 is used in most states.
   3. Serologic titers usually fall below diagnostic levels before the first calving.
   4. It provides protective immunity in about 65 percent of the animals vaccinated. The range of protection depends on

vaccination age and challenge dose.
  a. Calfhood vaccination results in significant protection
      from, but not the elimination of, infection and abortion.
C. Adult vaccination
  1. When older calves and adults are vaccinated with reduced-dose
      vaccine, the vaccinal titers usually decline to negative status
      after 4 to 6 months; however, the vaccine will cause persistent
      infections in 1 to 2 percent of the animals.

80	Campylobacteriosis

I. ETIOLOGY
    A. *Campylobacter fetus* ss *venerealis* is a microaerophilic, gram-negative
        bacillus.

II. TRANSMISSION
    A. Obligate parasite
        1. The natural habitat for *C. fetus* ss *venerealis* is the bovine
            reproductive tract.
            a. The sites of infection in heifers and cows are the mucosal
                surfaces of the uterus, oviducts, cervix, and vagina.
            b. In bulls, the organism colonizes the epithelial surface of
                the preputial cavity, and in particular the mucosa of the
                glans penis, prepuce, and distal portion of the urethra.
    B. Breeding
        1. Under natural conditions, transmission of infection occurs
            during coitus.
        2. Heifers and cows also can be infected by artificial insemination
            with infected semen.
    C. Mechanical
        1. Bulls occasionally are infected by mechanical transmission from
            contaminated bedding.

III. CLINICAL FEATURES
    A. Clinical signs
        1. Temporary infertility caused by early embryonic death or failure
            to conceive is the principal clinical sign, but abortions

occasionally occur in the fourth through the eighth month of gestation. The placenta is seldom retained in cows that abort.

    a. Infected females usually conceive 2 to 8 months after the initial infection and deliver full-term calves; however, they may remain carriers.

2. Bull susceptibility to campylobacteriosis varies from animal to animal.

    a. Most bulls less than 6 years old are difficult to infect and may carry the infection for only a few weeks after exposure. These young bulls can mechanically carry the bacterium between cows.

    b. Bulls more than 6 years of age are relatively easy to infect and are more likely to become permanent carriers. Their increased susceptibility is related to the deep crypts in the prepuce that develop with advancing age. The infection in bulls does not interfere with reproductive behavior or fertilization ability of semen.

B. Herd history

1. Campylobacteriosis is frequently introduced into a susceptible herd by a single infected cow or bull.

2. The history of an infected herd depends on the duration of the infection and the season of the year the disease is first observed.

    a. In susceptible herds with no immunity, an acute infertility is observed for 2 to 4 months before successful conception occurs.

        (1) A low calving rate of 25 to 50 percent may be the first observed evidence of the disease.

        (2) Bulls in acutely infected herds often show a decreased libido due to the increased number of breedings required to settle the cows.

    b. In chronically infected herds with some immunity, a vague infertility is observed and abortions are rare.

        (1) Most chronically infected beef herds are composed of cows and bulls of all ages, and the immune status of females and the number of carrier bulls are variable. The conception rate for the older cows returns to normal, and only first calf heifers and susceptible females introduced into the herd demonstrate the acute form of the disease.

        (2) Campylobacteriosis is self-limiting in females, but cows that have recovered from the infection may become reinfected during a subsequent breeding with an infected bull. Although the incidence of carrier cows that retain the infection from one gestation to the next is very low, it is often sufficient to permit the disease to persist in large beef herds.

IV. PATHOGENESIS
  A. Heifers and cows
  1. When susceptible females are bred to an infected bull, *C. fetus* ss *venerealis* is introduced into the female genital tract.
    a. The bacterium becomes established in the cervicovaginal (CV) area but is cleared from the uterus within 3 days after infection.
      (1) Neutrophils are numerous in the uterus at estrus and play a major role in preventing colonization.
    b. Repopulation of the uterus from the CV area begins after approximately 7 days. The uterine horns are successfully colonized after 12 to 14 days.
      (1) The colonization occurs during the progesteronal phase of the estrus cycle, when both the number and bactericidal competency of the neutrophils are decreased.
      (2) Few bacteria penetrate beneath the endometrium, and the infection generally does not stimulate an increase in serum antibody titers.
    c. From 1 to 2 weeks after infection, acutely infected females have a marked endometritis characterized by focal and diffuse infiltration of mononuclear cells with some necrosis.
      (1) The duration of the infection and endometritis correlates closely with the period of infertility. Fertilization usually occurs, but the fertilized ova die due to a histotrophic nutritional deficiency caused by a necrotic epithelium and are absorbed or expelled within a few weeks of conception.
      (2) When abortions occur in the second and third trimester of pregnancy, the bacteria are located in the placenta, chorion, and allantoic fluids.
  2. Protective immunity starts to develop between 6 and 12 weeks following infection.
    a. Antibodies to the superficial antigenic components of the bacterium are important in the clearance of the organisms from the infected animals.
      (1) Opsonization is important because *C. fetus* ss *venerealis* is easily killed by phagocytic cells, and immobilization of the bacterium prevents its penetration into the cervix and colonization of the uterine mucosa.
      (2) The bacteria are gradually eliminated from the uterus and fallopian tubes within 6 months but may persist in the cervix and vagina for up to 2 years.
    b. Females that have recovered from infection generally have a period of convalescent immunity but eventually become susceptible to reinfection.

    c.   The resistance to infertility and abortion and the persistance of CV infection in the presence of specific antibody indicate that different mechanisms are responsible for uterine clearance of the bacterium than are operative in the CV area.

        (1) Immunoglobulin G_1 and sIgA are the predominant immunoglobulins in the uterus and CV area, respectively. Immunoglobulin G_1 is obtained by transudation from the serum when inflammation occurs, and like IgM, it immobilizes and opsonizes the bacteria. The sIgA is produced due to local infection of the genital tract but will only immobilize the bacteria.

        (2) Since the bacterium possesses extremely labile surface antigens, the successful destruction of a major portion of the bacterial population by an antibody-mediated response leaves a residual population of bacteria with different antigenic determinants. The residual population will multiply and be largely eliminated by a second immune response, leaving a residual population of a third antigenic type. This process can be repeated indefinitely, and as the specific antibody response to a particular antigen wanes, the bacterium may reutilize these antigens. The marked antigenic variability of the bacterium may, in part, explain the persistence of the asymptomatic CV carrier state.

B.   Bulls

    1. Infection of the epithelial surface in the preputial cavity of the bull by *C. fetus* ss *venerealis* does not induce any pathological changes.

        a.   Young bulls are often refractory to reinfection for some months after the infection is eliminated; however, without treatment older bulls often remain permanent carriers.

        b.   The age susceptibility and persistence of infection in bulls is anatomically rather than immunologically related, as in females.

V.   PATHOLOGY

    A.   Aborted fetuses

        1. Aborted fetuses are often autolysed when expelled, which suggests that fetal death occurred several days before the abortion. Fetal and placental lesions are nonspecific.

    B.   Cows

        1. Cows that have aborted usually have only a mild endometritis provided other microorganisms have not secondarily invaded the uterus.

C. Bulls
   1. Infected bulls fail to exhibit any pathology.

VI. DIAGNOSIS
   A. Heifers and cows
      1. Culture, fluorescent antibody (FA) and cervical mucus agglutination (CMA) tests, and serum antibody (SA) titers are used to diagnose campylobacteriosis in the female.
         a. The duration and stage of the estrous cycle should be considered when interpreting the results of these tests.
      2. Diagnostic tests
         a. Culture
            (1) Culture and identification of *C. fetus* ss *venerealis* from the CV mucus is the method of choice. Most cultures are positive for *C. fetus* ss *venerealis* during the first 2 months after susceptible females are bred to infected bulls. Thereafter the number of positive cultures progressively declines until only about 20 percent are positive at 6 months. A marked decline in the rate of isolation of the bacterium from pregnant animals is observed, and bacteriologic examination of the stomach contents, lungs, and liver of aborted fetuses is the only practical method of confirming the diagnosis late in gestation.
         b. Fluorescent antibody test
            (1) The FA test compares favorably with culture; however, the FA conjugate does not differentiate between *C. fetus* ss *venerealis* and *C. fetus* ss *fetus*, which cross react serologically.
         c. Cervical mucus agglutination test
            (1) The CMA test is often unsatisfactory, since both false-positive and false-negative tests occur. It takes approximately 2 months after service by an infected bull for the mucus to test positive. The duration of positive titers range from 4 months to 1 year with a mean of 7 months. The abundant CV mucus secretions at estrus dilute agglutinins so false-negative reactions may occur at this time.
         d. Serum agglutination titers
            (1) The SA titers to *C. fetus* ss *venerealis* are generally not significantly increased during the course of infection. Since infection in females is self-limiting, the persistence of demonstrable serum antibodies is transient when it does occur. False-positives also can occur because antibodies against the O antigens of *C. fetus* ss *venerealis* are usually present in the serum of cattle. Formation of these

antibodies may be stimulated by *C. fetus* ss *fetus* or
other antigenically cross-reactive organisms.
  B. Bulls
     1. Bacteriologic examination of preputial and semen samples and FA
          examination of preputial scrapings are effective methods of
          diagnosing the carrier state in bulls.
          a. Culture
               (1) Preputial samples are generally heavily contaminated
                     with many nonpathogenic bacterial species, and
                     infected bulls are often culture-negative for *C. fetus*
                     ss *venerealis*.
          b. Fluorescent antibody test
               (1) The advantage of the FA test is that it is effective
                     for highly contaminated samples and samples containing
                     only nonviable organisms.
     2. The use of virgin heifers for testing suspected carrier bulls is
          effective but time-consuming and expensive.
          a. Virgin heifer test
               (1) Suspect bulls are bred to several virgin heifers from
                     which a diagnosis is made on the basis of positive
                     cultures from the heifers 3 to 6 weeks after breeding.

VII. IMMUNIZATION
  A. Commercial killed bacterins are effective both prophylactically and
       therapeutically and produce high titers of serum antibodies against
       both homologous and heterologous strains of *C. fetus* ss *venerealis*.
     1. Prophylactically, susceptible heifers and cows should be
          vaccinated 1 to 4 months prior to breeding and boostered
          approximately 10 days before breeding. Annual boosters are
          recommended.
          a. Vaginal immunity depends on high serum antibody titers,
               principally IgG, at the time of exposure.
     2. In infected females, the termination of infection depends on the
          outcome of the dynamic interplay between antibody concentration,
          time response of these antibodies in the genital secretions, and
          the opportunity for antigenic variation.
          a. The amount of plasma-derived antibody is greater in the
               uterus than in the CV area. This may explain, in part, the
               variable conception rate and persistence of the CV
               infection.

81	Contagious Pyelonephritis

I. ETIOLOGY
    A. *Corynebacterium renale* is a facultative anaerobic, gram-positive bacillus.

II. TRANSMISSION
    A. *C. renale*, an obligate parasite of the urinary mucosa, can be spread by direct contact from infected to susceptible cattle.

III. CLINICAL FEATURES
    A. Contagious bovine pyelonephritis is the most common cause of renal disease in cattle and is characterized by pyelonephritis, urethritis, and cystitis.
        1. It is more common in females than in males and usually affects only one kidney.
            a. Clinical disease is most commonly seen in mature cows and is predisposed to by pregnancy and parturition.
        2. The morbidity rate in infected herds is low, but the mortality rate in clinically infected animals is high.
    B. Clinical signs are often exhibited late in the course of the disease. Affected cattle exhibit a loss of condition, painful urination, and blood and purulent material in urine.
        1. On rectal palpation, the affected kidneys and ureters are greatly enlarged.

IV. PATHOGENESIS
    A. Pyelonephritis is an ascending urogenous infection from the lower urinary tract.
        1. *C. renale* has a predilection for the medulla of the kidney.
            a. The bacterium adheres by fimbriae to the cells lining the renal medulla.
            b. The high urease activity of *C. renale* splits the urea in the urine into ammonia and carbon dioxide. Alkalinization of the urine decreases the resistance of the renal epithelium to bacterial penetration.
    B. The site of the urinary tract infection determines the level of acquired immunity.
        1. Kidney and ureter infections
            a. Animals with chronic pyelonephritis and ureteritis produce high levels of serum antibodies.
        2. Urinary bladder infections
            a. Animals with only cystitis fail to produce serum antibodies.

V. PATHOLOGY
  A. The kidneys are enlarged and tan.
    1. Because of the usual long duration of infection, the
       interstitial fibrosis is extensive.

VI. DIAGNOSIS
  A. Clinical signs (above)
  B. Pathology (above)
  C. Culture
    1. Isolation and biochemical identification of *C. renale*

VII. IMMUNIZATION
  A. Commercial *C. renale* vaccines are not available.

82	Foot Rot

I. ETIOLOGY
  A. Bovine foot rot is caused by a synergistic infection of *Fusobacterium
     necrophorum* and *Bacteroides melaninogenicus*, both obligate anaerobic
     gram-negative bacilli.

II. TRANSMISSION
  A. Environmental
    1. *F. necrophorum* and *B. melaninogenicus* are normal flora of the
       bovine digestive tract and occur in the environment as fecal
       contaminants.
  B. Predisposing factors
    1. Bovine foot rot can occur in all seasons and weather conditions
       but is most frequently associated with wet conditions.
      a. Mud, dung, frozen mud, stones, and stubble are predisposing
         factors that can soften and macerate the interdigital
         epidermis, bruise the tissues, and create anaerobic
         conditions that render the feet susceptible to invasion by
         F. necrophorum and *B. melaninogenicus*.

III. CLINICAL FEATURES

    A.   Foot rot is seen in cattle of all ages and breeds and is responsible for 40 to 60 percent of the bovine foot diseases.

        1.   It usually occurs sporadically within a herd, but epizootics can occur in feedlot cattle.

    B.   Three clinical forms of bovine foot rot are observed: acute foot rot, chronic foot rot, and foot abscesses.

IV. PATHOGENESIS

    A.   Moisture and other predisposing factors compromise the integrity of the interdigital skin. This permits the colonization of the lesion with various bacteria, including *F. necrophorum* and *B. melaninogenicus*.

        1.   The interdigital lesions, which are the primary site of infection, are usually located on the posterior aspect of the hoof over the bulbs of the heels and may extend both medially and laterally between the claws.

    B.   Within 48 hours, the lesions can extend from the posterior to anterior aspects of the interdigital space and proximal to the fetlock.

        1.   The acute foot rot lesions are characterized by a suppurative necrosis of the subcutaneous connective tissues.

            a.   *F. necrophorum* is primarily responsible for the suppurative necrosis associated with the infection.

            b.   *B. melaninogenicus* produces proteolytic and collagenolytic enzymes that attack the subcutaneous connective tissue and tendons.

    C.   Clinical disease does not stimulate a solid or lasting immunity. Even cattle that have recently recovered from foot rot are susceptible to reinfection.

V. PATHOLOGY

    A.   Acute foot rot

        1.   The lesions can extend from the posterior to anterior aspects of the interdigital space and proximal to the fetlock and are characterized by a suppurative necrosis of the subcutaneous connective tissues.

    B.   Chronic foot rot

        1.   Foot abscesses, tendonitis, septic synovitis, arthritis, osteitis, and ankylosis of the coffin joint are common sequelae in chronically affected animals.

VI. DIAGNOSIS

    A.   Clinical signs

        1.   Diagnosis is usually based on clinical signs.

            a.   Acutely affected animals may have a temperature rise accompanied by swelling of tissues above the coronet and lameness in affected feet.

        b.   Foot rot exudates have a characteristic foul odor.

B.   Direct smears
    1.   Microscopic examination of gram-stained exudate is a valuable
       diagnostic aid.

C.   Culture
    1.   Isolation and identification of the causative bacteria are
       seldom necessary to confirm the clinical diagnosis.

VII. IMMUNIZATION

A.   Commercial vaccines for *F. necrophorum* and *B. melaninogenicus* are not available.

| 83 | Infectious Keratoconjunctivitis |

I. ETIOLOGY
A. *Moraxella bovis* is an obligate aerobic, gram-negative bacillus.
B. Cellular antigens and virulence factors
1. Cellular antigens
   a. Capsular antigens
      (1) A polysaccharide capsule may or may not be present.
      (2) Fimbrial presence and length varies with the strain and cultural conditions.
   b. Cell wall antigens
      (1) The lipopolysaccharide is a dermonecrotic endotoxin.
2. Virulence factors
   a. Hemolysin
      (1) Most pathogenic strains are hemolytic; however, not all hemolytic strains are pathogenic.
   b. Proteases
      (1) Proteases are important in causing corneal damage.
3. Colony characteristics
   a. Rough colonies are commonly pathogenic. They are usually beta hemolytic and fimbriated.
   b. Smooth colonies are frequently nonpathogenic. They are usually nonhemolytic and nonfimbriated.

II. TRANSMISSION
A. Seasonal incidence
1. The incidence of infectious bovine keratoconjunctivitis (IBK) is highest during periods of high solar radiation, when ultraviolet rays are direct. The highest incidence occurs in the summer.
B. Modes of transmission
1. Direct contact between cattle
2. Fomites contaminated with ocular and nasal discharges
3. Insect vectors
   a. Face flies, house flies, and stable flies can serve as mechanical vectors. *Musca autumnalis*, the face fly, is a very common vector.

III. CLINICAL FEATURES
A. IBK (pinkeye) is highly contagious among susceptible cattle.
B. Clinical signs are restricted to the eye and adjacent tissues and include photophobia, conjunctivitis, lacrimation, corneal opacity, and ulceration. The infection can be unilateral or bilateral.
1. Incidence is greater in cattle under 2 years of age.

IV. PATHOGENESIS
    A.   Bacterial factors
        1.   IBK is a localized infection of the eye.
        2.   Fimbriae provide attachment to the cornea.
        3.   *M. bovis* produces a dermonecrotic endotoxin, and most pathogenic
            strains produce hemolysins.
            a.   The modes of action of these virulence factors in the
                pathogenesis of IBK are not completely understood.
    B.   Host factors
        1.   The lack of eye pigmentation is significant.
            a.   Cattle with very little eye pigment are more severely
                affected.   Hereford cattle are very susceptible.
            b.   Calves and yearlings are often the most severely affected.
    C.   Contributing factors
        1.   High solar radiation is a predisposing factor.
        2.   Other eye infections, particularly infectious bovine
            rhinotracheitis viral infections, are common predisposing
            factors.
    D.   Immunity
        1.   Protective antibodies develop in most infected cattle, but this
            resistance is not complete.
            a.   Recovered animals often remain carriers.
                 (1) *M. bovis* is maintained in nature by chronic infections
                     of the conjunctival and nasal mucous membranes.
                 (2) Recovered animals that are either carriers or
                     reinfected with *M. bovis* may develop mild symptoms
                     with increased sunlight in the summer.
        2.   Role of lacrimal and serum antibodies
            a.   In the noninfected bovine eye, sIgA is the predominant
                 immunoglobulin present in the lacrimal secretions, which
                 bathe the eye and conjunctiva.
                 (1) It has been postulated that specific antibodies to the
                     fimbrial antigen of *M. bovis* help protect the eye
                     from colonization and infection of virulent *M. bovis*
                     strains.
                 (2) The levels of sIgA in the lacrimal fluids is
                     independent of the serum IgA levels.
            b.   During the inflammation caused by *M. bovis* infections,
                 there is a transudation of serum into the lacrimal
                 secretions.
                 (1) There is a positive correlation of the lacrimal and
                     serum levels of IgM and IgG_1. As the severity of the
                     infection increases, the tear immunoglobulin ratios of
                     IgM and IgG become more like the serum ratio.
            c.   The antibody response, which follows natural IBK
                 infections, is often insufficient to protect against
                 subsequent infection and disease unless the infection is
                 particularly severe.

V. PATHOLOGY
    A. Ocular lesions include corneal opacity and ulceration.

VI. DIAGNOSIS
    A. Clinical signs are diagnostic.
    B. Culture
        1. Isolation and biochemical identification of *M. bovis*
            a. Virulent *M. bovis* strains on blood agar are usually
                hemolytic and pit the agar.

VII. IMMUNIZATION
    A. Bacterins and live bacterial vaccines may be effective if given in
        multiple doses to young calves before pinkeye season.
        1. Immunization will decrease the severity caused by homologous
            challenge and to a lesser extent by heterologous infections.
            The nature of the immunity resulting from vaccination is not
            completely understood.

84	Infectious Necrotic Hepatitis

I. ETIOLOGY
    A. *Clostridium novyi* is an obligate anaerobic, gram-positive,
        sporeforming bacillus.

II. TRANSMISSION
    A. Ingestion
        1. *C. novyi* is ingested, passes through the intestinal wall, and
            lodges in the liver. The spores remain as a latent infection
            until an anaerobic environment is created by hepatic injury.
            a. The organism is widely distributed in soil and a frequent
                inhabitant of the intestinal tract.
    B. Predisposing factors
        1. *Fasciola hepatica*, the common liver fluke, is a primary
            initiating factor of the disease. The adult fluke is found in
            the liver, bile ducts, and gall bladder.
            a. The migration of the liver fluke in the hepatic parenchyma

causes necrosis with an anaerobic environment, which allows
the bacterium to proliferate and produce exotoxins.

III. CLINICAL FEATURES
A. Clinical signs
  1. Cattle with clinical infectious necrotic hepatitis die suddenly,
     often without premonitory signs.
B. Geographic distribution
  1. In the United States, the disease occurs primarily in areas
     where liver flukes are present, including the northwestern
     states, southern states, and Wisconsin.

IV. PATHOGENESIS
A. Infectious necrotic hepatitis is an intoxication following an
   infection.
  1. Primary liver damage by liver flukes or other causes predispose
     the liver to infection with *C. novyi*, which proliferates and
     produces a number of exotoxins.
     a. Alpha toxin is the principal toxin involved. It has a
        phospholipase activity that affects membrane permeability,
        possibly by disruption of the lipoprotein layers in the
        endothelial cell walls.
     b. *C. novyi* type B strains also produces beta toxin, which is
        both necrotizing and hemolytic, and zeta toxin, which has
        hemolytic activity.
B. Clinically affected animals die before protective immunity develops.

V. PATHOLOGY
A. Infectious necrotic hepatitis is often called black disease, due to
   the dark discoloration of the skin and subcutis that results from
   extensive subcutaneous congestion.
  1. Characteristic liver lesions consist of multiple foci of hepatic
     necrosis.

VI. DIAGNOSIS
A. Clinical signs
  1. Sudden death
B. Pathology
  1. Liver infarcts
C. Culture
  1. Isolation and biochemical identification of *C. novyi*

VII. IMMUNIZATION
A. Commercial *C. novyi* bacterins provide solid protective immunity.

85 | Leptospirosis

I. ETIOLOGY
A. *Leptospira hardjo* and *L. pomona* are obligate aerobic, gram-negative spirochetes. These two serovars are responsible for most of the clinical leptospirosis in cattle.

II. TRANSMISSION
A. Leptospires can penetrate intact mucous membranes and skin.
1. Urine-contaminated soil and water are the primary sources of infection.
   a. Cattle are the reservoir host of *L. hardjo* and the primary source of infection for susceptible cattle.
   b. Cattle, sheep, and swine are common sources of *L. pomona*.

III. CLINICAL FEATURES
A. Cattle of all ages may be affected with leptospirosis, but calves are usually more severely affected than are adults.
B. The severity and clinical manifestations are largely dependent on the serovar involved.
1. The pathogenic effects of *L. hardjo* are limited to lactating or pregnant cows. *L. hardjo* causes an atypical mastitis in which the udder secretions become thick and yellow. Most abortions occur in the last trimester of gestation, but some stillborn and weak calves will also result from these infections. Retained placentas may occur.
2. Acute infections of *L. pomona* often cause a hemolytic anemia and occasionally induce abortions. Clinically affected animals exhibit fever, anemia, and hemoglobinuria that imparts a port wine color to the urine. Acutely infected animals may die within 4 days after clinical signs are manifested.

IV. PATHOGENESIS
A. Ingestion of either *L. hardjo* or *L. pomona* results in a transient bacteremia, followed by localization of the leptospires in the kidneys and liver and sometimes the placenta, in which the leptospires produce fetal disease and abortion.
1. Acute systemic disease with *L. pomona* is often exhibited after an incubation period of 2 to 10 days, whereas abortion induced by either *L. hardjo* or *L. pomona* may occur during either the acute phase of the infection or during convalescence. *L. hardjo* has a greater affinity for the pregnant uterus than does

L. pomona, and most abortions occur from 6 to 12 weeks after the dams are infected.

V.   PATHOLOGY

A.   Acute systemic leptospirosis
1.   Cattle that die from *L. pomona* infections have a severe anemia, mild icterus, and occasionally hemoglobinuria. Nonspecific ecchymotic hemorrhages may be present on the serous membranes and in the subcutis.

B.   Abortions
1.   Aborted fetuses usually die in utero and undergo mild autolysis before being expelled from the uterus. Many infected fetuses will have mild interstitial nephritis.

VI. DIAGNOSIS

A.   Herd history and clinical signs (above)
B.   Isolation and identification of the *Leptospira* serovars
1.   The pathogenic serovars are indistinguishable by morphology and biochemical activity.
2.   Serovars are identified by microscopic agglutination and agglutinin adsorption tests with serovar-specific rabbit antiserum.

C.   Serology
1.   Serologic tests are often used to detect subclinical infections.

VII. IMMUNIZATION

A.   Commercial *L. pomona* and *L. hardjo* bacterins provide protective humoral immunity for 6 months to 1 year.

86 | Listeriosis

I. ETIOLOGY
  A. *Listeria monocytogenes*, a facultative anaerobic, gram-positive bacillus, is a facultative intracellular pathogen.

II. TRANSMISSION
  A. Ingestion of *L. monocytogenes*, which is present in soil, vegetation, and feces, is the primary mode of transmission.
    1. High numbers of bacteria are found in poor-quality, high-pH silage, particularly during cold weather.
    2. Normal animals commonly shed the bacterium in their feces.

III. CLINICAL FEATURES
  A. Four syndromes
    1. Subclinical infections are the most common form of infection.
      a. *L. monocytogenes* is frequently isolated from apparently normal animals.
    2. Neonatal infections are characterized as visceral infections with a septicemia.
      a. Adults may have a bacteremia but are asymptomatic.
      b. Clinical signs in neonatal animals include septicemia and often gastroenteritis and bilateral meningitis.
        (1) Deaths are frequent in neonatal animals.
    3. Listerial abortion is a sporadic condition in cattle.
      a. Abortion in the last trimester of pregnancy is the principal clinical sign. Retained placentas are common.
    4. Neural listeriosis, which is characterized as a unilateral meningoencephalitis, is the most commonly diagnosed type of clinical illness.
      a. Clinical signs of neural listeriosis include unilateral facial paralysis, unidirectional circling, corneal opacity, prostration, coma, and death.

IV. PATHOGENESIS
  A. Clinical listeriosis is usually related to the number of bacteria ingested.
    1. *L. monocytogenes* has a high infectivity but a low pathogenicity.
    2. Poor-quality silage frequently contains large numbers of *L. monocytogenes.*
    3. Silage-fed animals may be more susceptible to listeriosis because these animals have high serum iron levels, which

stimulate the extracellular growth of the bacterium.
B.   The bacteria proliferate in the digestive tract.
1.   Neonatal animals may have a clinical gastroenteritis with areas of focal necrosis.
2.   The bacteria penetrate through the mucous membranes of the digestive tract with a subsequent visceral infection and a neutrophil-associated bacteremia/septicemia.
a.   The visceral infections are usually asymptomatic.
b.   Clinical signs of a septicemia are seen frequently in neonatal animals.
c.   Clinical meningoencephalitis results if the bacteria penetrate the oral mucosa and affect the cranial nerves, especially the trigeminal and facial nerves, with unilateral localization in the brain stem.
C.   Immunity to natural infection is predominantly cell-mediated.
1.   Infected animals develop an enhanced cellular immunity. Humoral immunity is not considered to be significant.

V.   PATHOLOGY
A.   Neonatal listeriosis
1.   There are areas of focal necrosis in the gastrointestinal tract, liver, and spleen, as well as lesions of a septicemia.
B.   Listerial abortion
1.   Placentitis with lesions of a septicemia in the fetus are present.
C.   Neural listeriosis
1.   Gross lesions in the brain are seldom evident.
2.   Microscopic lesions are primarily in the brain stem.
a.   Microabscesses are often unilateral and are characterized by perivascular cuffing with mononuclear cells. Bacteria can be demonstrated in the lesions.

VI.   DIAGNOSIS
A.   Herd history and clinical signs (above)
B.   Pathology (above)
C.   Culture
1.   Isolation and biochemical identification of *L. monocytogenes*
a.   Visceral tissues can be cultured directly on blood agar.
b.   The cold enrichment technique is often required to isolate the bacterium from brain tissue. A ground suspension of neural tissue is refrigerated at 4^{0}C for 1 to 12 weeks with weekly attempts at isolation on blood agar.

VII. IMMUNIZATION
A.   Commercial *L. monocytogenes* vaccines are not available.

87 | Paratuberculosis

I. ETIOLOGY
   A. *Mycobacterium paratuberculosis*, an obligate aerobic, gram-positive, acid-fast bacillus, is a facultative intracellular pathogen.

II. TRANSMISSION
   A. Ingestion
      1. Ingestion is the primary mode of transmission.
         a. Fecal contamination of the dam's teats is the major source of infection.
            (1) The organisms present in the intestinal mucous membranes are excreted with the feces of both asymptomatic shedders and clinically ill animals.
            (2) The bacterium is highly resistant in the environment and remains viable for prolonged periods of time in feed, water, and on pasture.
         b. Excretion of *M. paratuberculosis* in the milk of clinically affected cows can occur but is relatively rare and probably only occurs when the cow has a fulminating type of infection.
   B. Intrauterine
      1. Intrauterine infection of fetuses from cows that have or subsequently develop clinical paratuberculosis is an infrequent mode of transmission.
   C. Herd infection
      1. *M. paratuberculosis*, an obligate parasite of ruminants, is frequently introduced into a herd by the purchase of replacement animals that are infected but do not exhibit clinical signs.

III. CLINICAL FEATURES
   A. Host range
      1. Paratuberculosis (Johne's disease) is a chronic enteric infection of ruminants.
         a. It primarily affects cattle and occasionally sheep, as well as numerous other ruminant species.
   B. Clinical signs
      1. Clinical disease is manifested as a chronic intestinal infection and is characterized by progressive weight loss, decreased milk production, diarrhea, emaciation, and eventually death.
         a. The diarrhea is initially intermittent but in time becomes more protracted. The feces are dark, semifluid, and

excreted in a steady stream with no signs of straining.
   b. Affected cattle often have a variable appetite and exhibit
       a gradual weight loss.
   c. Intermittent increases in body temperature are observed.
   d. Affected cows can live from a few weeks to many months;
       however, bulls often die within 1 week.
       (1) In most herds, the morbidity rate of clinical cases is
             usually between 1 and 10 percent per annum.
       (2) The mortality rate of clinically affected cattle
             approaches 100 percent.
   e. Asymptomatic carrier cattle have an increased incidence of
       mastitis and infertility.
   f. Clinical signs most frequently arise in thin cows within a
       few weeks after parturition of their second or third
       calves.
C. Infection and clinical status of affected herds
   1. Cattle in infected herds fall into four categories: clinically
       ill animals, asymptomatic shedders, infected cattle that are
       neither ill nor shedding, and uninfected cattle. The number of
       cattle in each category varies with husbandry practices and age
       when infected.
       a. When calves are raised separately from mature cattle and
           good husbandry practices prevail, few calves are exposed to
           infection. A majority of the calves will contract the
           infection, however, when they are raised with infected
           adults in conditions of poor sanitation.
       b. Animals infected with *M. paratuberculosis* as calves have a
           prolonged stage where they are apparently healthy. The
           transition from a subclinical to a clinical infection may
           occur at any age, but it is unusual to encounter clinical
           infections in cattle less than 2 years or more than 8 years
           of age. The peak age incidence is 3 to 6 years.
       c. Although adult cattle are the primary source of the
           organisms, they are difficult to infect, or if infected,
           they develop transient subclinical infections.
       d. In most herds, clinical disease occurs sporadically so that
           there are seldom more than one or two clinically ill
           animals at a given time.
D. Economic significance
   1. Bovine paratuberculosis causes serious economic loss in affected
       herds.
       a. The disease is widely distributed in the United States and
           has increased significantly in the last three decades.

IV. PATHOGENESIS
   A. Latency period
       1. The period from exposure to clinical disease is rarely less than
           a year and often extends for many years. It depends on the age

of the animal at exposure, virulence of the infective *M. paratuberculosis* strain, and level of exposure.

B. Intestinal infection

    1. The primary site of penetration after ingestion is the wall of the intestine at, or adjacent to, the ileocecal junction.

        a. The bacteria proliferate in the intestinal mucosa for 2 or 3 months. The host's reaction to the infection is characterized by a massive infiltration of macrophages. The microscopic lesions are characterized by intracellular and extracellular acid-fast bacilli, macrophages, epitheloid cells, multinucleated giant cells, eosinophils, lymphocytes, and plasma cells.

    2. The natural resistance of the animal largely determines the outcome of the infection. The majority will spontaneously recover, some will become chronic carriers, and a few will eventually develop clinical infections.

    3. In persistent infections, the lesions in the terminal ileum gradually extend anteriorly to the jejunum and duodenum, posteriorly to the colon, and in some cases as far as the rectum.

    4. Dissemination from the primary infectious foci in the intestine and mesenteric lymph nodes is rare, but the udder, supramammary lymph nodes and uterus in cows, and the testicles and accessory sex organs in bulls are occasionally infected.

C. Immunity

    1. Three immunological reactions to *M. paratuberculosis* or its products have been postulated to be responsible for the illness and its clinical signs.

        a. Type I reactions in the infected intestine can result in the degranulation of mast cells with histamine release and consequent diarrhea.

        b. Type III reactions are initiated by antigen-antibody complexes. Complement activation with the formation of chemotactic factors attracts leukocytes to the infectious foci, where they release enzymes and possibly other agents that injure the tissues.

        c. Type IV reactions that involve antigens of *M. paratuberculosis* and lymphocytes to these antigens can cause the release of lymphokines that may be involved in the leukopenia, anemia, and muscular atrophy of the disease.

    2. Little natural immunity can be demonstrated to the mycobacteria in animals.

        a. Antibodies and delayed hypersensitivity can be demonstrated in some infected animals but are not directly correlated with protective immunity.

        b. Cattle with paratuberculosis frequently exhibit cutaneous anergy.

V. PATHOLOGY
   A. Intestinal
       1. The affected intestine is characterized by a chronic catarrhal
           inflammation. In advanced cases, the affected intestine is
           greatly thickened and has a corrugated appearance. Petechiae on
           the crests of the ridges give a hemorrhagic appearance.
       2. In cattle that do not have gross changes in the intestine,
           microscopic lesions are most prevalent in the terminal 15 cm of
           the ileum and proximal 15 cm of the cecum.
   B. Mesenteric lymph nodes
       1. Mesenteric lymph nodes are often swollen and edematous, and
           microscopic lesions are usually situated adjacent to the
           capsule.

VI. DIAGNOSIS
   A. The reliability of the diagnostic procedures to identify infected
       animals varies markedly during the different stages of infection.
       1. Tests commonly employed include the complement-fixation (CF)
           test, intradermal (ID) johnin test, the intravenous (IV) johnin
           test, fecal smears, and fecal cultures.
           a. Johnin, an extracted antigen from *M. paratuberculosis*, has
               been used to elicit allergic responses in infected animals.
               The specificities of the johnin tests have been increased
               with the use of johnin purified protein derivative (PPD),
               which is prepared in a manner analogous to tuberculin PPD.
               Although improved, johnin PPD will still detect
               sensitization to other acid-fast bacteria, including both
               avian and mammalian tubercle bacilli.
   B. Diagnostic tests
       1. Complement-fixation test
           a. The CF test is the best serologic test available and is
               most accurate when intestinal lesions are well advanced in
               the preclinical suspect animal.
               (1) Complement-fixing antibodies generally are not
                    detectable during the first year after exposure but
                    become detectable as the lesions grow more extensive.
                    The CF titers decrease and often disappear before or
                    during the early signs of illness.
       2. ID johnin test
           a. The ID johnin test is performed by inoculating johnin PPD
               into the skin of the neck. The delayed hypersensitivity
               reactions are measured after 48 hours.
               (1) Peak responses usually occur a month or so after
                    infection and thereafter fluctuate between some degree
                    of reaction and no reaction until the intestinal
                    lesions become extensive when the response is likely
                    to be minimal. This test will identify most infected
                    cattle before clinical signs develop; however, cattle
                    with clinical infections frequently exhibit cutaneous
                    anergy.

3. IV johnin test
    a. The IV johnin test reactions are measured by increases in body temperature. A temperature rise of 1.5°F or more over the preinjection temperature is considered positive provided the pretest temperature of the animal is less than 103°F.
        (1) The IV johnin test will detect approximately 80 percent of the cattle with clinical signs and is considered more reliable than either the CF test or ID johnin test for diagnosing heavily infected cattle.

4. Fecal smears
    a. A presumptive diagnosis in asymptomatic shedders and clinically ill animals can be made if clumps of acid-fast bacilli are seen in fecal smears.
        (1) The examination of fecal smears from asymptomatic shedders is often unreliable due to intermittent shedding and to the relatively low number of mycobacteria excreted in the feces. In clinically affected animals, the bacterium can be demonstrated in 30 to 60 percent of the fecal smears.

5. Fecal cultures
    a. Isolation and identification of *M. paratuberculosis* from fecal culture is used as a definitive diagnosis.
        (1) Fecal cultures are often incubated for 16 weeks and examined periodically for growth typical of *M. paratuberculosis*. Suspect colonies are subcultured onto appropriate media with mycobactin and media without mycobactin. Subcultured specimens yielding colonies that are acid-fast and mycobactin-dependent are presumptively identified as *M. paratuberculosis*.

VII. IMMUNIZATION
   A. A federally licensed and controlled heat-killed *M. paratuberculosis* bacterin for immunization of calves less than 1 month of age can aid in controlling paratuberculosis in herds with high morbidity rates.
       1. The bacterin is administered in the brisket, and frequently fibrocaseous nodules develop at the vaccination site. The nodules are usually 2 to 5 cm in diameter but may enlarge to 10 to 15 cm. The nodules often persist and occasionally rupture and discharge an exudate.
       2. Vaccinates develop a hypersensitivity to johnin, avian tuberculin, and mammalian tuberculin. In comparative tests with these antigens, the allergic response to johnin and avian tuberculin are greater than the response to mammalian tuberculin; however, vaccination in tuberculosis-free cattle will not unduly interfere with tuberculin testing.
       3. Vaccination provides protection against clinical disease and decreases fecal excretion but does not eliminate infection.

88 | Rumenitis–Liver Abscess Complex

I. ETIOLOGY
   A. *Fusobacterium necrophorum*, an obligate anaerobic, gram-negative bacillus, is the primary etiologic agent of bovine liver abscesses.
      1. Biovars of *F. necrophorum*
         a. Of the three biovars of *F. necrophorum* (A, B, and C), only biovars A and B have been implicated in the rumenitis-liver abscess complex.
            (1) Biovar B is the predominant biovar isolated from the ruminal lesions.
            (2) Biovar A is the predominant biovar isolated from the liver abscesses.
      2. Liver abscesses
         a. Biovar A is usually found in pure culture, whereas biovar B is always found in mixed culture with either biovar A or with other bacterial species.
            (1) From mixed cultures, *Actinomyces pyogenes*, *Bacteroides* species, *Staphylococcus* species, and *Streptococcus* species are the most prevalent bacteria recovered.

II. TRANSMISSION
   A. *F. necrophorum* and other bacteria isolated from liver abscesses are considered to be components of the endogenous rumen flora.

III. CLINICAL FEATURES
   A. Liver abscesses can occur in all ages and breeds of cattle. The highest prevalence is in feedlot cattle where liver abscesses have been reported in as many as 95 percent of fattened cattle.
   B. Clinical signs
      1. Cattle with liver abscesses seldom exhibit clinical signs.
      2. A few cattle have liver abscesses that rupture and drain into the peritoneal cavity, the hepatic blood vessels, or the caudal vena cava.
         a. Two clinical syndromes are associated with ruptured abscesses. Approximately 60 percent of the cattle die suddenly, and the remaining 40 percent have vague digestive disturbances and varying degrees of respiratory distress.
   C. Economic significance
      1. Liver abscesses are responsible for economic losses to beef packers when affected livers are condemned as unfit for human consumption and to cattle producers when the abscesses reduce

the efficiency of feed utilization. It has been estimated that 10 percent of the livers of all cattle slaughtered in the United States are condemned.

IV. PATHOGENESIS
   A. Rumenitis and liver abscesses in cattle constitute a disease complex. The ruminal lesions are the primary foci of infection, and liver abscesses are the secondary foci of infection.
      1. Rumenitis in feedlot cattle is usually associated with the ingestion and rapid intraruminal fermentation of dietary carbohydrate with a subsequent increased acidity of the ruminal fluid.
         a. Feedlot cattle develop significantly more rumenitis when they are immediately transferred from a roughage ration to a fattening ration.
      2. *F. necrophorum*, alone or with other bacterial species, colonize the ulcerated rumen wall.
         a. Bacterial emboli in the lesions invade the hepatic portal venous system and are transported to the liver, where some of the emboli will establish foci of the hepatic necrobacillosis.
      3. The average duration of an *F. necrophorum* culture-positive abscess is 3 to 4 months.
         a. The majority of the abscesses will resolve as a sterile fibrous scar. This can occur anytime after 45 days.
   B. Although antibodies to *F. necrophorum* develop during the course of the infection, protective immunity does not develop.

V. PATHOLOGY
   A. Hepatic necrobacillosis lesions of less than 6 days duration have a pale yellowish color and are spherical with irregular outlines.
   B. Abscesses of more than 6 days duration may enlarge up to 6 cm in diameter. The majority will eventually resolve as sterile fibrous scars.
      1. Affected livers usually have from 3 to 10 abscesses but may have up to 100.

VI. DIAGNOSIS
   A. Postmortem lesions
      1. Most liver abscesses are observed at slaughter.

VII. IMMUNIZATION
   A. Commercial *F. necrophorum* vaccines are not available.

89 | Thromboembolic Meningoencephalitis

I. ETIOLOGY
   A. *Haemophilus somnus*, a facultative anaerobic, gram-negative bacillus, is considered to be an obligate parasite of cattle and possibly of other ruminants.

II. TRANSMISSION
   A. Inhalation of aerosols contaminated with *H. somnus* from cattle with respiratory infections is the primary mode of transmission.

III. CLINICAL FEATURES
   A. Four clinical syndromes
      1. Subclinical infections
         a. This is the most common form of infection. Serologic surveys indicate that almost 100 percent of the feedlot cattle in some areas have antibodies to *H. somnus* but with no clinical history characteristic of the disease.
         b. Clinical signs are not observed.
      2. Acute respiratory infections
         a. *H. somnus* may cause primary respiratory infections.
         b. Clinical signs are fever, a dry hacking cough, and dyspnea.
         c. Other bacteria, particularly *Actinomyces pyogenes*, *Pasteurella haemolytica*, and *P. multocida*, can invade secondarily, causing more serious disease.
      3. Septicemic and thromboembolic meningoencephalitis (TEME) infections
         a. TEME is the classic disease associated with *H. somnus*. It is usually associated with prior respiratory problems in the herd.
            (1) Animals with septicemia but no encephalitis are febrile and may show lameness or other symptoms associated with septicemia and a vasculitis.
            (2) Animals with TEME show symptoms of central nervous system disturbance and have high mortality rates.
      4. Chronic infections
         a. Chronic infections often are sequelae to the acute respiratory syndrome.
         b. Clinical signs
            (1) Respiratory symptoms, chronic tracheitis with a dry hacking cough
            (2) Lameness due to the joint infections and arthritis

(3) Chronically infected animals, frequently catagorized as "poor doers"

IV. PATHOGENESIS
A. Inhalation of *H. somnus*
   1. Respiratory infections are either subclinical or clinical.
      a. The upper respiratory infections are characterized by laryngitis and tracheitis, and if the lower respiratory tract is involved, by pneumonia and pleuritis.
   2. The septicemia disseminates the infection to other tissues, including the central nervous system.
B. Immunity to natural infection is poorly understood.

V. PATHOLOGY
A. Respiratory lesions are nonspecific and include laryngitis, tracheitis, pneumonia, and fibrinous pleuritis.
B. Septicemic infections cause hemorrhages in the heart, kidney, skeletal muscle, gastrointestinal tract, and serosal surfaces. If the joints are infected, the synovial fluid is cloudy.
C. Neural infections cause multiple foci of hemorrhage and necrosis. Rusty brown spots in the brain are pathognomonic.

VI. DIAGNOSIS
A. Clinical signs and herd history
   1. Concurrent respiratory disease, lameness, and encephalitis
B. Postmortem lesions
   1. Brain lesions are pathognomonic.
C. Culture
   1. Isolation and biochemical identification of *H. somnus*
      a. *H. somnus* will grow on blood agar under an atmosphere of 5 to 10 percent carbon dioxide and air. The bacterium does not require either factors X or V for growth.

VII. IMMUNIZATION
A. Commercial *H. somnus* vaccines are effective in preventing TEME, but it is debatable if they significantly reduce the incidence of respiratory disease.

90 | Tuberculosis

I. ETIOLOGY

A. *Mycobacterium bovis*, an obligate aerobic, gram-positive, acid-fast bacillus, is the primary agent of bovine tuberculosis. The bovine is the primary host.
1. Cattle are also susceptible to *M. tuberculosis*, although man is the primary host.
2. *M. bovis* and *M. tuberculosis* are facultative intracellular pathogens.

II. TRANSMISSION

A. Inhalation
1. Inhalation of infected aerosols is the most common mode of transmission. The lungs are the primary site of infection.
B. Ingestion
1. Ingestion of contaminated feed and water is an infrequent mode of infection. The intestinal tract is the primary site of infection.

III. CLINICAL FEATURES

A. Bovine tuberculosis is a chronic disease that is often present in cattle without symptoms.
B. It is a relatively uncommon disease in the United States. This has largely resulted from the successful efforts of a national eradication program for the disease.
1. The federal program is based on the test and slaughter of cattle with tuberculosis. Most infected cattle herds are identified by the traceback of animals with lesions at slaughter to the herds of origin. The tubercle lesions found at slaughter are cultured by either state or federal laboratories to confirm the diagnosis. All animals in the herd of origin are tuberculin-tested, and the positive reactors are slaughtered. The whole herd is eliminated if possible.

IV. PATHOGENESIS

A. Tubercles, the characteristic lesion of tuberculosis, can form in any organ in which reticuloendothelial tissue is present.
1. The lungs are the primary foci of infection following inhalation of the organisms.
2. The pulmonary and tracheobronchial lymph nodes, which drain the

lymphatics from the lungs, are common secondary foci of infection.
3. Miliary tuberculosis with multiple lesions in multiple organs can result from the erosion of a primary lesion into a blood vessel with hematogenous spread throughout the body.
B. Immunity
1. Cellular immunity is the primary mechanism of host resistance.
2. Humoral immunity plays little, if any, role in immunity to tuberculosis.

V. PATHOLOGY
A. The tubercle is the characteristic granulomatous lesion of tuberculosis.
1. In cattle, calcification of these lesions is common, particularly in the lymph nodes.

VI. DIAGNOSIS
A. Market traceback program
1. Postmortem lesions are cultured for *M. bovis* to confirm the diagnosis.
B. Tuberculin tests
1. Tuberculin tests measure the delayed hypersensitivity of infected cattle.
   a. Tuberculin is administered intradermally, and the reactions are measured at 48 to 72 hours.
   b. Cattle with severe terminal tuberculosis may be anergic.
2. Two types of tuberculin tests are used in cattle.
   a. The caudal fold test uses *M. bovis* PPD, which is inoculated into skin of the caudal fold.
   b. The comparative cervical test uses both *M. bovis* PPD and *M. avium* PPD, which are inoculated into the skin of the neck.
      (1) It is more sensitive and definitive than the caudal fold test and is used to clarify the status of suspects. In *M. bovis*-infected cattle, the reactions to *M. bovis* PPD are greater than those to *M. avium* PPD, whereas in cattle sensitized to *M. avium* or saprophytic mycobacteria, the reactions to *M. avium* PPD are greater than those to *M. bovis* PPD.

VII. IMMUNIZATION
A. Federal regulations prohibit the vaccination of cattle.
1. BCG (bacillus of Calmette and Guerin) vaccine is a live avirulent bovine strain of *M. bovis*. The vaccine is used in some countries to immunize cattle. Only cattle that are negative tuberculin reactors should be vaccinated.

PART **2**	Ovine Diseases

91	Caseous Lymphadenitis

I. ETIOLOGY
A. *Corynebacterium pseudotuberculosis*, a facultative anaerobic, gram-positive bacillus, is a facultative intracellular pathogen.

II. TRANSMISSION
A. Mechanical
1. Most infections are transmitted mechanically from animal to animal via fomites. Draining abscesses are a primary source of the organisms.
   a. Shearing of sheep with contaminated shears is a common mode of mechanical transmission.
   b. Abscesses that result from mechanical transmission are usually found in the superficial lymph nodes.
B. Ingestion
1. Ingestion of exudate with *C. pseudotuberculosis* has been postulated as the mode of transmission when internal abscesses develop in lymph nodes draining the respiratory and gastrointestinal tracts.

III. CLINICAL FEATURES
A. Clinical signs
1. Ovine caseous lymphadenitis is usually characterized by abscessation of one or more superficial lymph nodes. Progressive debilitation occurs in sheep with chronic infections, particularly if internal abscesses are present. Internal abscesses are most prevalent in the bronchial and mediastinal lymph nodes.
   a. Abscesses that ulcerate discharge a thick cream-colored purulent material.

B. Incidence
1. The incidence of caseous lymphadenitis is much higher in older sheep.

IV. PATHOGENESIS
A. Infection
1. A skin wound or some other mode of traumatic inoculation is considered necessary for *C. pseudotuberculosis* to penetrate the skin.
2. The bacteria spread from the initial skin infection to the contiguous lymph nodes.
   a. *C. pseudotuberculosis* has a cell wall lipid that is toxic for the host phagocytes and helps protect the bacterium from the antibacterial enzymes of host phagocytes, thus permitting intracellular survival.
   b. The bacterium also produces a phospholipase exotoxin that degrades the sphingomyelin of the vascular endothelial cells. This results in an increased permeability of the local vascular bed, leading to intense fluid and cellular exudation.
3. Lesions in the lymph nodes have dry caseous centers and eventually form concentric laminations around the abscess core.
B. Immunity
1. Antibodies to the exotoxin neutralize its permeability effects and are effective in reducing the bacterial spread from the initial skin infection; however, cellular immunity is considered to be responsible for the protective immunity induced in natural infections.

V. PATHOLOGY
A. Caseous abscesses with concentric laminations are characteristic lesions.

VI. DIAGNOSIS
A. Clinical signs (above)
B. Pathology (above)
C. Culture
1. Isolation and biochemical identification of *C. pseudotuberculosis*

VII. IMMUNIZATION
A. Autogenous *C. pseudotuberculosis* bacterins have shown some efficacy in preventing abscesses.

92 | Dermatophilosis

I. ETIOLOGY
   A. *Dermatophilus congolensis* is a facultative anaerobic, gram-positive bacillus.
      1. The bacterium has two characteristic morphologic forms: nonmotile filamentous hyphae and motile zoospores. The zoospores are the infective form.

II. TRANSMISSION
   A. Infected animals
      1. Infected animals are the reservoir of infection.
         a. Dermatophilosis is ubiquitous among domestic herbivores. The bacteria survive during dormant periods in chronically affected animals. The bacterium exists in a quiescent form in the integument until exacerbation occurs when climatic conditions are favorable for its infectivity.
         b. Dermatophilosis is contagious only in the sense that any reduction in the general or local resistance of an animal favors establishment of infection and subsequent disease.
   B. Predisposing factors
      1. To establish infection, the zoospores must overcome the protective barriers of the skin.
         a. Factors such as prolonged wetting by rain, high humidity, high temperature, and various ectoparasites that reduce or permeate the natural barriers of the integument influence the development, prevalence, seasonal incidence, and transmission of dermatophilosis.
         b. The spread of infection also may follow shearing, dipping, or the introduction of infected animals into a flock.
   C. Modes of transmission
      1. Direct contact with infected animals
      2. Biting insects, such as ticks and flies, which are mechanical vectors of zoospores
         a. Insect vectors can play a significant role in the persistence and spread of infection.

III. CLINICAL FEATURES
   A. Dermatophilosis is an acute or chronic bacterial infection of the epidermis characterized by an exudative dermatitis with scab formation.

1. The disease occurs in all ages but is most prevalent in young animals.
2. The dermatitis on an individual animal can vary from the acute to the chronic form, but all lesions usually are not at the same stage of progression.
3. The incidence in flocks will vary due to husbandry practices, time of year, and ectoparasite populations.
   a. Epidemics usually occur during wet periods, when protective skin barriers are damaged or deficient.

B. Clinical signs
   1. The condition is called mycotic dermatitis or lumpy wool when the wooled areas of the body are affected and strawberry foot rot when the distal portions of the limbs are affected.
      a. Lumpy wool resulting from chronic *D. congolensis* infection is characterized by the continuous production of scab material over a period of months or years. The scab material is bound by wool fibers and forms dense, pyramid-shaped masses over the back, flanks, face, and head.
      b. Strawberry foot rot is a proliferative dermatitis that initiates at the coronet region of the feet but can develop into an ulcerative dermatitis affecting the skin of the legs from the coronet to the carpus or hock.
   2. Few affected sheep exhibit pruritus.
   3. Sheep with severe generalized infections often lose condition and have difficulty in movement and in prehension of food if the lips and muzzle are severely affected. Deaths occasionally occur due to generalized disease with or without secondary infection.
   4. Most affected sheep will recover spontaneously during dry weather.

IV. PATHOGENESIS
A. Acute infections
   1. Moisture facilitates the release of zoospores from the lesions and their subsequent penetration of the epidermis.
      a. Zoospores are most active in the first hours after their release from the hyphae, when they are independent of external nutrient sources.
      b. Water provides a medium of transport for the zoospores.
   2. Zoospores initiate new foci of infection.
      a. The respiratory efflux of carbon dioxide from the skin is of optimal level to attract the zoospores to susceptible areas on the skin surface.
      b. The zoospores adhere to the skin and then germinate to produce hyphae, which penetrate into the living epidermis. The hyphae subsequently spread in all directions from the initial focus of infection.

   3. The invaded epidermis is eventually separated from its dermal
      matrix, and finally the epithelium is cast off and separates
      from the skin in the form of a scab.
      a. New layers of scab are added, thus causing a gradual
         increase in the size of the scab.
         (1) The infected tissues separate as a crust or scab after
             10 to 14 days.
B. Chronic infections
   1. In chronic infections, the initial process of tissue invasion
      and host reaction are similar to the acute lesion.
      a. The infection persists because of the continued invasion of
         new epidermis.
C. Immunity
   1. Natural resistance to acute infection with *D. congolensis* is due
      to the phagocytosis of the infective zoospores by neutrophils,
      but once infection is established, there is relatively little
      movement of leukocytes into the epidermis and little, if any,
      phagocytosis.
   2. Previously infected animals do not develop a significant
      immunity to reinfection.

V. PATHOLOGY
   A. Gross lesions are characterized by scab material bound by wool fibers
      that form dense, pyramid-shaped masses.
   B. Microscopic lesions reveal that the epidermis is covered with an
      exudate of keratinized epithelial cells, leukocytes, and inspissated
      serum.
      1. The organisms, which appear as branching hyphae with
         multidimensional septations and as individual coccoid cells and
         zoospores, are present throughout the epidermis but are more
         numerous on the outer edge of the lesions.

VI. DIAGNOSIS
   A. Clinical signs
      1. Presumptive diagnosis of dermatophilosis depends largely on the
         appearance of lesions in clinically diseased animals.
   B. Direct smears
      1. Giemsa-stained smears of lesions demonstrate the characteristic
         morphology of the hyphae in the epidermis.
   C. Microscopic examination
      1. Histopathological sections of scabs
   D. Culture
      1. Isolation and biochemical identification of *D. congolensis*

VII. IMMUNIZATION
   A. Commercial *D. congolensis* vaccines are not available.

93 | Enterotoxemia

I. ETIOLOGY

A. *Clostridium perfringens* is an obligate anaerobic, gram-positive, sporeforming bacillus.

1. Clinically, *C. perfringens* types A, B, C, and D produce different forms of enterotoxemia in sheep. The clinical disease and lesions produced by each toxigenic type are largely dependent on the major lethal toxins of each type of *C. perfringens* and on the amounts of each toxin produced (Table 93.1).

Table 93.1. Major lethal toxins of *C. perfringens*

Type	Toxins			
	Alpha	Beta	Epsilon	Iota
A	++	–	–	–
B	+	++	+	–
C	+	++	–	–
D	+	–	++	–

Note: ++ = large amount; + = small amount; – = none produced.

II. TRANSMISSION

A. Ingestion

1. Clinical infections tend to recur on the same premises, and the spores of *C. perfringens* can be isolated from soil in endemic areas. Clinically affected sheep also can contaminate soil with large numbers of *C. perfringens*. However, the ingestion of vegetative cells or spores rarely results in clinical disease.

B. Endogenous flora

1. *C. perfringens* is often found in small numbers in the intestinal tracts of healthy sheep. These endogenous bacteria produce disease only when conditions permit a dramatic increase in their population and the intestinal environment becomes favorable for toxin production.

   a. In healthy animals, *C. perfringens* is present only in the large intestine, but in disease, the bacteria colonize the small intestine, particularly the ileum and jejunum.

III. CLINICAL FEATURES

A. The enterotoxemias produced by *C. perfringens* type A, B, C, and D are acute, noncontagious diseases that originate in the lower small and large intestines. Apparently healthy sheep on full feed are often affected.

1. *C. perfringens* type A
   a. It primarily affects lambs under 3 months of age.
   b. This form of enterotoxemia is characterized by severe anemia, icterus, and hemoglobinuria. Almost all of the clinically affected lambs will die with a rapid course from onset to termination.
2. *C. perfringens* type B
   a. It affects neonatal lambs less than 10 days of age.
   b. This form of enterotoxemia is characterized by an extensive hemorrhagic enteritis of the small and large intestines. The disease is commonly called lamb dysentery. Affected lambs are depressed, exhibit abdominal pain, and have dark-colored semifluid feces. Death may occur without premonitary signs, and mortality approaches 100 percent of the affected lambs.
3. *C. perfringens* type C
   a. It can affect both neonatal lambs and adult sheep.
   b. In lambs, there is an acute hemorrhagic enteritis with diarrhea. Affected lambs often die within 12 hours of exhibiting clinical signs.
   c. In adult sheep, terminal convulsions and sudden death are primary clinical manifestations. Diarrhea rarely occurs.
4. *C. perfringens* type D
   a. It primarily affects feedlot sheep on a full grain ration.
   b. Peracute infections are the rule, and the animals are often found dead without premonitory clinical signs. Terminal convulsions occasionally are observed.

IV. PATHOGENESIS
   A. *C. perfringens*, which is frequently present in the large intestine in low numbers, proliferates rapidly and colonizes the ileum and jejunum and produces large amounts of the exotoxins. The concentration of the toxins in the intestine needs to be maintained at high levels for a period of time for intoxication to occur, because only small amounts of the toxins reach the bloodstream.
      1. Clinical and pathological changes are due to the amount of each toxin produced, particularly the major lethal toxins.
         a. Alpha toxin causes intravascular hemolysis and intestinal hemorrhages.
         b. Beta toxin causes intestinal necrosis and has a lethal effect on the nervous system.
         c. Epsilon toxin causes edema and hemorrhages and has a lethal effect on the nervous system.
   B. Acquired immunity
      1. Sheep exposed to sublethal levels of toxin develop antibodies that provide protective immunity to subsequent intoxication.

V. PATHOLOGY

A. Enterotoxemia affects primarily the intestinal tract and the nervous system, but lesions vary considerably with the toxigenic type and duration of illness.

1. *C. perfringens* type A
   a. The necropsy findings are severe anemia, icterus, hemoglobinuria, and multiple hemorrhages on the viscera.

2. *C. perfringens* type B
   a. There is usually extensive hemorrhagic enteritis of both the small and large intestine. Intestinal ulceration occurs primarily in the small intestine.

3. *C. perfringens* type C
   a. Most intestinal lesions are found in the jejunum and ileum and can range from hyperemia to hemorrhage and necrosis. The large intestine is usually normal in appearance.

4. *C. perfringens* type D
   a. The intestinal lesions tend to be minimal. The brain lesions are foci of liquefactive necrosis.

VI. DIAGNOSIS

A. Clinical signs and pathology
   1. Clinical diagnoses are often based on history, enteric and neurological clinical signs, and gross intestinal lesions.

B. Direct smears and culture
   1. Presumptive microbiological diagnoses are often based on finding large numbers of gram-positive bacilli in smears of intestinal contents and on the cultural isolation and identification of *C. perfringens*.
      a. When *C. perfringens* is cultured on blood agar under anaerobic conditions, the colonies are moderate to large in size, gray, glistening, and surrounded by a double zone of hemolysis. The inner zone of complete hemolysis is due to the hemolytic activity of theta toxin and the outer zone of partial hemolysis to alpha toxin.
      b. In litmus milk, *C. perfringens* produced a characteristic clot, which is formed due to the production of acid and large amounts of gas from carbohydrate fermentation. This reaction is often referred to as "stormy" fermentation.

C. Toxin type identification
   1. To confirm a diagnosis of enterotoxemia, the major lethal exotoxins must be demonstrated in the intestinal contents.
   2. Nagler reaction
      a. The Nagler reaction is used to identify *C. perfringens* by neutralization of alpha toxin by specific antitoxin.
         (1) A colony of *C. perfringens* is streaked on an egg yolk agar plate, where half of the plate has been spread with antitoxin. A zone of opacity is produced adjacent to the *C. perfringens* colonies on the

untreated half of the plate but no opacity on the area
with the antitoxin, because the antibody in the
antitoxin neutralizes the lecithinase activity of
alpha toxin.

VII. IMMUNIZATION
    A. Passive immunity
        1. Commercial-type specific antitoxins are available.
    B. Active immunity
        1. Commercial-type specific toxoids provide protective immunity.

94	Enzootic Abortion

I. ETIOLOGY
    A. *Chlamydia psittaci* is an aerobic, gram-negative, obligate
intracellular bacterium.
        1. It can infect a variety of nucleated cell types, where the
bacterium proliferates in cytoplasmic vacuoles.
        2. The bacterium has two characteristic morphologic forms:
elementary bodies and reticulate bodies. The elementary bodies
are the infective form.

II. TRANSMISSION
    A. Ingestion
        1. Ingestion of elementary bodies is the primary mode of
transmission.
            a. During abortion epidemics, large numbers of chlamydiae are
shed in the uterine fluids and fetuses when ewes abort.
            b. During interepidemic periods, fecal shedding from
asymptomatic carriers appears to be important in the spread
and maintenance of *C. psittaci* within a flock.
               (1) Cattle also can serve as intestinal carriers of the
infection and are potential reservoirs for sheep.
    B. Arthropod vectors
        1. *C. psittaci* has been isolated from numerous arthropods; however,
these arthropods play little, if any, role in the transmission
of ovine enzootic abortion.

III. CLINICAL FEATURES
A. Clinical signs
 1. Infection of a pregnant ewe may result in abortion, a stillbirth, or a weak lamb. Most ewes abort in the last month of gestation.
  a. Ewes are often latently infected and asymptomatic.
  b. After ewes abort, their fertility and subsequent pregnancies are not affected.
B. Incidence
 1. The abortion rate may be as high as 33 percent in a flock when it is initially exposed to *C. psittaci* infection.
 2. In subsequent years, when the infection becomes endemic in a flock, only 1 to 5 percent of the ewes will abort. First gestation ewes are most likely to abort.

IV. PATHOGENESIS
A. Sheep acquire the infection by ingesting elementary bodies. The elementary bodies infect a variety of nucleated cell types, which are transformed into reticulate bodies that subsequently proliferate in cytoplasmic inclusions.
 1. Most ewes are latently infected until the last trimester of gestation, when the bacteria induce a placentitis, resulting in abortion or a stillborn or weak lamb.

V. PATHOLOGY
A. Aborted fetuses
 1. Gross lesions are minimal and nonspecific.
 2. Microscopic lesions include splenic lymphoid follicular necrosis and a granulomatous pneumonia with neutrophils and necrotic cellular debris in the alveoli.
B. Placenta
 1. Chlamydiae-infected placentas often show thickening of the intercotyledonary areas and some clay-colored material in these areas as well as on cotyledons. The remainder of the placenta may have a normal gross appearance.

VI. DIAGNOSIS
A. Culture
 1. The stomach contents and liver from aborted fetuses are the specimens of choice for chlamydial isolation, whereas in placentas that are often heavily contaminated with other bacterial species, it is usually more difficult to isolate *C. psittaci*.
 2. Four procedures are commonly used to cultivate *C. psittaci*.
  a. Inoculation of specimens into the yolk sac of developing chicken embryos
  b. Intracerebral or intraperitoneal inoculation into 3-week-old mice

   c. Intraperitoneal inoculation of guinea pigs
   d. Inoculation of cell cultures, particularly McCoy cell
    monolayers
  B. Direct examination
   1. Microscopic examination of impression smears for chlamydial
    cytoplasmic inclusions and extracellular elementary bodies
    a. Giemsa's method stains chlamydiae a bluish-purple, and
     Gimenez and Macchiavello methods stain a bright red.
   2. Specific immunofluorescent staining for chlamydial antigens

VII. IMMUNIZATION
  A. Commercial *C. psittaci* vaccines for sheep are not available.

---

95 | Epizootic Abortion

I. ETIOLOGY
  A. *Campylobacter fetus* ss *fetus* is a microaerophilic, gram-negative
  bacillus.

II. TRANSMISSION
  A. Ingestion
   1. *C. fetus* ss *fetus* can be carried in the intestinal tract and the
    gall bladder of previously infected sheep, which spread the
    infection through fecal contamination of feed and water. This
    mode of transmission is probably responsible for maintaining the
    organism endemically within a flock.
    a. Cattle are often intestinal carriers of *C. fetus* ss *fetus*
     and may introduce the infection into a flock.
   2. In abortion epidemics, the ingestion of large doses of the agent
    from aborted fetuses and placentas is the primary mode of
    transmission.

III. CLINICAL FEATURES
  A. Clinical signs
   1. Ovine epizootic abortion is characterized by abortion during the
    last trimester of pregnancy and by the birth of dead and weak

         lambs. It is generally a flock condition, and the abortion rate is about 25 percent in most epidemic outbreaks but may be as high as 70 percent.

    2. Retained placentas are uncommon in ewes that have aborted. A ewe occasionally will die as a result of metritis, but most postparturient ewes exhibit only a mild endometritis. Postinfection infertility is rare, and the majority of the ewes will have normal lambs during subsequent pregnancies.

         a. *C. fetus* ss *fetus* is the most common cause of ovine abortion.

    3. Infection of nonpregnant sheep is asymptomatic.

IV. PATHOGENESIS
  A. Infection
    1. After the ingestion of *C. fetus* ss *fetus*-contaminated material, there is an intermittent bacteremia for 1 to 2 weeks.
       a. If the ewe is in the third trimester of pregnancy, the placenta and eventually the fetus will become infected. There is necrosis of the fetal and maternal placentome. Most fetuses are aborted, some are born dead, and a few are expelled alive but die soon after birth.
       b. The bacterium does not localize in the uterus prior to the third month of pregnancy or in the nonpregnant uterus.
  B. Immunity
    1. Following clinical infection, a convalescent immunity often persists for 2 or 3 years. Most ewes that abort lamb normally the next season.
       a. Humoral antibodies provide the protective immunity.

V. PATHOLOGY
  A. Fetuses
    1. Aborted fetuses have characteristic liver lesions 1 to 2 cm in diameter, light-colored, and randomly distributed on the surface of the organ.
    2. Placental lesions are more pronounced over the placentomes than in the intercotyledonary areas. A yellowish brown exudate often covers the surface of the enlarged cotyledons.

VI. DIAGNOSIS
  A. Herd history and clinical signs (above)
  B. Pathology (above)
  C. Culture
    1. Isolation and biochemical identification of *C. fetus* ss *fetus*

VII. IMMUNIZATION
  A. Commercial *C. fetus* ss *fetus* bacterins produce good humoral immunity and are highly effective in the control of the disease.

96 | Infective Bulbar Necrosis

I. ETIOLOGY
   A. Ovine infective bulbar necrosis (heel abscess) is caused by a synergistic infection of *Fusobacterium necrophorum* and *Actinomyces pyogenes*.
      1. *F. necrophorum* is an obligate anaerobic, gram-negative bacillus, and *A. pyogenes* is a facultative anaerobic, gram-positive coccobacillus.

II. TRANSMISSION
   A. *F. necrophorum* and *A. pyogenes* are normal flora of the ovine digestive tract and occur in the environment as fecal contaminates.

III. CLINICAL FEATURES
   A. Ovine infective bulbar necrosis can occur in all ages and breeds of sheep but is most common in pregnant ewes.
   B. The heel abscesses manifest themselves 1 to 4 weeks following the primary interdigital dermatitis.
      1. One or more feet can be infected, and the severity of the infection can vary from foot to foot.
      2. The medial digits of the hind feet are most frequently affected.
      3. Healing in untreated sheep is slow and may take up to 3 months.
   C. Economic significance
      1. Ovine infective bulbar necrosis is the most destructive infection of the ovine foot, and next to ovine contagious foot rot it causes the largest economic loss among sheep.

IV. PATHOGENESIS
   A. Interdigital dermatitis
      1. *F. necrophorum* and *A. pyogenes* establish a mixed infection in the primary interdigital lesions that can later penetrate the heel.
   B. Heel abscesses
      1. Lesions are most common in the medial digits of the hind limbs of pregnant ewes.
         a. It has been postulated that in late pregnancy the increased weight on the hind feet causes a vascular stasis and a reduced oxygen tension in the digital cushion, thereby predisposing it to *F. necrophorum* invasion.
         b. *F. necrophorum* is the predominant bacterium in the early necrotizing lesions, which are characterized by narrow

            pockets of necrosis extending into the fibrous tissue of
the digital cushion.

    c. *A. pyogenes* is the predominant bacterium in the older more
suppurative lesions that frequently form abscesses.

  2. Permanently deformed digits are a frequent sequela.

C. Synergistic factors

  1. *F. necrophorum* produces a leukocidal exotoxin that protects *A.
pyogenes* from phagocytosis and thus enables it to proliferate in
the tissues.

  2. *A. pyogenes* produces a diffusible factor that stimulates the
proliferation of *F. necrophorum* in the tissues.

D. Immunity

  1. Infection does not stimulate protective immunity, so sheep that
have recovered are susceptible to reinfection.

V. PATHOLOGY

A. Abscesses on heels of the digits

VI. DIAGNOSIS

A. Clinical signs

  1. Diagnosis is usually based on the lesions.

B. Microscopic examination and culture

  1. Gram-stained smears of exudate are a valuable diagnostic aid.

  2. Isolation and biochemical identification of the etiologic agents
occasionally are done to confirm the diagnosis.

VII. IMMUNIZATION

A. Commercial *F. necrophorum* vaccines are not available.

97 | Ovine Contagious Foot Rot

I. ETIOLOGY
   A. Ovine contagious foot rot is caused by a synergistic infection of *Bacteroides nodosus* and *Fusobacterium necrophorum*, both obligate anaerobic, gram-negative bacilli.
      1. *Actinomyces pyogenes* and motile fusiforms are commonly found in the hoof lesions but do not play a primary role in the pathogenesis of the disease.

II. TRANSMISSION
   A. Environmental
      1. Infected sheep serve as reservoirs of *B. nodosus*, an obligate parasite of the digital epidermis.
         a. Pastures are contaminated from the infected sheep. Under normal conditions, *B. nodosus* will not survive on pasture for more than 2 weeks.
      2. *F. necrophorum*, normal flora of the ovine digestive tract, occurs in the environment as a fecal contaminant.
   B. Predisposing factors
      1. Ovine foot rot can spread rapidly through a susceptible flock when environmental conditions are favorable for transmission.
         a. Abundant moisture, warm weather, and the presence of infected sheep are usually required for transmission.
            (1) Transmission ceases or is markedly decreased during periods of hot dry weather or when the average ambient temperatures are below 10°C.
         b. Other predisposing factors, such as hoof cracks, skin scratches, overgrown hoofs, and foreign matter between the digits, can alter the integrity of the interdigital skin and hoof, rendering the feet susceptible to bacterial invasion.

III. CLINICAL FEATURES
   A. Ovine foot rot is manifested as a painful and debilitating disease.
      1. Sheep with acute infections or mild chronic lesions frequently show pain when walking and may have a reduced rate of weight gain and wool growth due to reduced food consumption.
      2. Chronically affected sheep with severe lesions may walk on their knees, suffer considerable weight loss through failure to graze, and have an increased susceptibility to pregnancy toxemia.

IV. PATHOGENESIS
  A. Foot rot is usually initiated when the feet are subjected to prolonged wetness.
      1. The moisture-induced hyperkeratosis of the soft horn in the region of the skin horn junction causes a thickening and maceration of the interdigital skin.
  B. Bacteria present in the feces-contaminated environment colonize the interdigital skin and initiate a bacterial dermatitis.
      1. In the interdigital dermatitis lesions, *F. necrophorum* is the primary pathogen. *F. necrophorum* is dermonecrotic and produces a leukocidal exotoxin that protects itself and other bacteria from phagocytosis. When present, *A. pyogenes* produces a factor that stimulates the growth of *F. necrophorum*.
      2. The inflammation, anaerobiosis, and hyperkeratosis associated with the bacterial colonization of the interdigital skin facilitates the secondary infection of *B. nodosus*.
  C. *B. nodosus* is the primary pathogen in the hoof lesions.
      1. The fimbriae of *B. nodosus* adhere to the epidermal matrix of the horn, and the proteases produced by *B. nodosus* damage the horn.
      2. *F. necrophorum* is responsible for most of the necrosis and purulent exudate in the infected horn.
      3. If present, motile fusiforms increase the severity of the condition.
  D. Clinical disease does not stimulate a solid or lasting immunity. Even sheep that have recently recovered from foot rot are often susceptible to reinfection.

V. PATHOLOGY
  A. Interdigital lesions
      1. The interdigital dermatitis lesions frequently heal after a brief course, but they may slough and leave an erosion.
  B. Hoof lesions
      1. Acute foot rot
          a. The gross lesions are nondescript.
      2. Chronic foot rot
          a. The gross lesions are characterized by an undermining of the hoof with purulent exudate. The lesions eventually will extend under the axial wall and then under the sole of the hoof.

VI. DIAGNOSIS
  A. Clinical signs
      1. Clinical diagnosis is usually based on a flock history of chronic involvement of the feet with outbreaks of the disease, occurring during periods of warm moist weather.
          a. An affected animal may not be lame at all times, and the only way to detect every case is to examine all the feet of each sheep.

    B.   Direct smears
        1.   Microscopic examination of gram-stained exudate from the lesions
            a.   *B. nodosus* is a large gram-negative barbell or club-shaped bacterium and is etiologically specific for foot rot.
            b.   Fusiforms, gram-positive coccobacilli of *A. pyogenes*, and gram-negative filamentous rods of *F. necrophorum* are commonly observed, but these bacteria are not etiologically specific for foot rot.
    C.   Culture
        1.   The cultural and identification procedures for *B. nodosus* are difficult and seldom used to confirm the clinical diagnosis.

VII. IMMUNIZATION
    A.   Commercial bacterins
        1.   Commercial *B. nodosus* bacterins are prophylactically and therapeutically effective.
            a.   Prophylactically, it is desirable to vaccinate sheep just prior to anticipated periods of transmission so that the flock is most resistant when subjected to challenge. This reduces the number of new cases and the severity of the disease in newly affected sheep.
            b.   Therapeutically, vaccination accelerates healing, which is generally demonstrated as a progressive improvement within 4 to 5 weeks. The response may range from an increased body weight to complete resolution of clinical signs and lesions.
    B.   Autogenous bacterins
        1.   Autogenous bacterins prepared from field strains of *B. nodosus* are often preferred to the commercial bacterins due to the diversity of the fimbrial and cell wall antigens.

| PART 3 | Porcine Diseases |

| 98 | Atrophic Rhinitis |

I. ETIOLOGY

A. *Bordetella bronchiseptica* is an obligate aerobic, gram-negative bacillus.

1. *Pasteurella multocida* type D can also induce rhinitis in pigs.

2. Other microorganisms, including *Haemophilus parasuis* and cytomegalovirus have been associated with porcine atrophic rhinitis; these microorganisms, however, are not considered to play a major role in the pathogenesis of the condition.

II. TRANSMISSION

A. Inhalation

1. Droplet transmission from symptomatic infected and asymptomatic carrier swine to susceptible swine is the primary means of transmission.

2. Aerosols from nonporcine carriers is a mode by which bordetellae can be introduced into a herd of susceptible swine. Cats are common carriers.

B. Environmental

1. Bordetellae can survive in the soil for up to 6 weeks.

III. CLINICAL FEATURES

A. Atrophic rhinitis is an inflammation of mucous membranes of the nasal cavity with hypoplasia of the nasal turbinates.

1. Three conditions are required for severe turbinate damage to occur.

a. The pigs must be infected at less than 8 weeks of age.

b. The infections must be present for at least 3 to 5 weeks.

c. The infections must be with a virulent strain of *B. bronchiseptica.*

B. Incidence
1. In the major swine-producing areas in the United States, an estimated 5 to 10 percent of slaughtered swine have turbinate atrophy.

IV. PATHOGENESIS
A. Infection of nasal epithelium
1. The bordetellae adhere to the epithelium.
2. The bacteria release an exotoxin that diffuses into the newly ossifying tissues in the nasal turbinates.
a. There is degeneration of osteoblasts with subsequent hypoplasia of the nasal turbinates. The ventral turbinates are most severely affected.
B. Age susceptibility
1. All ages of swine are susceptible to *B. bronchiseptica* infection of the nasal mucous membranes (Table 98.1). Only pigs less than 8 weeks of age will develop hypoplasia of the nasal turbinates. Pigs over 8 weeks are apparently resistant to the detrimental effects of *B. bronchiseptica* and exhibit only a mild rhinitis or asymptomatic infections.

Table 98.1. Clinical syndromes of *B. bronchiseptica* infection

| Age of Piglet | Rhinitis | Atrophic Rhinitis | |
		Mild	Severe
<3 wk	+	+	+
3-8 wk	+	+	-
>8 wk	+	-	-

C. Sequelae to atrophic rhinitis
1. Pigs with clinical atrophic rhinitis lesions have an increased incidence of respiratory disease due to loss of filtering action of the nasal turbinates.
a. Opportunistic bacteria in the genera *Bordetella*, *Haemophilus*, *Mycoplasma*, and *Pasteurella* are commonly isolated from secondary pneumonias.
D. Immunity
1. Elimination of infection is slow, ranging from 4 weeks to 3 years. After 1 year, only 10 to 20 percent of swine remain carriers.
2. Local immunity is probably due to sIgA.

V. PATHOLOGY
A. Facial deformity, in which the snout is twisted, may occur in severe cases.
B. The gross nasal turbinate lesions vary from mild to severe. The scrolls of the ventral turbinates are first reduced in size, and as

the disease progresses, producing more severe disease, there is hypoplasia of the scrolls of the dorsal turbinates.
  1. The hypoplasia of the nasal turbinates is best demonstrated by making a cross section of the snout at the second premolar tooth.

VI. DIAGNOSIS
  A. Clinical signs and pathology
    1. Mild infections
      a. Rhinitis may be the only sign of infection.
    2. Severe infections
      a. The snout is often twisted with hypoplasia of the nasal turbinates.
  B. Culture
    1. Isolation and biochemical identification of *B. bronchiseptica*

VII. IMMUNIZATION
  A. Commercial bacterins are commonly used.
    1. Pig bacterin is usually given to piglets at 7 days of age with a booster at 28 days of age.
    2. Sow bacterin is usually given to sows from 2 to 4 weeks prior to farrowing.
      a. The two bacterins used together provide maximum protection.
  B. Autogenous bacterins have proven effective.

99	Colibacillosis

I. ETIOLOGY
  A. *Escherichia coli* is a facultative anaerobic, gram-negative bacillus.

II. TRANSMISSION
  A. Enteric flora and ingestion
    1. *E. coli*, a normal intestinal flora of pigs, is found in the environment as a fecal contaminant.
      a. Although there are innumerable serovars of *E. coli* in a herd, only a few serovars possess the necessary virulence factors to cause clinical colibacillosis.
      b. Enteric infections caused by pathogenic *E. coli* strains can

either be part of the normal intestinal microflora and proliferate within the intestinal tract to attain an infective dose level or be acquired by the ingestion of feces-contaminated material, particularly food and water.

B. Intestinal homostasis
1. Two main mechanisms help control the population size of *E. coli* in the intestinal tract.
a. The competitive antagonistic interaction with other bacterial species as well as between *E. coli* strains helps restrict the intestinal proliferation of pathogenic strains of *E. coli*.
b. Local intestinal immunity helps prevent the colonization of the intestinal epithelial cells, protecting against potential bacterial invasion.

C. Factors associated with colibacillosis
1. Establishment of the intestinal flora in the neonatal pig
a. At birth, the intestinal tract is sterile but rapidly is colonized from the mouth and rectum. The initial microflora is acquired from the dam's vaginal and perianal flora as well as from the environmental microbiota. Within hours after birth, the neonate's gastrointestinal tract becomes colonized by coliforms, lactobacilli, and obligate anaerobes.
b. The balance of the gastrointestinal flora is then controlled by numerous factors, including the acid secreted in the stomach, the ingestion of immunoglobulins and other protective factors in the colostrum and milk, and the establishment of lactobacilli as the dominant organisms in the stomach and upper small intestine. Obligate anaerobic bacterial species comprise the major flora of the ileum and large intestine.
(1) The *Lactobacillus* species produce acid, which causes a decreased pH in the small intestine. The low pH inhibits the growth of *E. coli* in the upper small intestine and thereby helps prevent potentially lethal diarrhea or scouring in young pigs.
(a) *Lactobacillus* species are facultative anaerobic, gram-positive bacilli and are normal nonpathogenic intestinal flora.
(2) Colostrum and milk can contain antibodies specific for a pathogenic *E. coli* strain as well as other nonspecific factors that inhibit the growth of *E. coli* within the intestinal tract. These factors can prevent *E. coli* from colonizing the intestinal epithelium and/or help restrict the bacterium to the intestinal tract.
(3) Dietary changes can alter the digestive tract physiology and set up conditions for the proliferation of *E. coli*.

2.   Sanitation and stress
     a.   Poor sanitation allows the environmental buildup of
          pathogenic *E. coli* strains to infective dose levels.
     b.   Various stress factors, including overcrowding and weather
          changes, can predispose the animals to clinical infections.

III. CLINICAL FEATURES
A.   Porcine colibacillosis comprises several disease syndromes in which
     the primary site of the *E. coli* infection is the digestive tract
     (Table 99.1). The virulence factors of the causative *E. coli*
     strains and the predisposing factors for each syndrome are considered
     to be different.

Table 99.1. Porcine colibacillosis syndromes

Syndromes	Age of Swine Usually Affected
Neonatal enterotoxic colibacillosis	1-8 days
Neonatal septicemic colibacillosis	1-8 days
Milk scours	10 days-3 wk
Postweaning colibacillosis	4-8 wk
Edema disease	6-16 wk

B.   Clinical disease syndromes
     1.   Neonatal enterotoxic colibacillosis
          a.   It is caused by enterotoxigenic *E. coli* (ETEC) strains that
               possess specific fimbrial (K88, K99, and 987P) antigens for
               the colonization of the small intestine and heat-labile
               and/or heat-stable enterotoxins that cause a loss of fluid
               and electrolytes into the intestinal lumen by active
               hypersecretion.
          b.   The disease is an enterotoxicosis, not an enteritis.
          c.   Clinical disease is characterized by dehydration and
               diarrhea. Deaths are caused by dehydration and electrolyte
               imbalances. A secondary bacterial septicemia occasionally
               is observed in agonal piglets, but it is not part of the
               pathogenesis of the disease.
          d.   On necropsy, the stomach and small intestine are distended
               with fluids and gas. There is little, if any, inflammation
               present in the gastrointestinal tract in uncomplicated
               infections.
     2.   Neonatal septicemic colibacillosis
          a.   Neonatal *E. coli* septicemias are considered to be
               opportunistic infections possibly resulting from low
               specific antibody levels in colostrum and milk.
               (1) The serovars and pathogenic mechanisms of the *E. coli*
                    strains associated with septicemia in neonatal piglets
                    are poorly understood.

    b.   Clinical disease is manifested as a septicemia with or
without a concurrent endotoxemia.

    c.   On necropsy, an enteritis is present, but the principal
lesions are those of a septicemia (Table 99.2).

Table 99.2. Comparison of neonatal enterotoxic and septicemic colibacillosis

Neonatal Colibacillosis	Small Intestine		Systemic Infection	
	Enteritis	Fluid Accumulation	Septicemia	Endotoxemia
Enterotoxic[a]	−	+	−	−
Septicemic	+	−	+	±

[a]Uncomplicated ETEC infection.

   3.   Milk scours

    a.   Milk scours, an enteritis that occurs in the best-doing
pigs from 10 days to 3 weeks of age, is characterized by a
yellow pasty diarrhea.

      (1) *E. coli* and concurrent viral intestinal infections are
involved in a large percentage of cases.

        (a) Coronavirus and rotavirus infections are
frequently implicated.

      (2) Large numbers of *E. coli* are found in the intestine
during the acute phase of the disease.

      (3) The immunologic status of piglets at the time of
infection is an important predisposing factor.

        (a) Colostral antibody levels are low.

        (b) The antibody in milk is being diluted by an
increased consumption of feed.

        (c) The animal is just beginning antibody production;
thus the serum levels of IgM and IgG and the
intestinal levels of sIgA are low.

   4.   Postweaning colibacillosis

    a.   This condition is often associated with weaning and a
dietary change, which alters the digestive tract physiology
and intestinal microflora.

      (1) There is an intestinal hypomotility that allows the
proliferation of *E. coli*.

    b.   Clinically, there is a severe diarrhea, and affected
animals often have a terminal septicemia.

   5.   Edema disease

    a.   Selected *E. coli* serovars that produce an edema-inducing
exotoxin are responsible for this specific disease, which
primarily affects feeder pigs on a full ration.

    b.   Clinically, the disease is characterized by a mild
enteritis, neurological disorders, and sudden death.

IV. PATHOGENESIS
  A. Neonatal enterotoxic colibacillosis
    1. Enterotoxigenic *E. coli* strains must be able to colonize the mucosal surface of the epithelial cells of the small intestine and produce enterotoxins.
      a. The genetic determinants controlling the production of the adhesive factors and heat-labile (LT) and/or heat-stable (ST) enterotoxins are carried on plasmids, which may be transferrable. The plasmids may simultaneously carry genes for both an adhesive factor and enterotoxin(s).
      b. The first adhesive factor found to be important in porcine *E. coli* strains was the K88 fimbrial antigen. This antigen binds to the villous bases of the intestinal epithelial cell receptors, thereby preventing the expulsion of the bacteria from the small intestine.
        (1) Three major fimbrial adhesins have been recognized on porcine ETEC, including K88, K99, and 987P. The K88 and 987P adhesins have been found only in porcine isolates, but the K99 adhesin also has been isolated from calves and lambs with neonatal enterotoxigenic *E. coli*.
          (a) Three antigenic variants of K88 have been described: K88ab, K88ac, and K88ad.
        (2) The glycoprotein receptors for the fimbrial antigens are determined by a single dominant genetic locus inherited in a simple Mendelian manner. Pigs lacking these receptors are resistant to clinical disease.
      c. The LT and ST enterotoxins are responsible for the physiological loss of electrolytes and water into the lumen of the small intestine. The LT and ST can be distinguished by heat treatment. The heat-labile enterotoxin is destroyed at $60^{\circ}C$ for 30 minutes, while the heat-stable enterotoxin is stable at $100^{\circ}C$ for 30 minutes but is destroyed when heated at $121^{\circ}C$ for 30 minutes.
        (1) The LT consists of two polypeptide subunits and resembles the enterotoxin of *Vibrio cholerae* both pharmacologically and immunologically. The B subunit is responsible for binding to the Gm_1 ganglioside of the epithelial cells of the small intestine, while subunit A carries out ADP-ribosylation of a GTP-binding protein with concomitant activation of adenylate cyclase, thereby increasing the concentration of the cAMP. The increased level of cAMP both inhibits the absorption of Na^+ and increases Na^+ secretion with a subsequent loss of Cl^- and water.
        (2) The ST, a polypeptide with 18 to 19 amino acids, activates guanylate cyclase with a subsequent increase

in cGMP levels in the intestinal cells. The mechanism
by which increased cGMP leads to a net secretion of
electrolytes and water is not well understood. The
mode of action of ST appears to be antiabsorptive.
There are two types of ST: ST_A and ST_B. ST_A is active
in both pigs and infant mice, whereas ST_B is only
active in pigs. These low-molecular-weight toxins are
nonimmunogenic.

(3) A given strain of *E. coli* may produce one or both of
the enterotoxins.

(4) The production of enterotoxin(s) is relevant in the
induction of diarrhea only when *E. coli* has
proliferated sufficiently to produce a high local
concentration of the exotoxins in the small intestine.

(5) Virulence factors are summarized (Table 99.3).

Table 99.3. Plasmid-mediated virulence factors of ETEC

Virulence Factor	Factors Necessary for Disease	Induces Intestinal Hypersecretion
Hemolysin	−	−
Fimbrial antigens[a]	+	−
Enterotoxins		
LT	+[b]	+
ST	+[b]	+

[a]K88 and K99 adhesins are controlled by plasmic DNA, but the
987P adhesin can be controlled by chromosomal DNA.
[b]LT, ST, or both are necessary for clinical disease.

B. Neonatal septicemic colibacillosis, milk scours, and postweaning
colibacillosis

1. Although the predisposing factors of these diseases are
recognized and at least partially understood, the serovars and
virulence factors of the enteroinvasive and enteropathogenic *E.
coli* associated with these conditions are not well understood at
this time.

C. Edema disease

1. Edema disease is caused by several *E. coli* serovars that adhere
and proliferate in the small intestine and produce a heat-labile
edema-inducing exotoxin. The toxin is absorbed from the
intestine and causes necrosis of the smooth muscle cells of the
arterioles and small arteries, resulting in ischemia and focal
encephalomalacia of the brain and edema in other tissues.

2. Clinical disease is most frequently seen in pigs during the
first few weeks after weaning, when they are on a high
nutritional level or after there has been a change in ration.
The mortality in affected pigs approaches 100 percent, and many
pigs will die without premonitory signs. In acute deaths, gross
lesions may be subtle or absent. After several days duration,

the swine will exhibit various nervous system signs and have a characteristic subcutaneous edema of the eyelids and the greater curvature of the stomach.

V. PATHOLOGY
  A. Neonatal enterotoxic colibacillosis
    1. The intestines are distended with fluid and gas, and the animals are dehydrated. There is little, if any, inflammation of the intestine.
  B. Neonatal septicemic colibacillosis, milk scours, and postweaning colibacillosis
    1. These conditions have an enteritis of varying severity and lesions of a septicemia are often present.
  C. Edema disease
    1. The enteritis is usually mild. The edema of the eyelids and intestine is characteristic. Lesions are found in the brain.

VI. DIAGNOSIS
  A. Clinical signs and pathology
    1. The different colibacillosis syndromes are diagnosed on the basis of the ages of the animals affected, clinical signs, and postmortem lesions.
  B. Culture and serotyping
    1. Cultural isolation and biochemical identification of *E. coli* is used to confirm the diagnosis. Most pathogenic strains are beta hemolytic.
      a. The organisms are found in high numbers in the small intestine and are often in pure culture.
      b. In septicemias, *E. coli* can be recovered from the liver, spleen, kidneys, and lungs.
    2. Different serovars are frequently correlated with the different colibacillosis syndromes.
      a. The ETEC strains require adhesive fimbrial antigens for the small intestine, such as K88.
      b. Many serovars of EIEC and EPEC have been isolated from porcine colibacillosis; however, the correlation between serovar and pathogenicity is not well documented.
  C. Laboratory techniques for detection of enterotoxins from ETEC
    1. Detection of heat-labile enterotoxins
      a. Tissue culture methods, using Y1 mouse adrenal cells, Chinese hampster ovary cells, and occasionally Vero monkey kidney cells are used for the detection of LT. In these tests, the tissue culture cells are exposed to bacterial culture supernatants. When LT is present, the intracellular level of cAMP increases leading to a morphological response that can be seen microscopically.
      b. Ligated ileal loops of rabbits are injected with bacterial culture supernatants. A positive test is indicated by the

accumulation of fluid in the section of ligated loop. This test cannot distinguish between LT and ST, unless the enterotoxin preparations are heat-treated to inactivate the LT (Table 99.4).

Table 99.4. Tissue culture test results of ETEC enterotoxins

Enterotoxin	Heat-treated[a]	Fluid Accumulation
LT and ST	−	+
LT and ST	+	+
LT only	−	+
LT only	+	−
ST only	−	+
ST only	+	+

[a]The culture supernatant preparation is heated at 60°C for 30 minutes.

2. Detection of heat-stable enterotoxins
   a. The infant mouse test is used for the detection of ST. In this test the cultural supernatants are injected directly into the milk-filled stomach of infant mice. After 4 hours, the mice are killed and their intestines examined for dilation due to fluid accumulation.

VII. IMMUNIZATION
   A. Neonatal enterotoxic colibacillosis
      1. Passive immunization of piglets
         a. Immunizing sows with *E. coli* K88 antigens during gestation results in the production of anti-K88 antibodies in the colostrum and milk. This protective immunity obtained from sows is due to the blocking of the adhesive capacity of K88 antigen on the bacteria by antibody in the colostrum and milk.
         b. Types of sow immunization
            (1) Parental immunization
               (a) Three types of immunization products are live *E. coli* bacteria with K88 antigen (oral vaccine), killed *E. coli* bacteria with K88 antigen (bacterin), and bacteria-free K88 antigen (subunit vaccine).
               (b) The immunization schedule usually includes three doses during gestation with the last dose given approximately 10 days before farrowing.
            (2) Oral immunization
               (a) Autogenous oral live vaccines of *E. coli* with K88 antigen are given to pregnant sows to stimulate the intestinal sIgA response and the seeding of anti-K88 antibody-producing lymphocytes in the udder. These cells then produce specific

antibodies in the colostrum and milk that provide
protection for suckling piglets.

   2.   Active immunization of piglets

       a.   Oral immunization

          (1) After weaning, piglets are fed live *E. coli* with K88
antigens to induce intestinal sIgA. These antibodies
are of some value in protecting against ETEC in
piglets, which are susceptible for only a short period
when the supply of maternal antibody is removed.

B.   Colibacillosis, other than neonatal enterotoxic colibacillosis

   1.   Commercial and autogenous *E. coli* bacterins have demonstrated
limited ability to protect swine.

---

100 | Enzootic Pneumonia

I. ETIOLOGY

   A.   *Mycoplasma hyopneumoniae* is an aerobic, cell wall-free bacterium.

II. TRANSMISSION

   A.   Inhalation of infected aerosols from carrier swine is the most common
mode of transmission. The lungs are the primary site of infection.

      1.   Transmission usually occurs from infected sows to newborn
piglets.

III. CLINICAL FEATURES

   A.   History

      1.   Pneumonia caused by *M. hyopneumoniae* was known as "viral pig
pneumonia" until 1963, when the mycoplasmal agent was first
isolated from the disease.

   B.   Clinical signs

      1.   Uncomplicated pulmonary disease

         a.   When *M. hyopneumoniae* is the only pulmonary pathogen, there
is little, if any, clinical illness. Affected pigs have a
subclinical pneumonia and a chronic, dry, nonproductive
cough.

         b.   Enzootic pneumonia may affect over 50 percent of the pigs

in a herd; however, in uncomplicated cases the mortality
rate is often less than 1 percent.
   2. Complicated pulmonary disease
      a. Epidemics of acute bacterial pneumonia frequently occur in
herds in which there is secondary bacterial invasion of the
lungs with species in the genera *Bordetella*, *Haemophilus*,
Mycoplasma, and *Pasteurella*.
  C. Economic losses
    1. Pigs with chronic enzootic pneumonia have reduced weight gains
of from 5 to 15 percent when compared with disease-free pigs.
      a. Surveys have shown over 50 percent of marketed swine carry
lesions of this disease.

IV. PATHOGENESIS
  A. Susceptible swine inhale infected aersols from carrier swine.
    1. The infection of the lungs causes a nonpurulent lobular
pneumonia.
      a. The lesions develop primarily in the apical and cardiac
areas of the lungs.
         (1) Autoantibodies to *M. hyopneumoniae* may cross react
with the pig lung, but the extent to which these
autoantibodies contribute to the disease is not known.
    2. Swine eliminate the infection after about 1 year due to the
development of immunity, and the pulmonary lesions resolve.
Thus, second and third litter sows do not carry the disease.
  B. Secondary bacterial pathogens often invade the damaged lungs during
periods of stress and climatic changes. The effects of these
secondary bacterial infections may include a purulent
bronchopneumonia, pleuritis, pericarditis, and polyserositis.

V. PATHOLOGY
  A. Gross lung lesions
    1. In primary *M. hyopneumoniae* infections, there are characteristic
well-demarcated plum-colored or grayish pneumonic areas in the
apical and cardiac areas of the lungs. In the absence of
secondary bacterial infection, the remainder of the lung appears
normal.
    2. Pleuritis with a serofibrinous or fibrinous exudate may occur.
  B. Microscopic lung lesions
    1. Histopathology is necessary for disease confirmation. The
microscopic lesions are characterized by a parabronchiolar and
perivascular lymphoid hyperplasia.

VI. DIAGNOSIS
  A. History and clinical signs
    1. The herd has a chronic respiratory disease.
  B. Pathology
    1. Gross and microscopic lesions are characteristic.

C. Culture
1. Isolation and identification of *M. hyopneumoniae*
D. Serology
1. The complement-fixation test is often used as a diagnostic aid; however, many infected animals do not have detectable antibodies so false-negative tests are common.

VII. IMMUNIZATION
A. Commercial *M. hyopneumoniae* vaccines are not available.

101	Eperythrozoonosis

I. ETIOLOGY
A. *Eperythrozoon suis* is an aerobic, gram-negative bacterium.
1. The bacterium is cell-associated with porcine erythrocytes and is generally found adhered to the surface of erythrocytes.

II. TRANSMISSION
A. Arthropod vectors
1. The pig louse, *Hematopinus suis*, has been implicated as an arthropod vector of *E. suis*.
2. The highest incidence of infection occurs during the summer months, suggesting bloodsucking insect vectors.
B. Fomites
1. Blood-contaminated needles, syringes, and surgical instruments, which are used to bleed, vaccinate, and castrate pigs, may mechanically transmit *E. suis*.

III. CLINICAL FEATURES
A. Clinical signs
1. The majority of *E. suis* infections are asymptomatic; therefore the presence of *E. suis* in blood smears should be interpreted with caution.
2. Eperythrozoonosis (porcine icteroanemia) as a clinical entity is manifested as anemia, fever, and icterus.

      a. Pigs less than 1 week of age are the most likely group in a herd to exhibit clinical signs. These neonatal infections are frequently fatal.

      b. Clinical infections in weaned pigs are generally less severe than in nursing piglets. These clinically affected swine also may exhibit weakness, increased susceptibility to other infections, and decreased rate of weight gain.

      c. Subclinical infections in sows may result in various reproductive problems, including delayed estrus and embryonic death.

B. Immunity
  1. Pigs that acquire *E. suis* infections often remain asymptomatic carriers.

IV. PATHOGENESIS
  A. *E. suis* infected erythrocytes are removed by the reticuloendothelial system, resulting in anemia as the number of circulating erythrocytes are decreased. Icterus occurs if excessive bilirubin is released from the destroyed erythrocytes.

V. PATHOLOGY
  A. Clinical pathology
    1. Low hematocrit values, bilirubinemia, and the demonstration of bacteria associated with the surface of erythrocytes in Giemsa-stained blood smears is diagnostic.
  B. Gross pathology
    1. The postmortem appearance is dominated by anemia, icterus, splenomegaly, and serous effusions.
  C. Serology
    1. The indirect hemagglutination (IHA) test is frequently used to determine the prevalence of *E. suis* infection in herds.
      a. Significant IHA titers are usually detectable after the febrile and bacteremic period; however, pigs less than 12 weeks of age, boars, and carrier sows often fail to develop significant titers.

VI. DIAGNOSIS
  A. Clinical signs (above)
  B. Pathology (above)
  C. Direct blood smears
    1. In Giemsa-stained blood smears, *E. suis* is found adhered to the surface of erythrocytes and free in the plasma with about equal frequency.
  D. Serology (above)

VII. IMMUNIZATION
  A. Commercial *E. suis* vaccines are not available.

102	Erysipelas

I. ETIOLOGY

A. *Erysipelothrix rhusiopathiae* is a facultative anaerobic, gram-positive bacillus.

1. The numerous serovars of *E. rhusiopathiae* are based on both heat-labile and heat-stable surface antigens, which are qualitatively homogenous but differ quantitatively. Serovars 1 and 2 account for approximately 80 percent of the *E. rhusiopathiae* isolates from porcine erysipelas.

2. The strains of *E. rhusiopathiae* vary markedly in virulence.

II. TRANSMISSION

A. Ingestion

1. Most erysipelas infections are acquired from the ingestion of *E. rhusiopathiae*-contaminated feces and soil.

   a. The bacterium can survive in the tonsils, gall bladders, and gastrointestinal tracts of immune swine, which excrete the organisms in the feces. Animals other than swine also may contain *E. rhusiopathiae* in their gastrointestinal tracts.

   b. The bacterium can survive for several weeks in alkaline soils.

B. Cutaneous contamination

1. Porcine erysipelas can be transmitted by the bites of infected flies and by the contamination of cutaneous wounds.

   a. The bacteria can persist for many months in the skin lesions of diseased pigs.

C. Carrier swine

1. *E. rhusiopathiae* can be maintained for years in a swine herd without clinical signs or in swine with chronic arthritis. When these swine are stressed, they may have a recrudescence of infections and then spread the infection to other swine.

III. CLINICAL FEATURES

A. Erysipelas occurs in pigs of all ages, but pigs from 2 months to 1 year of age tend to be the most susceptible to infection and clinical disease.

B. Clinical disease can be manifested as a highly fatal acute septicemia, a milder subacute form characterized by necrosis of the skin, or a chronic polyarthritis and valvular endocarditis.

1. Acute erysipelas
   a. In severe acute infections, the septicemia is characterized by high fever, depression, lameness, and high mortality. Sudden deaths may occur before clinical signs are manifested.
2. Subacute erysipelas
   a. In less severe infections, affected swine live for 3 or 4 days and pathognomonic cutaneous lesions develop on the skin of the abdomen, ears, and the extremities. The initial skin lesions are raised, rhomboid or square-shaped, and with a reddish to purplish color. In swine that survive for several weeks, the skin lesions undergo dry necrosis and occasionally coalesce over large areas of the skin, resulting in extensive cutaneous necrosis.
   b. Infected pregnant sows may abort or give birth to stillborn pigs.
3. Chronic erysipelas
   a. Bacterial localization in the joints and on the endocardium may occur as a sequela to an acute septicemic infection, after which the animal survives, or to a mild or inapparent systemic infection.
   b. Polyarthritis
      (1) Acute arthritis may occur in pigs as young as 3 weeks of age. The acute inflammatory response may last for up to 20 weeks.
      (2) Chronic arthritis is seen in pigs 10 weeks or older and may persist for several years. The hock and knee joints are most often involved, but the carpal and tarsal joints also may be severely affected.
   c. Valvular endocarditis
      (1) The mitral valves are most frequently involved; the conditon may result in valvular insufficiency and eventually congestive heart failure.
      (2) Most swine with valvular endocarditis are asymptomatic.
C. Epidemic and endemic erysipelas
   1. In epidemics of porcine erysipelas, the septicemic form predominates; however, in endemic areas the disease tends to be sporadic and all forms of the condition may be manifested simultaneously.

IV. PATHOGENESIS
   A. Septicemic erysipelas
      1. Virulent strains of *E. rhusiopathiae* are ingested by susceptible swine, penetrate the mucosa of the gastrointestinal tract, invade the bloodstream, and proliferate. The septicemia disseminates the organisms throughout the viscera and lymph nodes.

   B.   Diamond skin lesions
         1.   The cutaneous lesions are due to the suffusion and congestion of
              the dermal capillaries with thrombosis of the dermal arterioles,
              resulting in the necrosis of the skin.
   C.   Polyarthritis
         1.   *E. rhusiopathiae* can persist for up to 2 years in chronic
              arthritis despite a specific antibody response to the infection.
              The production of specific antibodies is a key factor in the
              pathogenesis of chronic proliferative changes that takes place
              in the synovium of infected joints. The articular proliferative
              changes are predominant when antibody titers are the highest.
              Localized immune complexes, which are made up of bacterial
              antigens, antibody, and complement, largely determine the level
              of chemotactic activity for neutrophils. The pathology
              associated with arthritis results from the accumulation of
              neutrophils, which subsequently release lysosomal enzymes that
              can damage cartilage and other joint tissues.
   D.   Valvular endocarditis
         1.   The bacteria colonize the heart valves, and eventually masses of
              fibrin and bacteria form on the valves.

V.   PATHOLOGY
   A.   Acute and subacute erysipelas
         1.   The generalized lesions of septicemia are petechial and
              ecchymotic hemorrhages on the epicardium, skeletal muscles, and
              serosa of the stomach. The spleen is enlarged and hyperemic.
         2.   Congestion and infarction of the gastric mucosa are often
              present.
         3.   The skin lesions are the only pathognomonic sign of acute
              erysipelas.
   B.   Chronic arthritis
         1.   The chronic arthritic lesions are characterized as
              nonsuppurative, proliferative, and erosive.
              a.   The joint fluid is not suppurative.
              b.   There is connective tissue proliferation of the affected
                   joints.
              c.   There are erosions of the articular cartilage.
   C.   Valvular endocarditis
         1.   There are cauliflowerlike masses of fibrin and bacteria on the
              involved heart valves.
              a.   Septic emboli from the valvular lesions often produce
                   randomly distributed abscesses and infarcts in the kidneys.

VI. DIAGNOSIS
   A.   Herd history (above)
   B.   Clinical signs
         1.   The diamond skin lesions are pathognomonic for porcine
              erysipelas.

C. Pathology
    1. The lesions induced during the acute septicemia cannot distinguish erysipelas from other infections with an acute septicemia, such as *Salmonella choleraesuis* infections.
    2. The arthritic lesions, which are nonsuppurative, proliferative, and erosive, will often distinguish erysipelas from other arthritic lesions caused by the streptococci, staphylococci, haemophili, and mycoplasmas.

D. Culture
    1. Isolation and biochemical identification of *E. rhusiopathiae*
       a. Colonies of *E. rhusiopathiae* can be either smooth or rough. After 24 hours incubation, smooth colonies are convex, circular, transparent, and smooth with an entire edge but are only about 1 mm in diameter. Rough colonies are flatter, opaque, and larger. Colonies on blood agar often produce a narrow zone of incomplete hemolysis.
         (1) Smooth colonies are usually recovered from acute infections, whereas rough colonies are recovered from chronic infections.
       b. The bacterium has only weak fermentative activity but will ferment both glucose and lactose and produce H_2S in triple sugar iron (TSI) agar. These reactions in TSI agar are characteristic for this gram-positive, nonsporing, bacillus.

VII. IMMUNIZATION

A. Passive immunity
    1. Swine erysipelas antiserum provides protective immunity for about 2 weeks and is frequently used to provide immediate protection during an outbreak of the disease.
       a. Swine erysipelas antiserum will often exacerbate a preexisting arthritis caused by the bacterium.

B. Active immunity
    1. Erysipelas bacterins and vaccines are often made from serovar 2, which also provides good protection for serovar 1. The potency of the bacterins and vaccines depend not only on the immunogenic properties of the antigen(s) used but also on the number of organisms used in the inoculum.
    2. Bacterins
       a. Formalized killed bacterins are usually administered to pigs from 4 to 6 weeks of age.
       b. Humoral immunity develops at 2 to 3 weeks after immunization and usually persists for 3 to 6 months.
       c. Bacterins provide protection against the septicemic form of the disease but not against arthritis.
    3. Vaccines
       a. Vaccines are composed of live avirulent strains of *E. rhusiopathiae* and are administered orally to pigs from 4 to

6 weeks of age. The virulence of these strains is not
fully fixed, and there is always a possibility of their
reconversion to the virulent form.
   b. Oral vaccines prevent the septicemic form of erysipelas and
       greatly reduce the incidence of arthritis but may not
       completely prevent chronic arthritis.

103	Salmonellosis

I. ETIOLOGY
   A. *Salmonella* serovars are faculative anaerobic, gram-negative bacilli.
       1. Over 50 serovars have been isolated from clinically affected and
           asymptomatic pigs. From pigs with clinical salmonellosis, *S.
           choleraesuis* is the most frequently isolated serovar and *S.
           typhimurium* the second most frequently isolated. Other
           important serovars are *S. anatum*, *S. derby*, *S. dublin*, *S.
           newport*, and *S. typhisuis*.
       2. Salmonellae are facultative intracellular pathogens.

II. TRANSMISSION
   A. Ingestion
       1. Ingestion of feed and water contaminated with salmonellae is the
           primary mode of transmission.
           a. Salmonellae in feces may survive in the environment for 1
               year or more.
       2. The majority of the epidemics of porcine salmonellosis result
           from the oral ingestion of feces contaminated with either *S.
           choleraesuis* or *S. typhimurium* from clinically affected or
           asymptomatic carrier swine.
           a. *S. choleraesuis* is highly host-adapted to swine, whereas *S.
               typhimurium* has a wide host range, including birds, wild
               and domestic animals, and man.
   B. Carrier swine
       1. Adult swine can become asymptomatic carriers of salmonellosis
           for indefinite periods of time. The bacteria can persist in low
           numbers in the intestine and be excreted in the feces, or the

feces can be seeded intermittently from the gall bladder, which is a common habitat of the bacterium. Salmonellae also can persist in the regional lymph nodes of the alimentary tract but not be excreted in the feces.

III. CLINICAL FEATURES
A. Age susceptibility
1. Swine of all ages may be affected, but clinical disease is most frequent in pigs 8 to 16 weeks of age.
   a. Clinical salmonellosis is uncommon in nursing pigs.
   b. Adult swine are less likely to get systemic infections than are younger swine.
B. Serovars and clinical diseases
1. The serovar of *Salmonella* is important in the clinical and pathological manifestations of porcine salmonellosis.
   a. The major clinical manifestations are septicemia and enterocolitis. Usually one syndrome or the other will be manifested, but both can occur simultaneously.
      (1) The principal clinical manifestation of *S. choleraesuis* is an acute septicemia.
      (2) The principal clinical manifestation of *S. typhimurium* and most other serovars is an enterocolitis with diarrhea.
C. Clinical signs
1. The acute septicemic form of salmonellosis is characterized by high fever, depression, prostration, and acute death. It is usually fatal and death may occur quickly without premonitory signs.
   a. Nonspecific clinical signs can include red or purplish skin blotches, pneumonia, and neurological signs due to meningitis and/or encephalitis.
2. The enteric form of salmonellosis is characterized by fever, anorexia, mucohemorrhagic diarrhea, progressive emaciation, and eventually death. The diarrhea material often contains variable amounts of blood, fibrin, and sloughed necrotic mucosa.
   a. Many survivors of the enteric form will be unthrifty and remain carriers.

IV. PATHOGENESIS
A. The pathogenesis of salmonellae infections can be described in four sequential stages.
1. Infection and invasion of the gastrointestinal tract
   a. Most salmonellae infections are acquired by the ingestion of feces-contaminated feed and water, and some infections result from the recrudescence of the carrier state.
   b. Small numbers of ingested salmonellae invade the mucous membranes along the alimentary tract and colonize the lymphoid tissues, but the major route of invasion is from

the intestinal lumen into the lamina propria and Peyer's patches of the ileum, cecum, and colon.

c. The bacteria that invade the gastrointestinal mucosa evoke a fluid exsorption, multiply within the mucosa, and elicit an acute inflammatory reaction. Neutrophils are the predominant cell type in these initial infectious foci in the lamina propria, and many phagocytes will migrate into the intestinal lumen.

2. Proliferation in the intestinal wall and regional lymph nodes

a. The invasion and destruction of the epithelial cells and reticuloendothelial cells in the intestinal wall results in mucosal and serosal hemorrhages followed by thrombosis, necrosis, and ulceration of the mucous membranes. These lesions occur primarily in the ileum, cecum, and colon, which have high concentrations of lymphoid tissues.

b. The bacteria reach the regional lymph nodes via the lymphatics. Bacterial proliferation results in lymphadenopathy with hemorrhages.

3. Bacteremia/septicemia

a. Following a period of proliferation in the regional lymph nodes, the bacteria invade the bloodstream via the lymphatics and cause a septicemia or transient bacteremia. Some infections remain confined at their primary foci of infection and do not disseminate.

(1) The septicemia is usually rapidly fatal in young animals. Complications include pneumonia, meningitis, and enteritis.

(2) In bacteremias, the organisms are removed by the fixed reticuloendothelial cells, especially in the liver, spleen, and bone marrow. In these tissues, the bacteria proliferate, and in due course there is a second bacteremia phase, which may cause fatal septicemia or result in secondary localization in various organs and tissues.

4. Intestinal localization

a. The bacteria gain entry into the intestine via the liver and bile ducts; the result is enterocolitis with diarrhea.

B. Virulence factors of salmonellae

1. Heat-labile and heat-stable enterotoxins similar to the enterotoxins of *E. coli* have been described, but their role in the enteritis induced in salmonellae infections have not been resolved.

2. Salmonellae-induced enterocolitis may cause an increased synthesis and secretion of prostaglandins, which in turn stimulate mucosal adenyl cyclase activity. Adenyl cyclase enzymatically acts on ATP, converting it to a cAMP, which causes abnormal fluid, chloride, and sodium transport in the enterocytes.

   3. The lipopolysaccharides are considered to play a major role in the pathogenesis and clinical manifestations of salmonellosis.
- a. The O side chain polysaccharide antigens play a major role in host specificity and intestinal invasion.
- b. The potency of the endotoxins are responsible for many of the clinical manifestations.

V. PATHOLOGY
- A. Enteric lesions
    1. Intestinal lesions are primarily in the ileum, cecum, and colon. The duodenum and jejunum occasionally are affected.
        - a. Diphtheritic lesions probably result from a primary intestinal salmonellosis ulcerative lesion becoming secondarily contaminated with *Fusobacterium necrophorum*.
- B. Visceral lesions
    1. Lymphadenopathy, hepatomegaly, and splenomegaly are common.
- C. Septicemic lesions
    1. Meningitis, encephalitis, and pneumonia are common complications of septicemias.

VI. DIAGNOSIS
- A. Clincal signs (above)
- B. Pathology (above)
- C. Culture
    1. Isolation and biochemical identification of the genus *Salmonella* and serologic identification of the serovars

VII. IMMUNIZATION
- A. In general, salmonellae vaccines have not provided adequate protective immunity in swine.

104 | Tuberculosis

I. ETIOLOGY

A. *Mycobacterium avium* complex is composed of a group of obligate aerobic, gram-positive, acid-fast bacilli. Serovars 1, 2, and 3 can cause tuberculosis in swine.

1. Swine also are susceptible to infection with *M. bovis* and *M. tuberculosis*.

2. *M. avium*, *M. bovis*, and *M. tuberculosis* are facultative intracellular pathogens.

II. TRANSMISSION

A. Ingestion

1. Ingestion of infected material is the most common mode of transmission.

   a. Swine often become infected with *M. avium* after contact with chickens that have tuberculosis or with an environment previously occupied by poultry with tuberculosis.

B. Serovars

1. *M. avium* serovars 1, 2, and 3 are commonly acquired from poultry with tuberculosis.

   a. Since avian tuberculosis in domestic poultry has been drastically reduced due to the federal control program, swine are now only infrequently infected with these avian-adapted serovars.

2. Some serovars in the *M. avium* complex have been shown to adapt to swine and can be transmitted from pig to pig, while other serovars are noncommunicable among swine.

III. CLINICAL FEATURES

A. Tuberculosis and mycobacteriosis are difficult to diagnose clinically because the infected pigs are virtually asymptomatic.

1. The majority of these infections are found during meat inspections. The market traceback program, which determines the herd of origin, is the most common regulatory method used in detecting infected herds.

   a. Swine found to have tuberculosis are slaughtered.

IV. PATHOGENESIS

A. Tubercles, which are the characteristic lesion of tuberculosis, can form in any organ in which reticuloendothelial tissue is present.

      1.   The pharyngeal, cervical, and mesenteric lymph nodes are the primary foci of infection following ingestion of the organisms. The liver is a common secondary site of infection.

V.   PATHOLOGY

   A.   The granulomatous caseous lesions are most prevalent in the cervical and mesenteric lymph nodes.

VI.   DIAGNOSIS

   A.   Market traceback program

      1.   Postmortem lesions are cultured for mycobacteria to confirm the diagnosis.

   B.   Tuberculin tests

      1.   *M. avium* complex infection can be suspected with a positive skin test using *M. avium* PPD.

         a.   Tuberculin is injected intradermally at the base of the ear and evaluated 48 hours postinjection for the presence of necrosis, erythema, and induration.

         b.   The herd test is usually used, since some pigs may exhibit either false-positive or false-negative tuberculin reactions.

VII.   IMMUNIZATION

   A.   Swine are not immunized for tuberculosis in the United States.

| PART 4 | Equine Diseases |

| 105 | Actinobacillosis |

I. ETIOLOGY
   A. *Actinobacillus equuli* is a facultative anaerobic, gram-negative bacillus.

II. TRANSMISSION
   A. Umbilical infections
      1. Infections are acquired via the umbilicus in utero, during parturition, or shortly after birth.

III. CLINICAL FEATURES
   A. Foals
      1. Most foals infected at birth die within 3 days, but some may survive for a month or longer.
         a. Some foals may die within 24 hours of birth with a fulminating septicemic infection. These foals, which are weak and unable to stand or nurse, die before characteristic lesions develop.
         b. Foals that live for 2 or 3 days have a polyarthritis characterized by swollen hot joints with clinical signs similar to those that die of acute septicemia.
         c. Foals that live for several weeks have a polyarthritis and an unthrifty appearance.
   B. Adults
      1. Most adults infected with *A. equuli* have subclinical infections.

IV. PATHOGENESIS
   A. The bacteria establish a primary focus of infection in the umbilicus with a subsequent bacteremia/septicemia.
      1. The bacteria in the bloodstream lodge in the kidneys and joints to initiate suppurative nephritis and polyarthritis, which are

characteristic lesions of actinobacillosis in foals.
   a. The bacteria alone or as small septic emboli lodge mainly
       in the glomerular tufts. Neutrophils soon accumulate, and
       small foci of suppuration develop in the cortex of the
       kidney. The renal medulla is relatively free of abscesses.

V. PATHOLOGY
    A. Kidney abscesses
        1. Foals that survive a couple of days or more develop abscesses in
            the renal cortex that are 0.5 to 3 mm in diameter.
            Microscopically, the abscesses are composed of bacteria and
            neutrophils.
    B. Polyarthritis
        1. Infected joints contain a sanguineous or purulent exudate.

VI. DIAGNOSIS
    A. Clinical signs (above)
    B. Pathology
        1. The kidney abscesses are a pathognomonic lesion.
    C. Culture
        1. Isolation and biochemical identification of *A. equuli*

VII. IMMUNIZATION
    A. Commercial *A. equuli* bacterins are not available.

106	Contagious Equine Metritis

I. ETIOLOGY
    A. *Taylorella equigenitalis* is a facultative anaerobic, gram-negative
        bacillus.
        1. When this fastidious bacterium was first isolated from
            clinically infected mares in 1977, it was called the contagious
            equine metritis organism (CEMO). In 1978, the newly recognized
            pathogen was named *Haemophilus equigenitalis*. After further
            studies of the bacterium by numerous investigators, it was
            placed in a new genus and officially classified as *T.
            equigenitalis*.

II. TRANSMISSION

A. Contagious equine metritis (CEM) is a highly contagious venereal disease of horses.
  1. Venereal transmission is the primary mode of transmission.
      a. The stallion, which is an inapparent carrier of the disease, transmits it to mares during coitus. Likewise, infected mares can transmit the infection to stallions.
      b. Contaminated semen from stallions also will infect mares.
  2. Mechanical transmission can occur when contaminated instruments are used to examine the genitalia of mares and stallions.
  3. Vertical transmission to foals born to infected mares has been documented.

III. CLINICAL FEATURES

A. History
  1. The disease was not a recognized entity prior to 1977, when the CEMO was isolated from the first officially recorded outbreak among thoroughbred mares in England and the disease was experimentally reproduced in pony mares.
      a. In 1976, the condition was first recognized in Ireland and France by equine practitioners as a new venereal disease of horses, but the etiologic agent was not determined.
  2. CEM was first diagnosed in the United States on a thoroughbred horse farm in Kentucky in 1978, when a mare bred to a stallion imported from France showed clinical signs. The disease was again confirmed on a horse farm in Missouri in 1979. Since these initial disease outbreaks, CEM has not been reported in the United States.

B. Clinical signs
  1. Mares
      a. Acute infections are characterized by endometritis, cervicitis, and vaginitis with copious production of a mucopurulent exudate. The purulent vaginal discharge reaches a maximum volume about 96 hours after coitus with an infected stallion, but the exudate is barely visible after 7 to 10 days. The bulk of the discharge originates from the uterus, and it becomes encrusted on the vulvar lips and tail hairs.
      b. The majority of the mares will fail to conceive and return to estrus after a shortened diestrus. A few mares will conceive but abort during the first 60 days of pregnancy.
      c. The clinical course of most acute infections is less than 1 month.
      d. Subclinical infections may last 1 year or more. Poor reproductive performance is the primary manifestation of these inapparent infections.
      e. Pregnant mares may carry the infection in an inapparent state.

2. Stallions
   a. Infected stallions are asymptomatic but can remain carriers of the bacterium for years.

IV. PATHOGENESIS
A. Mares
   1. The primary pathology is confined to the uterus, where the infection is associated with necrosis and shedding of the endometrial epithelium.
      a. The causative agent appears to have a special affinity for the endometrial glands or for the secretions of these glands. There is a proliferation of the luminal epithelial cells as early as 2 days after infection.
      b. The early marked infiltration of the endometrium by neutrophils results in a copious purulent exudate by day 2 that rapidly subsides by day 10 despite the continuous presence of the causative organism. There also is infiltration of the uterine stroma by mononuclear cells, including plasma cells.
      c. Local antibody in the uterus, cervix, and vagina help eliminate the infection from these areas after the initial invasion and resultant pathology.
B. Stallions
   1. The bacteria colonize the epithelial surfaces of the penile sheath, urethra, and urethral fossa and sinuses but does not invade the tissues.

V. PATHOLOGY
A. Mares
   1. Lesions are confined to the uterus, cervix, and vagina. Occasionally the fallopian tubes are infected, but salpingitis is not considered a significant feature of the disease.
B. Stallions
   1. No lesions develop in infected stallions.

VI. DIAGNOSIS
A. Clinical signs
   1. A copious mucopurulent vaginal discharge is characteristic.
B. Serology
   1. The complement-fixation (CF) test is the most commonly used serologic test for the diagnosis of CEM in mares.
      a. The CF test is most reliable in mares when used between 2 and 6 weeks postinfection.
      b. The CF test will not detect most carrier mares and stallions.
C. Culture
   1. *T. equigenitalis* is a fastidious organism, but it will grow on chocolate agar with 10 percent horse serum when incubated at 37°C in an atmosphere of air and 10 percent carbon dioxide.

2. Mare culture sites
    a. The uterus, urethra, clitoral fossa, and clitoral sinuses are the preferred sites to culture in clinically infected mares. The clitoral fossa is the best site to culture in carrier mares.
3. Stallion culture sites
    a. The penile sheath, urethra, and urethral fossa are preferred sites in carrier stallions.

VII. IMMUNIZATION
A. Commercial *T. equigenitalis* vaccines are not available.

| 107 | Endometritis |

I. ETIOLOGY
A. Numerous bacterial pathogens have been isolated from equine endometritis (Table 107.1).

Table 107.1. A partial listing of aerobic bacteria that cause equine endometritis

Gram-positive cocci	Gram-positive rods	Gram-negative rods
Staphylococcus aureus	*Rhodococcus equi*	*Bordetella bronchiseptica*
Streptococcus zooepidemicus		*Escherichia coli*
Other streptococci		*Klebsiella pneumoniae*
		Other Enterobacteriaceae

II. TRANSMISSION
A. The bacteria enter the uterus via the cervix.
    1. The causative bacteria can be components of the mare's cervical and vaginal flora, from the flora of the stallion's prepuce and genitalia, or from exogenous sources, including the feces.

III. CLINICAL FEATURES
A. Bacterial endometritis is the most common cause of infertility in the mare and contributes significantly to fetal death.
    1. Mares can conceive while infected, but many will resorb the conceptus, abort the fetus, or produce infected foals.
        a. Mares with endometritis have their highest percentage of pregnancy loss during the first 35 days.

      2. The incidence of endometritis increases with age.

B. A variety of anatomical and congenital conditions predispose mares to endometritis.

    1. Pneumovaginitis and subsequent pneumouterus results from poor conformation that allows an inadequate vulvo-vestibular closure.

    2. Abortion and retained placenta are common predisposing factors to bacterial endometritis.

    3. Poor hygienic practices at breeding and during genital examinations can result in endometritis.

        a. A large number of bacteria normally enter the uterus at breeding when the cervix is relaxed. If these bacteria are not eliminated within 1 week after ovulation, when the embryo descends to the uterus, endometritis may result.

IV. PATHOGENESIS

A. The bacteria colonize the endometrium via the cervix, and a failure of the uterine defense mechanisms leads to prolonged inflammation and an endometritis.

    1. Normally the mare has highly efficient defense mechanisms that clear the uterus of bacterial contamination; these depend on the triad of phagocytosis, ovarian endocrine responses, and specific immunity.

        a. Ovarian hormones greatly influence the inflammatory and immune responses in the uterus. The uterus is most susceptible to bacterial infection during the progesterone phase of the estrous cycle and most resistant during the estrogen phase.

        b. Neutrophils are found in greatest number in the uterus and exhibit their greatest killing capacity during estrus.

        c. Specific immunoglobulins can be derived from the transudation of IgM and IgG into the uterus during inflammation and estrus and from locally synthesized immunoglobulins, mainly sIgA, in the uterus, cervix, and vagina.

    2. Anestrus often prediposes the uterus to infection.

        a. Mares are frequently in anestrus after embryonic loss, delaying the next estrus for a significant period of time and allowing the infection sufficient time to become established.

B. Metritis and pyometra are sequelae to endometritis.

    1. Although metritis and pyometra occasionally occur, their systemic manifestations are relatively mild when compared with those in the dog.

V. PATHOLOGY

A. Mucocatarrhal and purulent vaginal discharges with endometritis, cervicitis, and vaginitis are commonly observed.

VI. DIAGNOSIS
    A. Uterine cultures, uterine cytology, endometrial biopsies, and rectal palpations are used to diagnose endometritis in the mare.
        1. Uterine cultures should be collected during midestrus for the identification of bacteria.
            a. Approximately 75 percent of the mares are culture-positive for 72 hours after breeding. In breeding animals, numerous bacterial species have been recovered from the cervicovaginal area of the mare and from the prepuce and external genitalia of the stallion. The clinical significance of cultures that contain normal bacterial flora is often debatable.
            b. From 1 to 30 days after foaling, the majority of the mares will be culture-positive.
        2. Cytology evaluates the uterine response to any bacterial contamination.
            a. Bacteria associated with a significant inflammatory response, particularly a neutrophilia, indicates a correlation between endometritis and a positive culture.
        3. Endometrial biopsies are indicated in cases of metritis and pyometra to evaluate inflammatory changes in the endometrium.
        4. Rectal palpation evaluates uterine tone, conformation, and congenital defects.

VII. IMMUNIZATION
    A. Commercial and autogenous bacterins are seldom used either prophylactically or therapeutically.

108 | Neonatal Streptococcal Infections

I. ETIOLOGY
   A. *Streptococcus zooepidemicus* is a facultative anaerobic, gram-positive coccus.
      1. The majority of the neonatal streptococcal infections are caused by *S. zooepidemicus*; however, other *Streptococcus* species can induce similar types of disease.

II. TRANSMISSION
   A. The majority of the neonatal foal infections are contracted from environmental contamination through the umbilicus shortly after birth.
      1. *S. zooepidemicus* is part of the normal equine flora of the skin and upper respiratory tract.

III. CLINICAL FEATURES
   A. Neonatal *S. zooepidemicus* infections are characterized by a bacteremia/septicemia and a polyarthritis. Affected foals may die from the septicemia within a few days after parturition.
      1. Acutely affected joints are hot and painful.
   B. Predisposing factors and immunity
      1. Failure to acquire passive immunity (colostrum) is probably the most important factor in the pathogenesis of infection, predisposing to opportunistic infection.
         a. The equine placenta is epitheliochorial. There is no transplacental passage of immunoglobulin.
         b. The foal must receive antibodies through the colostrum.
      2. Passive immunity of the foal
         a. Colostral antibodies can only be absorbed by the foal during the first 24 to 48 hours after birth. IgG and IgM are absorbed, while sIgA is left in the intestine.
         b. A normal suckled foal's immunoglobulin level approaches that of the mare's within 12 to 18 hours. An unsuckled foal has extremely low levels of immunoglobulin in the serum.
         c. The passive antibody (colostral antibody blood levels in the foal) declines to less than half their original values by 4 weeks of age and completely disappears by 6 months of age.
         d. In presuckle colostrum, IgG is the predominant immunoglobulin, and sIgA is present in low concentrations.

      e.   In lactation milk, sIgA is the predominant immunoglobulin and IgG is present in low concentrations.

   3. Active immunity of the foal

      a.   The foal is immunologically competent at birth but does not produce appreciable levels of immunoglobulins until about 2 months of age.

      b.   The foal's immunoglobulin level is equivalent to that of an adult by 4 months of age.

   4. Reasons for hypogammaglobinemia in foals

      a.   Premature lactation with a steady drip of milk (colostrum) before parturition

      b.   Failure to nurse in the 24-hour period after birth

      c.   Premature foaling, with inadequate colostrum production

      d.   Lack of immunoglobulin in the colostrum

      e.   Intestinal malabsorption in the foal

IV. PATHOGENESIS

  A. Susceptible foals acquire the infection through the navel shortly after birth and develop a bacteremia or septicemia with localization in the joints, causing a suppurative polyarthritis.

  B. Bacterial virulence factors

    1. Capsular and cell wall antigens

      a.   The capsule is composed of hyaluronic acid, which is nonantigenic and antiphagocytic.

      b.   *S. zooepidemicus* is in Lancefield group C, which is determined by the group-specific carbohydrate antigen of the cell wall.

      c.   There are a multiplicity of *S. zooepidemicus* serotypes based on the M, R, and T protein antigens, which are type-specific.

    2. Extracellular virulence factors

      a.   The extracellular virulence factors of *S. zooepidemicus* are similar to those of *S. pyogenes* (group A) and *S. equi* (group C).

V. PATHOLOGY

  A. Gross lesions

    1. Petechial and ecchymotic hemorrhages, which are characteristic of a septicemia, are often present when foals die of acute infections.

    2. Acutely affected joints have suppurative synovial fluid. After several weeks, the arthritis is characterized as suppurative, proliferative, and erosive.

VI. DIAGNOSIS

  A. History (above)

  B. Pathology (above)

  C. Culture

    1. Isolation and biochemical identification of *S. zooepidemicus*

VII. IMMUNIZATION
 A. Vaccination of mares
  1. Since there are a multiplicity of types of *S. zooepidemicus*,
   immunization against one strain does not necessarily protect
   against other strains.
  2. Passive immunity is provided to the foal in the colostrum.

109	Strangles

I. ETIOLOGY
 A. *Streptococcus equi* is a facultative anaerobic, gram-positive coccus.

II. TRANSMISSION
 A. Inhalation and ingestion
  1. *S. equi* is transmitted in the respiratory aerosols and nasal
   discharges of clinically infected and carrier horses to
   susceptible horses, which acquire the infection either by
   inhalation or ingestion.
   a. *S. equi* is considered to be an obligatory pathogen on the
    mucous membranes of the upper respiratory tract of horses.

III. CLINICAL FEATURES
 A. Clinical signs of strangles
  1. Strangles is an acute contagious disease of horses characterized
   by inflammation of the upper respiratory tract and abscessation
   in the regional lymph nodes.
   a. The animals become febrile after a 3- to 6-day incubation
    period with a bilateral mucopurulent nasal discharge.
   b. The pharyngeal and mandibular lymph nodes often rupture and
    drain a purulent exudate.
   c. In severe infections, a septicemia gives rise to abscess
    formation in a variety of lymph nodes, organs, and tissues.
    These infections tend to be chronic with varied symptoms.
  2. The disease usually affects animals 1 to 2 years of age.
 B. Clinical signs of purpura hemorrhagica
  1. Purpura hemorrhagica is a post-*S. equi* immune complex disease.
   a. It is characterized by extensive subcutaneous edema of the

face, muzzle, and limbs, which pits on pressure, and by petechial and ecchymotic hemorrhages of the skin and mucous membranes.

IV. PATHOGENESIS
 A. The inhaled or ingested *S. equi* colonize the nasal and buccal mucous membranes.
   1. The bacteria adhere to the epithelial surfaces via M protein cell wall antigens, which extend through the capsule of the bacterium as hairlike fimbriae. The M protein also is antiphagocytic.
   2. The bacteria invade the mucous membranes, and the infection spreads via the lymphatic system to the regional lymph nodes, where abscesses develop.
   3. If a septicemia occurs, abscesses can form in a variety of lymph nodes, organs, and tissues. This condition is often referred to as "bastard strangles."
 B. Purpura hemorrhagica may develop several weeks after the primary infection. If antibodies to M protein form immune complexes, which can localize in the capillary beds and activate complement, there is an increased vascular permeability that allows the exudation of plasma and cells into the tissues.
 C. Immunity
   1. Recovery from natural disease confers lifelong immunity.

V. PATHOLOGY
 A. Catarrhal rhinitis and abscesses in the mandibular and pharyngeal lymph nodes are the primary lesions in uncomplicated strangles.

VI. DIAGNOSIS
 A. Clinical signs (above)
 B. Culture
   1. Isolation and biochemical identification of *S. equi*

VII. IMMUNIZATION
 A. Bacterins
   1. *S. equi* bacterins provide immunity for about 1 year.
 B. Subunit vaccine
   1. Purified M protein antigen will induce humoral immunity.
     a. There is only one antigenic type of M protein in *S. equi*.

| PART **5** | Canine Diseases |

| 110 | Anaerobic Bacterial Infections |

I. ETIOLOGY

A. Numerous obligate anaerobic and aerobic bacterial species have been associated with opportunistic polymicrobial infections in dogs.

1. The obligate anaerobic genera that contain species frequently recovered from polymicrobial infections are shown in Table 110.1.

Table 110.1. Genera of obligate anaerobes

	Gram-positive Genera			Gram-negative Genera	
	Nonsporeforming	Sporeforming			Nonsporeforming
Cocci	Rods	Rods	Cocci		Rods
Peptococcus	*Actinomyces* [a]	*Clostridium*	*Veillonella*		*Bacteroides*
Peptostreptococcus	*Bifidobacterium*				*Fusobacterium*
	Eubacterium				
	Propionibacterium				

[a]The genus *Actinomyces* is classified as facultative anaerobic, but some species are obligate anaerobes. *A. pyogenes* is a facultative anaerobe, and *A. viscosus* is a microaerophile.

2. Aerobic bacteria commonly isolated from polymicrobial anaerobic infections

a. Members of the family Enterobacteriaceae are the most commonly isolated gram-negative bacteria.

b. Species of *Staphylococcus* and *Streptococcus* are the most commonly isolated gram-positive bacteria.

II. TRANSMISSION

A. Endogenous sources

1. Obligate anaerobic bacteria are the majority population of the normal flora of the skin, mucous membranes, and gastrointestinal

tract. Most of these organisms involved in infectious processes have their sources from the normal flora.

2. Members of the family Enterobacteriaceae make up the majority of the facultative anaerobic flora of the gastrointestinal tract.

3. The staphylococci and streptococci are normal flora of skin and mucous membranes. The enterococci are normal enteric flora.

B. Exogenous sources

1. Many anaerobic bacteria and enterobacteriae are acquired from fecal contamination of the environment.

2. Some anaerobic bacteria are found in the soil, particularly the *Actinomyces* species and *Clostridium* species.

III. CLINICAL FEATURES

A. The clostridia tend to produce either a cellulitis or a necrotizing myositis.

1. The *Clostridium* species are the predominant pathogens in these conditions and are frequently recovered from the lesions in pure culture.

B. The *Actinomyces* species, except *A. pyogenes*, produce pyogranulomatous or granulomatous lesions and are frequently recovered from the lesions in pure culture.

1. *A. viscosus* is the most commonly isolated species.

C. The obligate anaerobic gram-positive cocci, gram-positive nonsporeforming rods, gram-negative cocci, and gram-negative rods are usually found in localized suppurative processes.

1. Two or more bacterial species are usually recovered from these opportunistic infections. Most of the anaerobic bacteria are of low virulence.

a. *F. necrophorum* is occasionally isolated in pure culture.

2. Types of infections

a. Abscesses

b. Fight wounds

c. Postsurgical wound infections

d. Fractures associated with trauma of soft tissues

e. Infections near or on mucous membranes

f. Aspiration pneumonias

g. Septic pleuritis and peritonitis

3. Tissue characteristics of anaerobic infections

a. Foul-smelling discharges

b. Necrotic tissue

c. Presence of gas in tissues or discharges

IV. PATHOGENESIS

A. Pathogenic factors that predispose tissue to infections with an anaerobic bacterial component are tissue injury, necrosis, and lowering of the oxidation-reduction potential from impaired blood supply.

1. When obligate anaerobes are in mixed infection with facultative anaerobes, the facultative anaerobes will utilize the oxygen

present in the tissues, thereby reducing the oxidation-reduction potential of the in vivo microenvironment to a level at which the obligate anaerobic bacteria can proliferate. Once the available oxygen is utilized in the lesions, the facultative anaerobes will shift from a respiratory metabolism to a fermentative metabolism.

V. PATHOLOGY
  A. The lesions vary with the anatomical site of infection and the etiologic agents involved.
    1. Cellulitis and myositis lesions
        a. *Clostridium* species are the predominant pathogen in these conditions.
    2. Pyogranulomatous and granulomatous lesions
        a. *Actinomyces* species are the primary obligate anaerobes that induce this type of host response.
            (1) Sulfur granules showing peripheral clubs with branched filamentous bacilli suggest either *A. bovis* or *A. israelii*.
    3. Suppurative lesions
        a. Obligate anaerobes frequently involved in suppurative lesions include numerous species of gram-positive cocci, gram-positive nonsporeforming rods, gram-negative cocci, and gram-negative rods.

VI. DIAGNOSIS
  A. Clinical signs
    1. The tissue characteristics and lesions are often highly suggestive of anaerobic bacterial infections.
  B. Culture
    1. Isolation and identification of the various bacterial species
        a. Although most deep abscesses and other necrotizing lesions containing anaerobes are polymicrobial, it is not uncommon to isolate a single species of an anaerobe in pure culture.
        b. Anaerobes, particularly the bacteroides and fusobacteria, have shown changing patterns in their susceptibility to three or four antimicrobial agents that have commonly been used to treat anaerobic infections during the past decade.

VII. IMMUNIZATION
  A. Commercial anaerobic bacterial vaccines are not available for dogs.

| 111 | Ehrlichiosis |

I. ETIOLOGY
  A. *Ehrlichia canis* is an aerobic, gram-negative, obligate intracellular bacterium.
    1. It infects selected leukocytes and reticuloendothelial cells.

II. TRANSMISSION
  A. Biological arthropod vectors
    1. *Rhipicephalus sanguineus*, the brown dog tick, is a biological vector of *E. canis*. Larval, nymphal, and adult stages of the tick feed on dogs.
      a. The bacterium has a transstadial transmission.

III. CLINICAL FEATURES
  A. Clinical signs
    1. Canine ehrlichiosis (canine tropical pancytopenia) is a febrile disease characterized by anorexia, emaciation, pancytopenia, peripheral edema, hemorrhage, and often death. Secondary bacterial infections are common in affected dogs.
      a. Epistatis is a predominant clinical sign in affected dogs.
      b. Death often occurs 1 to 7 days after the onset of hemorrhage.
  B. Latent infections
    1. Asymptomatic infections can be maintained in the dog for as long as 5 years.

IV. PATHOGENESIS
  A. Effect on leukocytes and platelets
    1. The pancytopenia and associated clinical signs that occur 50 to 100 days after initial infection are probably related to impaired production of blood leukocytes, whereas the severe hemorrhage is a result of a thrombocytopenia.
    2. Platelet toxicity occurs in the acute stage of the disease, prior to antibody formation.

V. PATHOLOGY
  A. Clinical pathology
    1. Affected dogs have an anemia, leukopenia, and varying degrees of thrombocytopenia.
      a. The bleeding time is prolonged; however, the coagulation and prothrombin times are normal.

   2. In Giemsa-stained blood smears, *E. canis* is found in
       cytoplasmic inclusions in monocytes. These inclusions have a
       mulberry appearance and are called morula.
   B. Gross pathology
   1. Ecchymotic hemorrhages are a predominant postmortem feature.

VI. DIAGNOSIS
   A. Clinical diagnosis
   1. Clinical signs and the presence of *R. sanguineus* on dogs are
       used as the basis of clinical diagnosis.
   B. Pathology (above)
   C. Serology
   1. Demonstration of anti-*E. canis* serum antibodies with an indirect
       fluorescence technique will confirm a diagnosis.

VII. IMMUNIZATION
   A. Commercial *E. canis* vaccines are not available.

| 112 | Respiratory Infections |

I. ETIOLOGY
   A. Bacteria isolated from canine respiratory infections
   1. Bacteria frequently isolated from canine respiratory infections
       include *Actinomyces viscosus*, *Bordetella bronchiseptica*,
       Escherichia coli, *Klebsiella pneumoniae*, *Pasteurella* species,
       Staphylococcus species, and *Streptococcus* species. Other
       aerobes occasionally isolated include *Actinomyces pyogenes*,
       Mycoplasma species, *Pseudomonas aeruginosa*, *Proteus* species,
       and other members of the family Enterobacteriaceae.
   2. The most frequently isolated obligate anaerobic bacteria are in
       the genera *Bacteroides*, *Fusobacterium*, and *Peptostreptococcus*.
       Occasionally species in the genera *Bifidobacterium*, *Eubacterium*,
       Clostridium, *Peptococcus*, and *Propionibacterium* are isolated
       from lower respiratory tract infections.

II. TRANSMISSION
    A. Inhalation
        1. The majority of the bacteria isolated from canine respiratory infections are acquired by inhalation or aspiration of mucus containing bacteria either from the endogenous upper respiratory tract flora or from exogenous sources, particularly soil and feces.
    B. Hematogenous dissemination
        1. Most of the remaining infections are acquired by hematogenous dissemination.
    C. Contiguity
        1. A few pulmonary infections are acquired by the extension of adjacent infections.

III. CLINICAL FEATURES
    A. Canine respiratory infections are often classified based on the anatomic site (Table 112.1).

Table 112.1. Anatomic sites of canine respiratory diseases

Anatomic Sites	Respiratory Diseases
Trachea and bronchi	Primary infectious tracheobronchitis Canine contagious cough complex
Lungs	Pneumonia Lung abscesses
Pleura	Pleural empyema

        1. Different microorganisms are associated with each anatomic type of infection, although considerable overlap occurs with some microorganisms.
        2. Canine respiratory infections frequently contain both viral and bacterial agents.
            a. Primary pulmonary infections are generally caused by viruses, and secondary infections are usually due to bacteria. Evidence of both viral and bacterial infection is often found in the canine cough complex and pneumonias.
        3. There are several pathogenic factors that contribute to the bacterial superinfection in viral respiratory disease.
            a. The most important is the impairment of normal host defense mechanisms, thus allowing the localization, colonization, and proliferation of bacteria. The epithelium of the upper airways is frequently damaged, and the normal mucociliary apparatus is greatly impaired. This leads to decreased removal of bacteria from the respiratory tract with a resultant increase of bacteria in the respiratory system.
            b. Viral respiratory infections that result in inflammation of the lung parenchyma with an increased transudation of

protein and fluid from the interstitial spaces provides a suitable culture medium for bacterial proliferation.
c. Some viral infections, such as canine distemper, can cause an immunosuppression that predisposes the animal to secondary bacterial infection.

IV. PATHOGENESIS
A. Primary infectious tracheobronchitis
1. *B. bronchiseptica*, canine adenovirus type 2 (CAV-2), and canine parainfluenza virus (PI) are individually capable of causing primary infectious tracheobronchitis. These infections are usually acquired by inhalation from clinically infected or carrier animals.
   a. *B. bronchiseptica* can cause a severe tracheobronchitis. The bacteria colonize the tracheobronchial epithelial cells by attaching to the cilia.
   b. Primary viral infections frequently produce a mild tracheobronchitis.
B. Canine contagious cough complex
1. Canine distemper virus (CD), PI, CAV-2, *B. bronchiseptica*, mycoplasmas, and numerous other bacterial pathogens have been implicated in the canine contagious cough complex.
   a. One or more of these viruses and bacteria may simultaneously infect a dog, producing a severe tracheobronchitis, cough, and in some cases pneumonia.
   b. The viral infections predispose the tracheobronchial and lung tissues to secondary microbial infections. These secondary opportunistic pathogens are frequently the upper respiratory bacterial flora. These microbes increase the tissue damage and hence the severity of disease.
C. Pneumonia
1. Viral respiratory infections of several days duration often precede and predispose the lung tissue to secondary bacterial infections.
   a. Canine distemper, PI, and CAV-2 are the most frequently implicated viruses.
   b. Aerobic bacteria commonly isolated are *Streptococcus* species, *Staphylococcus aureus*, *B. bronchiseptica*, and *Nocardia asteroides*. Aerobic bacteria less frequently isolated are *S. epidermidis*, *A. pyogenes*, *P. aeruginosa*, *Proteus* species, and other Enterobacteriaceae. Anaerobic bacteria commonly isolated include the *Bacteroides* species, *Fusobacterium* species, and *Peptostreptococcus* species. Less frequently isolated are *Bifidobacterium* species, *Clostridium* species, *Eubacterium* species, *Peptococcus* species, and *Propionibacterium* species. The majority of these bacteria are acquired by inhalation or aspiration.
2. The clinical syndromes produced by infection with different viruses, bacteria, or combined infections with these agents may

be quite similar; nevertheless, certain features are characteristic of particular bacterial agents.

a. Aerobic bacteria
    (1) Staphylococcal and streptococcal pulmonary infections tend to produce suppurative pneumonias. Lung abscesses frequently develop as sequelae.
    (2) *K. pneumoniae* produces suppurative necrotizing pneumonias. Lung abscesses frequently develop as sequelae.
    (3) *P. multocida* is frequently involved in severe fibrinopurulent pneumonias.
    (4) *B. bronchiseptica* and *N. asteroides* are frequently sequelae to canine distemper pulmonary infections.
    (5) *N. asteroides* alone causes relatively mild pneumonic processes; however, some infections eventually progress to an empyema.
    (6) *P. aeruginosa* is an opportunistic pulmonary pathogen. These infections are often associated with preexisting tissue damage, with diminished host responses, or as a superinfection in animals in which the initial pathogens have been eradicated with antibiotics.

b. Anaerobic bacteria
    (1) Anaerobic bacteria are commonly involved as etiologic agents in aspiration pneumonias, necrotizing pneumonias, lung abscesses, and empyema. The microbial composition of these anaerobic pulmonary infections usually contain one or more obligate anaerobic bacterial species and one or more facultative anaerobic bacterial species.
    (2) The anaerobic bacteria most commonly isolated include the gram-positive cocci and gram-negative bacilli. The majority of these anaerobic bacteria are of endogenous origin.
    (3) Clinical characteristics that suggest a possibility of anaerobic bacteria include foul-smelling discharges or exudates, necrotic tissue, and the presence of actinomycotic sulfur granules in exudates.
    (4) Pathogenic factors that predispose to pulmonary infections with an anaerobic bacterial component are the lowering of the oxidation-reduction potential due to impaired blood supply, tissue injury, tissue necrosis, and mixed infection with other obligate anaerobic or facultative anaerobic bacteria. Facultative anaerobic bacteria, such as *E. coli*, will metabolize and use available tissue oxygen, thereby reducing the oxidation-reduction potential of the in vivo microenvironment to a level at which obligate anaerobic bacteria can proliferate. These predisposing factors allow anaerobic bacteria to

colonize the lower respiratory tract, whereas normal lung tissue prevents the growth of anaerobic bacteria.

c. Host factors
   (1) Another significant factor in both predisposing and predicting the type, severity, and outcome of these infections, in addition to the causative microorganisms and their virulence, is the status of the host.
   (2) Primary bacterial pneumonias are common in dogs that are immunologically compromised.
   (3) Mycoplasmal agents commonly infect dogs with or without respiratory disease.

D. Lung abscesses
   1. The principal bacterial agents recovered from lung abscesses include *S. aureus*, *K. pneumoniae*, other Enterobacteriaceae, the anaerobic gram-positive cocci, and the anaerobic gram-negative bacilli.
   2. Predisposing factors and mode of infection greatly influence the bacterial flora of lung abscesses, which are rarely found in the canine.
      a. Lung abscesses caused by infection arising in, or spread by, the respiratory passages are the most common sources. This occurs when inhaled or aspirated bacteria become established in the lungs that have been predisposed to infection by concurrent viral infection or as a complication of pneumonia. *S. aureus* and *K. pneumoniae* have a tendency to develop infection in the consolidated areas of the lung. If untreated, these infections can develop into encapsulated abscesses.
      b. Lung abscesses due to septic emboli, which form septic pulmonary infarcts, are usually located peripherally in the pulmonary parenchyma. Staphylococci are commonly isolated from these abscesses, which can erupt into the pleural cavity, producing pleural adhesions and a localized or diffuse empyema. Less frequently, aseptic pulmonary emboli subsequently become infected by bacteria that later reach the site. These infections often contain a mixed bacterial flora.
      c. Lung abscesses are frequently sequelae to traumatic injury and develop in areas of pulmonary hemorrhage. The microbial flora of open chest wounds commonly contains bacteria of exogenous origin. The microbial flora of closed chest wounds is usually composed of endogenous respiratory flora.

E. Pleural empyema
   1. Empyema is an accumulation of purulent pleural fluid and often results from bacterial infection.
   2. Empyema may develop by any of six modes of infection.

   a. Complication of lung abscesses that rupture and drain into
       the pleural cavity
   b. Extension of diffuse suppurative infections from the lungs
   c. Penetrating chest wounds
   d. Complication of thoracic surgical procedures
   e. Contagious infection
   f. Complication of septicemia
3. Bacterial pathogens most commonly isolated include *N.
   asteroides*, *A. viscosus*, *Streptococcus* species, *S. aureus*, *K.
   pneumoniae*, other coliform bacteria, the anaerobic gram-positive
   cocci, and the anaerobic gram-negative bacilli.
4. Pulmonary actinomycosis and pulmonary nocardiosis are similar
   clinical diseases and are common causes of empyema in the
   canine.
   a. Primary pulmonary actinomycosis and nocardiosis are
       acquired by inhalation or aspiration. The *Actinomyces*
       species are frequently found as endogenous flora of the
       mouth and upper respiratory tract, whereas *N. asteroides* is
       of exogenous origin from the soil.
   b. The progression of the diseases is characterized by
       pneumonia, pyogranulomatous and granulomatous pulmonary
       tissue reactions, and empyema. Pleuritis and empyema often
       appear at an early stage in the disease. Later the
       bacteria transgress fascial planes and eventually produce
       abscesses and draining sinuses in the chest wall.
   c. *A. viscosus* is the most commonly *Actinomyces* species
       isolated from pulmonary actinomycosis, but occasionally *A.
       bovis* and *A. israelii* are isolated. The *Actinomyces*
       species may be recovered in mixed culture with facultative
       anaerobes or obligate anaerobes.
   d. *N. asteroides* is frequently isolated in pure culture from
       pulmonary nocardiosis.

V. PATHOLOGY
   A. The respiratory tract lesions vary with the etiologic agents
       involved, route of transmission, anatomical site of infection, and
       duration of the conditions.
       1. The isolation and identification of the bacterial species are
           generally required to confirm the diagnosis.

VI. DIAGNOSIS
   A. Clinical signs and pathology (above)
   B. Microbiological diagnoses
       1. Bacteria
           a. Isolation and biochemical identification of bacterial
               agents
       2. Viruses
           a. The laboratory diagnosis of canine viral respiratory

pathogens can be made by virus isolation or by
demonstrating a 4-fold increase from acute to
convalescent serologic titers (which is regarded as
significant).

VII. IMMUNIZATION
    A.   Bacterial vaccines
        1.   A commercial *B. bronchiseptica* bacterin is effective in
            preventing clinical primary tracheobronchitis disease but is
            seldom used prophylactically due to its adverse side effects.
        2.   Commercial canine bacterial vaccines for the other bacterial
            agents are not available.
    B.   Viral vaccines
        1.   Commercial CD, PI, and CAV-2 vaccines that provide protective
            immunity against homologous viral challenge are available.

---

113 | Rocky Mountain Spotted Fever

I.   ETIOLOGY
    A.   *Rickettsia rickettsii* is an aerobic, gram-negative, obligate
       intracellular bacterium.
        1.   The bacterium multiplies in both the cytoplasm and the nucleus
            of eucaryotic cells.

II. TRANSMISSION
    A.   Arthropod vectors
        1.   *R. rickettsii* is transmitted to dogs through the bite of
            infected ticks, which are biological vectors of the disease.
            a.   Rodents and dogs are mammalian reservoirs of *R. rickettsii*.
            b.   Ticks acquire the infection by feeding on an infected
                animal. When the rickettsiae in the bloodmeal reach the
                tick's gut, the organisms invade and multiply in the
                epithelial cells. The infected cells lyse and release
                large numbers of bacteria into the tick's intestinal
                contents. The ticks excrete the rickettsiae in their
                feces.

c.   Female ticks can transmit the bacterium transovarially to their offspring. These ticks provide a natural habitat for *R. rickettsii*.

2.   The geographic distribution of Rocky Mountain spotted fever (RMSF) is determined by the tick vectors.

a.   *Dermacentor variabilis*, the American dog tick, is the principal vector in the eastern United States, where the disease is most prevalent in North Carolina and Virginia.

b.   *D. andersoni*, the wood tick, is the principal vector in the western United States, where the disease is most prevalent in the Rocky Mountain states.

c.   *Amblyomma americanum*, the lone star tick, and *Rhipicephalus sanguineus*, the brown dog tick, and a few other tick species have been found naturally infected with *R. rickettsii*; however, their role in the transmission of RMSF to dogs has not been delineated.

3.   The seasonal incidence of canine RMSF is largely determined by the feeding patterns of *D. andersoni* and *D. variabilis*, which are three-host ticks. The larvae and nymphs feed on small mammals, particularly rodents, whereas the adults feed on dogs, man, and other large mammals.

a.   The larvae and nymphs often acquire *R. rickettsii* infection from infected rodents and subsequently serve as adult vectors for dogs.

b.   The adults of *D. andersoni* are most active in the spring and early summer, while the adults of *D. variabilis* are active from spring until early fall.

III. CLINICAL FEATURES

A.   The severity of canine RMSF varies; it can be asymptomatic, or mild and self-limiting, or fulminating and fatal.

1.   Clinical signs of acute infections are fever, depression, vomiting, and diarrhea within 2 or 3 days following infection. Most animals exhibit scleral injection, conjunctivitis, mucopurulent ocular and nasal discharges, and petechial and ecchymotic hemorrhages on the ocular, oral, and genital mucous membranes.

2.   Death can result from cardiovascular, renal, and neurological complications.

B.   Serologic surveys indicate that *R. rickettsii* infections are widespread among wild and domestic animals and that infection is much more frequent in dogs from endemic than from nonendemic areas.

1.   It is probable that most infected dogs survive the infections with mild disease.

IV. PATHOGENESIS

A.   Infected ticks inoculate the rickettsiae into the dermis, where the organisms subsequently invade the bloodstream.

1. The bacteremia disseminates the organisms through the cardiovascular system, where the rickettsiae have a predilection for the vascular endothelial cells lining the small blood vessels.
    a. The bacteria actively penetrate into the cytoplasm and proliferate. This stimulates the endothelial cells to swell and proliferate.
2. The hyperplasia and necrosis of the endothelial cells and localized thrombus formation are the primary pathology and are responsible for many of the clinical manifestations of RMSF.

V. PATHOLOGY
   A. Gross lesions
       1. Petechial and ecchymotic hemorrages occur in all tissues. Lymphadenopathy and splenomegaly are common necropsy findings.
   B. Microscopic lesions
       1. Necrotizing vasculitis and intracellular bacteria in the endothelial cells are found in affected tissues.

VI. DIAGNOSIS
   A. Clinical signs and pathology
       1. The diagnosis of RMSF is usually made on the basis of the clinical picture and a history of a tick bite in an area where the disease is endemic.
   B. Serology
       1. The complement-fixation, microscopic agglutination, and latex agglutination tests are used to diagnose RMSF in dogs.
           a. It normally requires 2 or 3 weeks following the attachment of an infected tick before significant serologic titers develop.
   C. Culture
       1. *R. rickettsii* can be grown in embryonated eggs and selected tissue cultures.
           a. The bacterium usually can be isolated from the blood for at least 2 weeks after infection.

VII. IMMUNIZATION
   A. There is no canine vaccine available for this disease.

114 | Salmon Poisoning

I. ETIOLOGY
  A. *Neorickettsia helminthoeca* is an aerobic, gram-negative, obligate intracellular bacterium.
    1. The bacterium multiplies within cytoplasmic vacuoles of eucaryotic cells.

II. TRANSMISSION
  A. Ingestion
    1. Dogs acquire the infection by ingestion of raw fish parasitized with metacercariae of the fluke *Nanophyetus salmincola*, which in turn are infected with the rickettsial organism *N. helminthoeca*.
      a. Fish in the family salmonidae, particularly salmon and trout, are susceptible to infection with cercariae of *N. salmincola*. The metacercariae are encysted in the musculature of the fish.
  B. Life cycle of the fluke vector
    1. *N. salmincola*, the fluke vector of *N. helminthoeca*, has a three-host life cycle involving snails, fish, and dogs. *N. helminthoeca* has been found in all stages (egg, miracidia, cercariae, and adult) of the trematode.
      a. The snail *Oxytrema silicula*, the first intermediate host of the fluke, is infected by the miracidia, which develop from the fluke eggs.
      b. Salmonid fish are the second intermediate host of the fluke. The fish ingest the snails, and the cercarial stage of the fluke encyst in the musculature of the fish.
      c. Dogs ingest the parasitized fish, and the metacercariae develop into the adult flukes in their intestinal tract. The dogs are infected with *N. helminthoeca* carried by the fluke.
      d. The life cycle of the fluke is completed when fluke eggs are passed in the dog's feces.

III. CLINICAL FEATURES
  A. Clinical signs
    1. Salmon poisoning is an acute febrile, often fatal infection that is characterized by vomiting and diarrhea. About 10 percent of clinically affected dogs recover from clinical infections.
  B. Geographic distribution
    1. Salmon poisoning is geographically restricted to the seaboard of the northwestern states.

IV. PATHOGENESIS
  A. Dogs ingest raw fish infested with the metacercariae of *N. salmincola.*
    1. *N. helminthoeca* are released from the fluke in the dog's intestinal tract. The incubation period is 5 to 7 days.
      a. The rickettsial organisms parasitize the lymphocytes and macrophages, and eventually the infection depletes the small lymphocytes and destroys the germinal centers of the lymph nodes.
      b. The intestinal infection causes a hemorrhagic enteritis.
  B. Immunity
    1. Dogs that survive the initial acute infections develop immunity to reinfection.

V. PATHOLOGY
  A. Gross lesions
    1. There is often a hemorrhagic enteritis, and the cervical and visceral lymph nodes are enlarged. The spleen and tonsils also may be enlarged, and a mild interstitial pneumonia may be observed.

VI. DIAGNOSIS
  A. Clinical signs
    1. Clinical symptoms are usually characteristic of the disease.
  B. Fecal examination
    1. Fluke ova in the feces are presumptive evidence of infection.
  C. Pathology
    1. Gross lesions (above)
    2. Demonstration of rickettsiae in macrophages of Giemsa- or Gimenez-stained smears of fluid aspirated from mandibular lymph nodes

VII. IMMUNIZATION
  A. Commercial *N. helminthoeca* vaccines are not available.

PART **6**	Feline Diseases

115	Extracellular Bacterial Diseases

I. SUSCEPTIBILITY OF CATS TO BACTERIAL DISEASES
   A. Cats that are not immunosuppressed tend to be highly resistant to the majority of the extracellular and facultative intracellular pathogens that commonly affect other domestic animals.
      1. Cats are the primary host for only a few bacterial species, particularly *Mycoplasma felis.*
      2. In nonimmunologically compromised cats, only a few bacterial species consistently produce severe and often debilitating infections, particularly *Pasteurella multocida.*

II. BACTERIAL INFECTIONS OF SELECTED TISSUES AND BODY SYSTEMS
   A. Skin and subcutaneous infections
      1. Dermatitis
         a. *Pseudomonas aeruginosa, Staphylococcus* species, and *Streptococcus* species are responsible for the majority of the bacterial dermatoses of cats.
      2. Abscesses
         a. Abscesses resulting from cat fights account for a significant number of clinical bacterial infections presented to the practicing veterinarian. These abscesses are especially frequent in intact males.
            (1) *P. multocida*, a component of the feline oral flora, is the most commonly isolated species. The staphylococci, streptococci, enterobacteria, and obligate anaerobes also are frequent etiologic agents.
            (2) *Nocardia asteroides* causes subcutaneous lesions, often with fistulous tracts. The abscesses and nodules frequently ulcerate and develop chronic draining tracts. The lesions are usually on the limbs, neck,

tail, ears, and abdomen. Some lesions may perforate
into the thorax, producing a pyothorax.

   3. Anal gland abscesses

      a. The anal glands become impacted with glandular material and
subsequently become infected with various bacterial
species.

B. Eye infections

   1. Conjunctivitis

      a. Various *Mycoplasma* and *Ureaplasma* species have been
isolated from the eyes of cats with conjunctivitis.

         (1) Most mycoplasmal species are considered to be
secondary or opportunistic pathogens; however, *M.
felis* can serve as a sole pathogen of feline
conjunctivitis.

C. Respiratory tract infections

   1. Cats are relatively resistant to bacterial infections of the
respiratory tract and lungs, even when prior tissue damage has
resulted from viral infections.

   2. Upper respiratory tract infections

      a. *Bordetella bronchiseptica* is a common upper respiratory
tract pathogen of kittens, but adults seldom exhibit
clinical signs.

   3. Pneumonias

      a. Bacterial pneumonias invariably occur secondarily to a
primary viral infection. Secondary bacterial pathogens
include *B. bronchiseptica*, *Escherichia coli*, other
coliforms, and mycoplasmas.

D. Gastrointestinal tract infections

   1. Salmonellosis

      a. *Salmonella typhimurium* is the most common serovar isolated
from cats. Several other *Salmonella* serovars, including
some pathogenic for domestic animals and man, also have
been isolated.

      b. Most clinical infections are acquired by ingestion;
however, stress-induced recrudescence of subclinical
salmonellae infections in carrier cats also has been
incriminated.

         (1) Clinical salmonellosis occurs more commonly in young
than in adult cats. Severe salmonellosis causes
gastroenteritis with vomiting and diarrhea and often
ends fatally in septicemia.

      c. Cats are common carriers of salmonellae. After clinical or
inapparent infection, many cats shed salmonellae in their
feces for months.

   2. Tuberculosis

      a. Cats are very susceptible to *Mycobacterium bovis* but are
highly resistant to *M. tuberculosis*. *M. avium* infections
in cats are uncommon.

(1) The incidence of feline tuberculosis is fairly high in areas in which there is a high incidence of *M. bovis* infections in man and animals.
  b. Most infections are acquired by ingestion.
     (1) Granulomatous lesions are often initiated along and adjacent to the digestive tract, including the oral pharynx.
E. Urinary tract infections
  1. Bacterial cystitis
     a. Infection of the urinary bladder invariably results from ascending bacteria from the urinary tract.
        (1) Cats appear to be highly resistant to clinical bacterial cystitis. When infections occur, *E. coli*, *Proteus* species, and *Staphylococcus aureus* are the most commonly isolated bacteria.

116	Haemobartonellosis

I. ETIOLOGY
  A. *Haemobartonella felis* is an aerobic, gram-negative bacterium.
     1. The bacterium is cell-associated with feline erythroctyes and is generally found firmly adhered to the surface of the erythrocytes.

II. TRANSMISSION
  A. Direct contact
     1. *H. felis* can be transmitted by the oral, intravenous, and intraperitoneal routes. The infection also can be transmitted during cat fights.
        a. *H. felis* does not persist in the environment.
  B. Insects
     1. Bloodsucking insects, particularly fleas, have been incriminated as mechanical vectors of *H. felis*.

III. CLINICAL FEATURES
  A. Clinical signs
     1. Feline haemobartonellosis (feline infectious anemia) is clinically manifested as an anemia, anorexia, depression,

intermittent fever, splenomegaly, and weight loss. Icterus may occur if the hemolysis of the red blood cells is sufficiently rapid during a hemolytic crisis.
  a. Most cats are asymptomatic, but various stress factors, particularly splenomegaly, can cause recrudescence of latent infection, resulting in recurrent episodes of clinical disease.
  b. Cats of any age may be infected and exhibit clinical disease.
  B. Immunity
    1. The immunity acquired during natural infections is poorly understood; however, the bacteria often persist in the blood of asymptomatic carriers after clinical recovery.

IV. PATHOGENESIS
  A. Within the cat, *H. felis* associates with the erythrocytes and reproduces by binary fission, forming chains of bacteria on the surface of erythrocytes.
    1. The bacteremia (*H. felis* associated with circulating erythrocytes) tends to be intermittent, and the bacteria are not always detectable in the blood on successive days.
    2. The *H. felis*-induced anemia is regenerative and characterized by a reticulocytosis.
  B. The infected erythrocytes are destroyed without the release of free hemoglobin; therefore hemoglobinuria is not seen in haemobartonellosis.

V. PATHOLOGY
  A. Clinical pathology
    1. The regenerative anemia is characterized by an increased number of reticulocytes and nucleated erythroid cells in the peripheral blood.
  B. Gross pathology
    1. The postmortem appearance is dominated by pallor, with or without icterus, enlargement of mesenteric lymph nodes, hyperplasia of bone marrow, and splenomegaly.

VI. DIAGNOSIS
  A. Clinical signs (above)
  B. Clinical and gross pathology (above)
    1. In Giemsa-stained blood smears, *H. felis* is identified based on its cellular morphology, arrangement, and association with the surface of erythrocytes. *H. felis* is seldom found free in the plasma.

VII. IMMUNIZATION
  A. Commercial *H. felis* vaccines are not available.

117 | Pneumonitis

I. ETIOLOGY

A. *Chlamydia psittaci* is an aerobic, gram-negative, obligate intracellular bacterium.
  1. The bacterium has two characteristic morphologic forms: elementary bodies and reticulate bodies. The elementary bodies are the infective form.

II. TRANSMISSION

A. Inhalation and direct contact
  1. Feline pneumonitis is highly contagious among cats and is transmitted by inhalation of infected droplets expelled by sneezing or by contaminated ocular discharges.
    a. In feline pneumonitis, *C. psittaci* primarily infects the epithelial cells of the conjunctiva and upper respiratory tract.

III. CLINICAL FEATURES

A. Clinical signs
  1. The clinical syndrome is characterized by absence of significant fever, anorexia, depression, droolings of saliva, and by serous discharges from the eyes and nose, which often become mucopurulent due to secondary bacterial infection. The disease is debilitating; it may linger for weeks without change in symptomology and then is followed by a slow recovery. The mortality rate is low.
  2. Complications of feline pneumonitis include bronchopneumonia, empyema, meningitis, and purulent otitis media. *Pasteurella multocida* is the organism chiefly responsible for the complications, although in kittens coliforms and the streptococci are not uncommon.
B. Age susceptibility
  1. Neonatal kittens are more susceptible than adults and generally have more severe disease. Infections in adult cats are often mild and subclinical.
C. Immunity
  1. The immunity produced in natural infections is not strong, and recovery from infection is characteristically associated with the persistence of subclinical infections in carrier cats.

IV. PATHOGENESIS

A. *C. psittaci* infects the epithelial cells of the conjunctiva and respiratory tract, producing a conjunctivitis and pneumonitis.

        1. The bacteria proliferate in cytoplasmic vacuoles forming
        inclusion bodies.

  B. Cats that recover from pneumonitis are often susceptible to
     reinfection with *C. psittaci*.

V. PATHOLOGY
  A. The lesions of uncomplicated pneumonitis consist of a catarrhal
     inflammation of the conjunctiva and upper respiratory tract.

VI. DIAGNOSIS
  A. Clinical signs (above)
  B. Pathology (above)
  C. Direct smears
     1. In Giemsa-stained conjunctival smears, the epithelial cells have
       intracytoplasmic inclusions containing large numbers of
       bacteria.

VII. IMMUNIZATION
  A. Commercial *C. psittaci* vaccine for feline pneumonitis have a
     questionable efficacy.

SECTION VI

Determinative Bacteriology

PART **1**	Aerobic Extracellular Bacteria

118	Diagnostic Procedures for Aerobic Extracellular Bacteria

I. SPECIMEN COLLECTION
   A. The proper collection of a specimen for culture is an important step in the recovery of bacteria responsible for disease.
      1. A poorly collected specimen is often responsible for the failure to isolate the causative bacterium or bacteria, while the recovery of contaminants can lead to an incorrect diagnosis.
   B. The success of specimen collection largely depends on the type, stage, and extent of the infection. When the specimens are obtained, they should be examined directly for bacteria and cytological features, cultured on appropriate media, and incubated at proper temperature and atmospheric conditions.

II. DIRECT EXAMINATION OF SPECIMENS
   A. Criteria that can aid in the presumptive identification of bacteria in stained preparations from clinical specimens include the Gram reaction, cellular morphology and arrangement, acid-fast properties of the mycobacteria and nocardiae, and endospores of the genera *Bacillus* and *Clostridium*.
   B. The presence and types of leukocytes and inflammatory cells observed in smears should correlate with the microorganisms present.
      1. The presence of bacteria without accompanying inflammatory cells should be interpreted with caution. This may represent a contaminated specimen, or it may represent colonized bacteria not associated with an invasive infection.
      2. Large numbers of neutrophils suggest an acute infection caused by extracellular bacteria.
         a. Pyogenic bacteria in the genera *Staphylococcus* and *Streptococcus* induce suppurative lesions that often progress to form abscesses.

     b.   Extraintestinal infections of most members of the family Enterobacteriaceae cause suppurative lesions.

     c.   Opportunistic infections with obligate anaerobes in the genera *Peptococcus*, *Peptostreptococcus*, *Bacteroides*, and *Fusobacterium* tend to be suppurative in nature.

3. Large numbers of macrophages indicate either chronic bacterial infections or infections caused by facultative intracellular bacteria.

4. Epithelioid cells and giant cells are often present in chronic granulomatous tissue reactions.

     a.   The extracellular pathogens in the genera *Actinomyces* and *Nocardia* induce pyogranulomatous or granulomatous lesions.

     b.   The facultative intracellular pathogens in the genera *Brucella* and *Mycobacterium* induce granulomatous lesions.

5. The number and morphologic forms of bacterial agents present in the direct smear should correlate with the number and morphologic forms of bacteria recovered in culture. When a microorganism is not recovered on culture, two factors frequently responsible are prior antimicrobial therapy and improper culture procedures. Prior antimicrobial therapy may affect the recovery of bacteria either by preventing growth or by prolonging the time before visible growth is evident. Also different types of bacteria may require specific culture media, unique incubations, or both for growth. The majority of the bacteria incriminated in domestic animal infections are not particularly fastidious in their growth requirements, and satisfactory growth is obtained on blood agar and/or MacConkey agar when incubated aerobically at 37°C. After 24 to 48 hours, blood agar plates should be observed for colonial morphologic features and hemolytic patterns, and MacConkey plates should be observed for the presence or absence of colony formation and lactose reaction.

III. BACTERIAL STAINS

  A. Gram stain

     1. The Gram stain is used to distinguish gram-positive from gram-negative bacteria. It is based on differences of their cell wall composition.

        a.   This procedure requires four steps: crystal violet is the primary stain, Gram's iodine is used to bind the crystal violet to the cell wall of gram-positive bacteria, an organic decolorizer removes the crystal violet stain from gram-negative bacteria and the unbound stain from gram-positive bacteria, and safranin is used as a counterstain.

        b.   Gram-positive bacteria retain the iodine-bound crystal violet and stain purple. Gram-negative bacteria are stained with safranin dye and appear pink.

B. Acid-fast stains
   1. Different acid-fast staining methods are used for the acid-fast mycobacteria and the partially acid-fast nocardiae.
      a. The Ziehl-Neelsen method is used to stain members of the genus *Mycobacterium*.
         (1) Carbolfuchsin is the primary stain, and heat is used to facilitate the penetration of the stain through the lipid-rich cell wall. An acid-alcohol solution is used as the decolorizer and methylene blue as the counterstain.
         (2) The mycobacteria resist decoloration with the acid-alcohol solution and retain the carbolfuchsin stain and appear red, whereas non-acid-fast bacteria and the nocardiae are decolorized and stain blue.
      b. The Kenyon modification of the acid-fast stain is often used to stain members of the genus *Nocardia*.
         (1) Carbolfuchsin is the primary stain, and tergitol, which is a surface active detergent, is added to the stain to facilitate penetration of the nocardial cell wall. An aqueous-acid solution is used as the decolorizer, and methylene blue is used as the counterstain.
         (2) *Nocardia* species retain the carbolfuchsin and appear red, whereas non-acid-fast bacteria stain blue.

IV. BACTERIOLOGIC MEDIA
   A. Nutrients
      1. Proteins
         a. Protein hydrolysates, including casein, meat infusion, peptones, and tryptones, provide a source of carbon and nitrogen. Most media will contain 1 to 2 percent protein.
            (1) Amino acids and low molecular weight peptides produced by the degradation of proteins by bacterial proteases are actively taken up and utilized for growth by most pathogenic bacteria.
      2. Carbohydrates
         a. Various carbohydrates are used to provide a source of carbon and energy. Most fermentation, oxidation, and differential media will contain 0.5 to 2 percent carbohydrate.
      3. Lipids
         a. The pathogenic leptospires and mycobacteria require various lipids for in vitro cultivation.
      4. Enrichments
         a. Blood, serum, vitamin supplements, and yeast extract are added to basal media for the support of fastidious organisms.

          (1) Blood agar will usually contains 5 percent
               defibrinated sheep or bovine blood.

B.   Agar, buffers, and salts
    1.   Agar, a gelatinous extract of red seaweed, is used as a
        solidifying agent in numerous bacteriologic media.
        a.   Plating media contain from 1 to 2 percent agar.
        b.   The different motility media contain from 0.05 to 0.4
             percent agar.
        c.   Agar is used in varying concentrations as needed in a
             variety of other media. Trace amounts of agar are added to
             some broth media.
    2.   Buffers are used to provide a stable pH for bacterial growth and
        to provide a standard pH reference for those media in which a
        shift in pH is used to detect bacterial metabolic products.
        a.   Monosodium phosphate, disodium phosphate, and potassium
             phosphate are frequently used as buffers.
    3.   A variety of salts are used to provide inorganic ions required
        by various bacteria.

C.   pH indicators
    1.   Purposes of pH indicators
        a.   Some pH indicators are used to measure the pH in test media
             resulting from bacterial enzymatic activity on a given
             substrate (Table 118.1).

Table 118.1. Indicators to measure pH

Indicators	pH Range	Acid Color	Basic Color
Bromocresol purple	5.2–6.8	Yellow	Purple
Bromothymol blue	6.0–7.6	Yellow	Blue
Litmus	4.5–8.3	Red	Blue
Methyl red	4.2–6.0	Red	Yellow
Neutral red	6.8–8.0	Red	Yellow
Phenol red	6.8–8.4	Yellow	Red

          (1) Bromocresol purple is often used in reactions that
               detect amino acid catabolism.
          (2) Bromothymol blue is used in the citrate utilization
               test.
          (3) Litmus, when incorporated into litmus milk broth, is
               both a pH indicator and a redox indicator. Some
               anaerobic bacteria are capable of reducing litmus to a
               white leuco base. Litmus milk is frequently used in
               identifying selected *Clostridium* species.
          (4) Methyl red is used in methyl red-Voges Proskauer
               (MRVP) medium.
          (5) Neutral red is used in MacConkey agar.
          (6) Phenol red is used in most carbohydrate fermentation
               media.

b. Some pH indicators selectively inhibit bacterial growth.
  (1) Eosin Y and methylene blue dyes are incorporated into eosin methylene blue (EMB) agar, which is both a selective and differential medium. Eosin Y is both a pH indicator and a selective inhibitor of bacterial growth. EMB agar markedly inhibits the growth of most gram-positive bacteria and fastidious gram-negative bacteria. It is used primarily in the identification of the members of the family Enterobacteriaceae.
  (2) Malachite green dye inhibits gram-negative and most gram-positive bacteria other than the mycobacteria. Malachite green has a yellow-green color at pH 2.0 or less and is colorless at pH 11.6 or higher.
c. Some pH indicators serve as redox indicators to monitor anaerobiosis (Table 118.2).

Table 118.2. Redox indicators to monitor anaerobiosis

Redox Indicator	Millivolt Potential	Oxidized State		Reduced State	
		mv	Color	mv	Color
Methylene blue	+11 mv	≥ +11	Blue	≤ +11	Colorless
Resazurin	-42 mv	≥ -42	Pink	≤ -42	Colorless
Phenosafranin	-252 mv	≥-252	Pink	≤-252	Colorless

  (1) Methylene blue is used as a redox indicator for oxygen-free conditions in anaerobic culture jars and chambers. It is seldom used as a redox indicator in culture medium.
  (2) Resazurin and phenosafranin are commonly used as a redox indicators in anaerobic bacteriologic culture media.

D. Inhibitors of bacterial growth
  1. Four groups of compounds are used in selective media to inhibit the growth of various types of bacteria and fungi.
    a. Antibiotics and antibacterial drugs
      (1) Bacitracin, carbenicillin, cephalothin, chloramphenicol, colistin, cycloserine, gentamicin, kanamycin, methicillin, neomycin, penicillin, streptomycin, sulfonamides, trimethoprim, and vancomycin are frequently incorporated into agar media to inhibit bacterial growth.
    b. Chemicals
      (1) Bile salts (sodium deoxycholate, sodium taurocholate, and oxgall), phenylalcohol, potassium cyanate, potassium thiocyanate, sodium azide, and sodium selenite are commonly employed in selective media.
    c. Dyes
      (1) Brilliant green, crystal violet, eosin Y, ethyl

violet, and methylene blue dyes are commonly employed
in selective media. Dyes that also act as pH
indicators include brilliant green, eosin Y, and
methylene blue.

    d.   Heavy metals

        (1) Several compounds containing heavy metals will inhibit
bacterial growth. These include bismuth sulfite,
cadmium sulfate, lithium chloride, and potassium
tellurite.

V.   AGAR MEDIA

    A.   Streaking technique

        1.   A primary function of agar media is the isolation of bacterial
colonies from clinical specimens or broth cultures (Fig. 118.1).

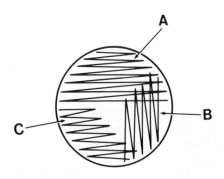

Fig. 118.1. Common streaking method for the isolation of bacteria on agar
media showing the primary streak area (*A*), the second streak area (*B*), and the
third streak area (*C*).

    B.   Nonselective agar media

        1.   Blood agar is a nonselective medium that will support the growth
of most commonly encountered bacterial pathogens.

           a.   Hemolytic reactions on blood agar

               (1) Alpha hemolysis is characterized by partial clearing
of blood around colonies, with greenish discoloration
of the medium.

               (2) Beta hemolysis is characterized by a complete clearing
of blood around colonies.

               (3) Double zone hemolysis has a zone of complete hemolysis
adjacent to colonies with a second zone of partial
hemolysis at the periphery.

b. Colony characteristics
   (1) The size, form, elevation, color, density, and surface appearance are used to describe colony morphology.
       (a) The diameter of colonies is measured in millimeters.
       (b) The elevations of most pathogenic bacteria are flat, raised, convex, or umbonate. The colony margins are entire, undulate, filamentous, or rhizoid (Fig. 118.2).

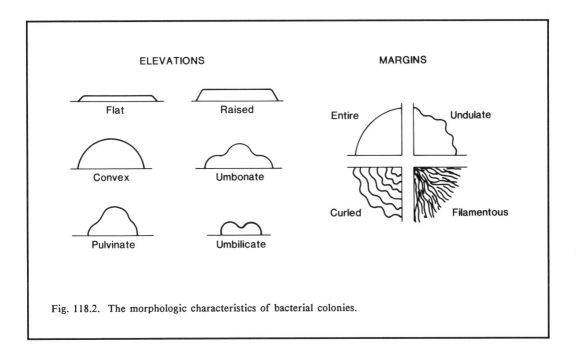

Fig. 118.2. The morphologic characteristics of bacterial colonies.

       (c) The color of most bacteria are white, buff, or yellow, but a few are orange, red, or black.
       (d) The density of colonies is usually described as opaque, translucent, or transparent and the surface appearance is either glistening or dull.
C. Selective agar media
   1. Selective media are designed to support the growth of certain bacteria while inhibiting the growth of others.
   2. Commonly used selective and/or differential media include sodium azide blood agar, brilliant green agar, eosin methylene blue agar, MacConkey agar, mannitol salt agar, and tergitol 7 agar.

VI. BIOCHEMICAL AND MOTILITY TESTS
A. Catalase and oxidase tests
   1. A catalase or oxidase test is frequently used as the initial

biochemical test in determinative identification schema for
aerobic gram-positive and gram-negative bacteria, respectively.

2. Catalase test

   a. Catalase is a iron-containing hemoprotein enzyme that
       decomposes hydrogen peroxide (H_2O_2) into water and oxygen.
       The colonies to be tested are removed from the agar sruface
       with an inoculation loop and placed on a glass slide. A
       drop of hydrogen peroxide (3 percent concentration or
       greater) is placed on the colony. Gas bubbles formed by
       the oxygen indicate a positive test (Fig. 118.3).

$$2H_2O_2 \xrightarrow[\text{catalase}]{} 2H_2O + O_2$$

Fig. 118.3. The catalase reaction.

   b. Catalase activity is present in most aerobic bacteria but
       in only a few anaerobic bacteria.
       (1) Aerobic gram-positive bacteria that are catalase-
            negative include *Actinomyces pyogenes*, *Erysipelothrix
            rhusiopathiae*, and *Streptococcus* species.
       (2) The majority of the bacteria classified in anaerobic
            genera are catalase-negative; however, catalase
            activity is present in *Bacteroides fragilis* and some
            Peptostreptococcus species.

3. Oxidase test

   a. The cytochrome system has iron-containing hemoproteins that
       transfer electrons or hydrogen to oxygen with the formation
       of water (Fig. 118.4).

   b. The oxidase test uses a fresh 1 percent solution of
       tetramethyl-*p*-phenylenediamine, which will substitute for
       oxygen as an electron acceptor. The dye in the reduced
       state is colorless but in the oxidized state forms a blue

$$4e^- + O_2 \xrightarrow[\text{cytochromes}]{} H_2O$$

Fig. 118.4. The cytochrome system reaction.

color. When 1 or 2 drops of the oxidase reagent is added onto a colony, a change in color indicates a positive reaction. The color change usually occurs within 10 to 15 seconds.

   c. The oxidase test is used primarily in the identification of aerobic gram-negative bacteria. Many gram-positive bacteria also have a detectable cytochrome system.

      (1) Oxidase-positive bacteria have cytochrome oxidase, while oxidase-negative bacteria lack cytochrome oxidase but may contain other cytochromes. Bacteria with low levels of cytochrome oxidase may give a slow or negative oxidase reaction.

   d. Commonly isolated aerobic gram-negative bacteria that are oxidase-negative include all genera in the family Enterobacteriaceae, as well as *Acinetobacter* species, *Francisella* species, and some *Haemophilus* species.

B. Nitrate reduction test

   1. The ability to reduce nitrate is useful in identifying bacteria in the family Enterobacteriaceae and the genus *Haemophilus*. All species in the genus *Haemophilus* and the family Enterobacteriaceae, except *Enterobacter agglomerans*, reduce nitrate to nitrite or other products.

      a. Oxygen derived from nitrate when it is reduced by bacteria to form nitrite reacts with electrons (hydrogen) to form water. The enzyme nitroreductase reduces nitrate only under anaerobic conditions or conditions of very low oxygen tension (Fig. 118.5).

   2. Nitrite in the test medium is detected by the addition of two test reagents, alpha-naphthylamine and sulfanilic acid, to form a red diazonium compound. If the nitrate is reduced to form compounds other than nitrite (ammonium, nitric oxide, nitrous oxide, or hydroxylamine), no color change is produced when the test reagents are added to the test medium and a false-negative test is observed. To determine if a false-negative reaction has occurred, zinc dust is added to the test medium. If nitrate is present, the zinc ions will reduce nitrate to nitrite and a red color will form, confirming a true-negative reaction; however, if no color develops it indicates a true-positive reaction.

$$NO_3 + 2e^- + H_2 \xrightarrow{\text{nitroreductase}} NO_2 + H_2O$$

nitrate   nitrite

Fig. 118.5. The reduction of nitrate to form nitrite.

C. Motility tests
    1. Direct examination method
        a. The motility of bacteria can be determined by light
            microscopic examination of a hanging drop preparation. A
            drop of broth culture is placed on a coverglass, which in
            turn is inverted on a glass slide with a central depressed
            area (Fig. 118.6).
    2. Soft agar motility media
        a. The agar concentration in media used to detect bacterial
            motility is generally less than 0.5 percent (Fig. 118.7).
        b. Types of motility media
            (1) Motility test medium with tetrazolium salts

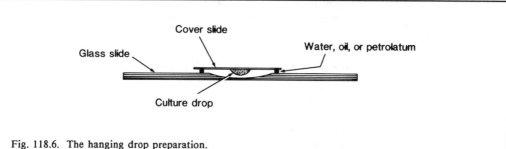

Fig. 118.6. The hanging drop preparation.

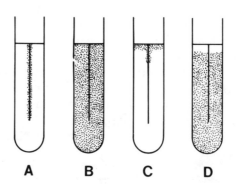

Fig. 118.7. Bacterial motility and oxygen requirements in a soft agar medium.
A nonmotile facultative anaerobe grows only along the line of stab inoculation
(A), a motile facultative anaerobe spreads from the line of inoculation
producing turbidity throughout the agar (B), a motile obligate aerobe spreads
from the line of inoculation only near the agar surface (C), and a motile
obligate anaerobe spreads from the line of inoculation except at the agar
surface (D).

(a) This medium is composed of protein, sodium chloride, 0.4 percent agar, and tetrazolium salts as an indicator. In this test, the media is inoculated by stabbing the medium with the microorganism to be evaluated. The tetrazolium salts are colorless in uninoculated media but are converted to an insoluble red formazan complex by the reducing properties of growing bacteria. The red color helps to trace the spread of bacteria from the inoculation line.

(2) Combination test media
    (a) Motility-indole-ornithine (MIO) medium
    (b) Sulfide-indole-motility (SIM) medium

D. Carbohydrate tests
  1. Saccharolytic bacteria utilize a variety of carbohydrates (monosaccharides, disaccharides, and trisaccharides), polyhedral alcohols, and cationic salts of organic acids as sources of carbon and energy (Table 118.3).

Table 118.3. Carbohydrates, polyhedral alcohols, and cationic salts of organic acids commonly used as substrate in determinative bacteriology

Carbohydrates				Polyhedral Alcohols	Cationic Salts of Organic Acids
Monosaccharides					
Hexoses	Pentoses	Disaccharides[a]	Trisaccharides[a]		
Glucose	Arabinose	Cellibiose	Raffinose	Adonitol	Acetate
Mannose	Xylose	Lactose		Dulcitol	Citrate
Rhamnose		Maltose		Glycerol	Malonate
		Melibiose		Inositol	
		Sucrose		Mannitol	
		Trehalose		Ribitol	
				Sorbitol	

[a]Each disaccharide and trisaccharide has one or more monomers of glucose.

  2. Carbohydrate fermentation media for individual substrates
    a. Individual carbohydrate substrates are added at a 1 percent concentration to a semisolid basal medium, which is usually composed of 2 percent protein, 0.5 percent agar, and sodium chloride. Most media are adjusted to a pH of 7.4. The pH indicator is phenol red.
    b. Carbohydrate fermentation produces acid or acid with gas. Aerogenic bacteria produce both acid and gas, but anaerogenic bacteria produce only acid. Gas production (carbon dioxide and hydrogen) is detected by the accumulation of gas in an inverted glass test tube (Durham tube), which is immersed in the medium (Fig. 118.8).
  3. Lactose fermentation and the orthonitrophenyl galactoside (ONPG) test
    a. The fermentation of lactose, a disaccharide of glucose and galactose with a glycoside bond, requires the enzymes beta-

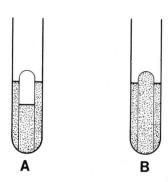

Fig. 118.8. Durham fermentation tubes. Tube *A* was inoculated with an aerogenic bacterium, which produces both acid and gas. Tube *B* was inoculated with an anaerogenic bacterium, which produces only acid. Note the presence of gas in the Durham tube in tube *A* and the absence of gas in *B*.

galactoside permease and beta-galactosidase. The permease is responsible for the transmigration of lactose in the culture medium across the cell wall, while the intra-cellular beta-galactosidase hydrolyzes the covalent glycoside bond with the formation of glucose and galactose (Fig. 118.9).

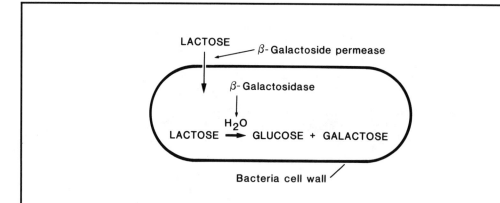

Fig. 118.9. Bacterial uptake and hydrolysis of lactose to produce glucose and galactose.

(1) Lactose-positive bacteria vary considerably in their
        rate of lactose fermentation. Strong lactose
        fermenters such as *Escherichia coli* possess adequate
        levels of both enzymes, whereas slow lactose
        fermenters such as *Klebsiella pneumoniae* usually
        possess adequate beta-galactosidase activity but show
        sluggish permease activity.

b. The ONPG test detects beta-galactosidase activity. The
      biochemical structure of ONPG is similar to lactose, except
      that the glucose has been substituted for by an
      orthonitrophenyl radical that is linked to galactose by a
      glycoside bond. Unlike lactose, the ONPG molecule is
      readily permeable through the cell wall and does not
      require permease. The intracellular ONPG is hydrolyzed by
      beta-galactosidase with the formation of orthonitrophenyl
      and galactose. ONPG is colorless, but its orthonitrophenyl
      radical is yellow, turning the test medium a bright yellow.
      This test is often used to detect slow or weak lactose-
      positive bacteria (Fig. 118.10).

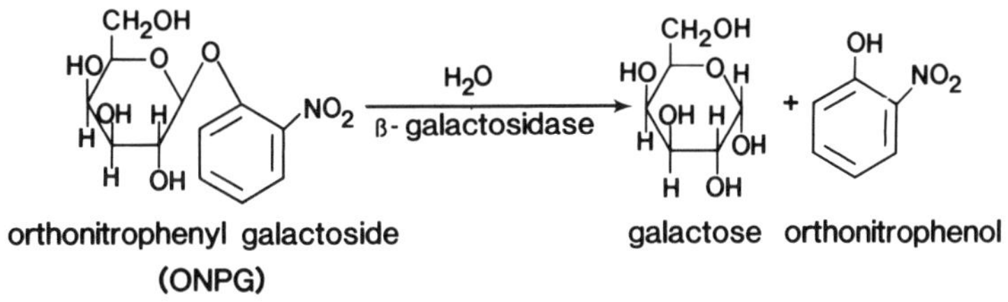

Fig. 118.10. The ONPG test.

4. Methyl red and Voges-Proskauer tests
    a. The methyl red (MR) test is a qualitative test for acid
          production from glucose via a mixed acid fermentation
          pathway. The Voges-Proskauer (VP) test is based on the
          fermentative degradation of glucose to acetoin as a major
          metabolic product. These tests are often conducted
          simultaneously in the same broth medium, which is composed
          of protein, 0.5 percent dextrose, a buffer, and a pH of
          6.9. The pH indicator is methyl red.
5. Citrate test
    a. Some bacterial species can utilize citrate as their sole

source of carbon and energy. Simmon's citrate agar is commonly used. The medium is composed of sodium citrate and ammonium phosphate. Bromothymol blue is the pH indicator. The sodium citrate serves as a source of carbon and energy, while ammonium phosphate serves as a source of nitrogen. In aqueous solution, ammonium hydroxide is formed, resulting in an alkalinization of the medium that turns the pH indicator a deep blue color.

6. Oxidation-fermentation (OF) test medium
   a. Individual carbohydrate substrates are added at a 1 percent concentration to a semisolid basal medium composed of 0.2 percent protein, 0.3 percent agar, sodium chloride, and dipotassium phosphate. It has a pH of 7.4. The pH indicator is bromothymol blue. Glucose is the standard carbohydrate substrate.
      (1) When compared with carbohydrate fermentation media, the OF medium has a lower protein:carbohydrate ratio, which reduces the formation of alkaline amines that can neutralize the small quantities of weak acids that may form from oxidative metabolism.
      (2) Two tubes of OF test medium are inoculated with the unknown organism, using a straight needle to stab the medium. One tube is covered with sterile mineral oil to provide an anaerobic medium, while the other tube is left open to the air, providing an aerobic medium. The metabolic utilization of a carbohydrate substrate produces acid and changes the color of the medium from blue to yellow (Fig. 118.11).

7. Triple sugar iron (TSI) agar
   a. TSI agar is used to detect H_2S production and the fermentation of glucose, lactose, and sucrose. The medium contains 2 percent protein, about 1 percent agar, 0.1 percent glucose, 1 percent lactose, and 1 percent sucrose. The medium has a pH of 7.4, and phenol red is the pH indicator. The agar is poured on a slant, which allows two reaction chambers within the same tube. The deep of the tube is protected from air and is relatively anaerobic, whereas the slant of the tube is exposed to atmospheric air. When the medium is inoculated with the test colony, an inoculating wire is stabbed to the deep of the tube; and the wire is then removed from the deep of the tube and used to streak the slant surface. The inoculated TSI tube is then incubated aerobically at $37^{\circ}C$ for 18 to 24 hours.
   b. Reactions on TSI agar
      (1) Alkaline slant/alkaline deep or no change
         (a) No carbohydrate fermentation
         (b) The alkaline reaction on the slant results from the oxidative decarboxylation of proteins and amino acids in the medium.

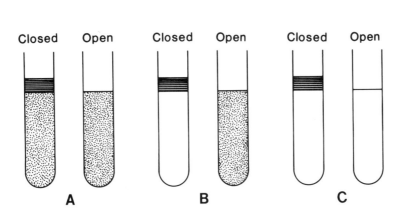

Fig. 118.11. Oxidative-fermentative tests. The fermentative bacterium produces acid in both the closed (anaerobic) and open (aerobic) tubes (*A*). An oxidative bacterium produces acid only in the open tube (*B*). An asaccharyolytic bacterium does not produce acid in either tube (*C*).

      (2) Alkaline slant/acid deep
         (a) Glucose is fermented, but lactose and sucrose are not fermented.
      (3) Acid slant/acid deep
         (a) Glucose is fermented, which turns the deep acid, and lactose and/or sucrose are fermented, which turns the slant acid.
      (4) Alkaline slant/acid deep with H_2S production
         (a) Glucose is fermented, and H_2S gas is produced.
E.   Amino acid and protein tests
    1.   Selected amino acids degraded by specific bacterial enzymes and their principal metabolic products are listed in Table 118.4.
    2.   Arginine dihydrolase test
        a.   Arginine dihydrolase removes the NH_2 group from arginine to form citrulline, which in turn is converted to ornithine. The ornithine undergoes decarboxylation to form putrescine with an alkaline reaction.

Table 118.4. Amino acids, degrading enzymes, and principal metabolic products

Amino Acids	Enzymes	Metabolic Product
Arginine	Arginine dihydrolase	Citrulline
Lysine	Lysine deaminase	Alpha-keto carboxylic acid
	Lysine decarboxylase	Cadaverine
Ornithine	Ornithine decarboxylase	Putrescine
Phenylalanine	Phenylalanine deaminase	Phenylpyruvic acid
Tryptophane	Tryptophanase	Indole

3. Deamination and decarboxylation tests
    a. Lysine deaminase removes the amine group from lysine with
        the formation of alpha-keto carboxylic acid with an acid
        reaction. Lysine decarboxylase, on the other hand, removes
        the carboxyl group from lysine with the formation of
        cadaverine with an alkaline reaction. Bromocresol purple
        is a commonly used pH indicator. The indicator turns yellow
        if a positive lysine deamination reaction occurs and purple
        if lysine decarboxylase is positive.
    b. Ornithine decarboxylase removes the carboxyl group from
        ornithine with the formation of putrescine with an alkaline
        reaction.
    c. Phenylalanine deaminase removes the amine group from
        phenyalanine with the formation of phenylpyruvic acid. The
        test is positive if a green color develops on the addition
        of a 10 percent ferric chloride solution.
4. Indole test
    a. Tryptophanase hydrolyzes and deaminates tryptophane with
        the production of indole, pyruvic acid, and ammonia.
        Reagents containing p-dimethylaminobenzaldehyde react with
        indole to form a red color (Fig. 118.12).
        (1) Ehrlich's reagent is more sensitive than Kovac's
             reagent and is preferred when testing asaccharolytic
             aerobic bacteria or when testing obligate anaerobic
             bacteria, in which indole production is often scant.
5. Casein hydrolysis test
    a. Casein is a protein that is hydrolyzed by proteolytic
        enzymes to form peptides and amino acids. Casein agar,
        tyrosine agar, and xanthine agar are used to differentiate
        N. asteroides and *N. brasiliensis*. The inoculated agar
        media are incubated at $30^{\circ}C$ for up to 2 weeks. A positive

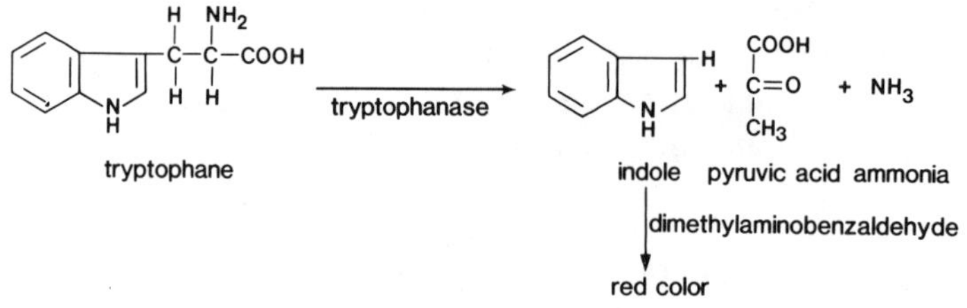

Fig. 118.12. The indole test.

hydrolytic reaction is indicated by a clearing of the medium around the colonies.

6. Gelatin liquefaction test
   a. Gelatin is derived from animal collagen. It has a poor nutritive value. Gelatinases are proteolytic enzymes capable of breaking down gelatin into peptides and amino acids. Those bacteria that secrete gelatinase can be detected by observing the liquefaction of the culture media containing gelatin, following inoculation of the test organism and incubation for an appropriate period of time.
   b. The test is used for identifing many nonfermentative gram-negative bacteria.

F. Urea test
   1. Bacteria with the enzyme urease hydrolyze urea with the release of carbon dioxide and ammonia. The ammonia reacts in solution to form ammonium carbonate, resulting in alkalinization of the medium. Phenol red is the pH indicator (Fig. 118.13).

$$NH_2-\overset{\overset{\displaystyle O}{\|}}{C}-NH_2 + 2H_2O \xrightarrow{urease} CO_2 + H_2O + 2NH_3 \rightleftharpoons (NH_4)_2CO_3 \ (\uparrow pH)$$

Fig. 118.13. The urea test.

G. Hippurate test
   1. Hippuric acid is hydrolyzed by the enzyme hippuricase to form sodium benzoate and glycine.
      a. Sodium benzoate is tested for using a ferric chloride solution. The formation of a precipitate indicates a positive test.
      b. Glycine is tested for using ninhydrin. The development of a deep purple color indicates a positive test.

H. Esculin test
   1. Esculin is composed of glucose and 7-hydroxycoumarin linked by a glycoside bond. The esculin is hydrolyzed to form glucose and esculetin. The esculetin is reacted with an iron salt, like ferric citrate, to form an insoluble black or brown precipitate.

I. Hydrogen sulfide tests
   1. Numerous bacterial species possess enzyme systems capable of producing hydrogen sulfide (H_2S) gas.

2. Bacteriologic media used for the production of H_2S, a colorless gas, must provide the essential nutrition requirements for the growth of the bacterium being tested, an acid environment (a requirement for an organism to produce H_2S) and a source of sulfur. Most media also contain iron salts that will react with the H_2S gas to produce ferrous sulfide, an insoluble black precipitate.

  a. Sources of sulfur atoms

    (1) Sulfur-containing amino acids (cysteine, cystine, and methionine) are commonly used substrates.

    (2) Sodium thiosulfate (NaS_2O_3) is the chemical most commonly incorporated in test media.

  b. H_2S detectors

    (1) Ferrous sulfate and ferric ammonium citrate are commonly incorporated in the test medium. The iron salts react with H_2S gas to produce ferrous sulfide, an insoluble black precipitate, which indicates H_2S production.

    (2) Lead acetate also reacts with H_2S, forming an insoluble black precipitate. Lead acetate, which inhibits the growth of many fastidious bacteria, may be incorporated into the test medium, or lead acetate-impregnated filter paper strips may be placed in the atmosphere of a closed test tube.

3. Sensitivity of H_2S detection methods

  a. Lead acetate-impregnated paper strips

    (1) This is the most sensitive method and is often used to detect bacteria that produce scant amounts of H_2S.

      (a) This method is often used to distinguish *Campylobacter fetus* ss *fetus*, which produces H_2S, from *C. fetus* ss *venerealis*, which is H_2S-negative.

  b. SIM medium

    (1) Sodium thiosulfate and ferric ammonium sulfate are incorporated in the medium. SIM medium is less sensitive than the lead acetate strip method but more sensitive than TSI agar.

  c. TSI agar

    (1) Sodium thiosulfate and ferric ammonium sulfate serve as the media's source of sulfur and H_2S indicator, respectively.

J. Lipid tests

  1. Tween 80 hydrolysis

    a. Tween 80, polyoxyethylene sorbitan mono-oleate, is hydrolyzed by a bacterial lipase into oleic acid and polyoxyethylated sorbitol.

      (1) Lipase activity on Tween 80 agar plates is detectable by the appearance of a precipitate of calcium oleate.

119 | Culture and Identification Procedures for Aerobic Extracellular Bacteria

The culture and identification criteria commonly used for identifing the genera and selected pathogenic species of domestic animals that will grow on blood agar and/or MacConkey agar when incubated aerobically at 37°C are briefly described. The culture and identification procedures for the aerobic extracellular bacteria with fastidious growth requirements have been previously described within their respective genera and will not be discussed further.

AEROBIC GRAM-POSITIVE BACTERIA

I. GENERA OF AEROBIC GRAM-POSITIVE COCCI
    A. The genera *Micrococcus*, *Staphylococcus*, and *Streptococcus* can be distinguished from one another on the basis of colony morphology and type of hemolysis on blood agar, growth on MacConkey agar, cellular morphology and arrangement in gram-stained preparations, catalase reactivity, and glucose metabolism (Table 119.1).

Table 119.1. Presumptive identification characteristics of genera *Micrococcus*, *Staphylococcus*, and *Streptococcus*

Characteristic	Genera		
	Micrococcus	*Staphylococcus*	*Streptococcus*
Motility	−	−	−,+[a]
Cellular arrangement			
Clusters of cells	−	+	−
Chains or pairs of cells	−	−	+
Growth on blood agar	+	+	+
Nonhemolytic	+	+	+
Alpha hemolysis	−	−	+
Beta hemolysis	−	+	+
Double zone hemolysis	−	+	−
Growth on MacConkey agar	−	−	−,+[b]
Catalase	+	+	−
Glucose fermentation	−	+	+

[a]Some group D streptococci are motile.
[b]Enterococci will grow on MacConkey agar.

1. Colony characteristics and hemolytic patterns on blood agar
    a. *Micrococcus* and *Staphylococcus* colonies are large, convex, and opaque. Their colonies are usually either white or yellow, but some micrococci have pink or red colonies. The micrococci are nonhemolytic, and the coagulase-negative staphylococci (CNS) are usually nonhemolytic. However,

most coagulase-positive staphylococci (CPS) produce either beta hemolysis or a double zone (complete-partial) hemolysis.

b. *Streptococcus* colonies are pinpoint size to less than 2 mm in diameter and translucent to semiopaque. The nonpathogenic streptococci are usually either nonhemolytic or produce alpha hemolysis, whereas most pathogenic streptococci are beta hemolytic. The enterococci that are occasionally isolated from pathologic processes are usually nonhemolytic, but some strains produce alpha hemolysis.

2. Growth on MacConkey agar
   a. MacConkey agar, which contains bile salts, inhibits the growth of the micrococci, staphylococci, and most streptococci except the enterococci, which are part of the intestinal microflora.

3. Selective and differential agar media
   a. Phenylethyl alcohol (PEA) blood agar is a selective medium for the isolation of gram-positive cocci from clinical specimens of mixed gram-positive and gram-negative flora.
      (1) The phenylethanol in the medium usually inhibits the growth of all gram-negative bacilli and the swarming phenomenon of *Proteus* species. The hemolytic patterns of the staphylococci and streptococci are often atypical on PEA blood agar.
   b. Mannitol salt agar is a selective and differential medium used for the isolation and presumptive differentiation of *Staphylococcus* species.
      (1) Mannitol salt agar is selective due to the high salt content and differential due to mannitol. The staphylococci will grow in the presence of 7.5 percent NaCl, which inhibits the growth of other pathogenic bacteria. Colonies of staphylococci that ferment mannitol produce a yellow halo in the surrounding agar, indicating the production of acid from mannitol and a color change of the phenol red indicator from red to yellow. Traditionally the medium has been used for the presumptive identification of human *S. aureus* isolates, which will usually ferment mannitol, whereas the CNS do not ferment mannitol. About 97 percent of human CPS will ferment mannitol, and therefore there is a high degree of correlation with the tube coagulase test. Many CPS isolated from domestic animals, however, do not ferment mannitol.
   c. Sodium azide blood agar is a selective medium frequently used for the isolation of streptococci from mixed microbial flora.
      (1) Sodium azide (NaN_3) inhibits the transfer of electrons through the cytochrome system by tying up the iron in

the cytochrome molecule in the ferric state, thus preventing the final electron transfer to molecular oxygen.
4. Cellular morphology and arrangement
   a. The cocci are approximately 1 um in diameter and are nonmotile except the group D streptococci.
   b. The cellular arrangement of the staphylococci and streptococci can be determined using Gram-stained preparations from either agar or broth cultures. The cellular arrangement is usually more clearly delineated when tryptose broth cultures incubated aerobically at 37°C for 18 to 24 hours are used. The staphylococci form grapelike clusters of cocci, but the streptococci form chains or pairs of cells.
5. Catalase reactions
   a. Micrococci and staphylococci are catalase-positive and the streptococci catalase-negative.
6. Glucose metabolism
   a. The obligate aerobic micrococci cannot ferment glucose but may utilize glucose oxidatively, whereas the facultative anaerobic staphylococci and streptococci ferment glucose.
B. Identification procedures for *Staphylococcus* species
   1. Coagulase test
      a. Traditionally the coagulase test has been used to distinguish the CPS from the CNS, but occasionally there is a need to determine the specific species of staphylococci isolated from pathologic processes.
      b. Coagulase is a protein enzyme with a prothrombinlike activity capable of converting the plasma protein fibrinogen to fibrin. Coagulase produced by the CPS can be present in two forms, bound and free, each having different properties, which requires the use of separate testing procedures.
         (1) The slide coagulase test is used to detect bound coagulase attached to the bacterial cells and not present in culture filtrates. In this test, fibrin strands are formed between the bacterial cells when suspended in plasma (fibrinogen) on a glass slide, causing them to clump into visible aggregrates. A positive agglutination reaction is usually detected within 15 to 20 seconds.
            (a) Most canine strains of *S. intermedius* are clumping factor-positive; however, some strains of *S. hyicus* and *S. intermedius* lack clumping factor.
         (2) The tube coagulase test will detect both bound and free coagulase. In this test, a suspension of the staphylococcal isolate is mixed with plasma in a test

tube. If the test is positive, a visible clot is formed in the tube. Strong CPS may produce a clot within 1 to 4 hours, and the test should be observed at 30-minute intervals for the first hours of the test, since some CPS strains also produce fibrinolysins, which may dissolve the clot soon after it is formed.   Traditionally rabbit plasma has been used. However, some animal CPS will not react with rabbit plasma but will react with plasma from other animal species. *S. intermedius* isolates from dogs may fail to clot rabbit plasma but will clot dog plasma.

C.   Identification procedures for *Streptococcus* species
   1.   Lancefield serologic procedures
      a.   The Lancefield groups are based on serologic differences in the C polysaccharides of the cell wall. These carbohydrate antigens are extracted from the streptococci before being reacted with absorbed antisera of known specificity. The precipitation test is most commonly performed with capillary tubes, in which antisera is layered over the antigen extract or vice versa. A precipitate at the interface of the antigen solution and plasma indicates a positive test.
   2.   Tests to identify Lancefield groups
      a.   Group A streptococci
         (1) The bacitracin susceptibility test is used to presumptively identify the group A streptococci. The growth of *S. pyogenes* is inhibited by bacitracin-impregnated paper disks on blood agar. A zone of bacterial growth inhibition adjacent to the disk is a positive test. Most other streptococci are not inhibited, but both false-positive and false-negative reactions may occur (Fig. 119.1).
      b.   Group B streptococci
         (1) The CAMP test is used to identify *S. agalactiae*, which produces an extracellular factor called the CAMP factor. CAMP factor enhances the hemolytic activity of staphylococcal beta toxin, which produces a zone of partial hemolysis around the staphylococcal colony on blood agar (Fig. 119.2).
      c.   Group D streptococci
         (1) The salt tolerance test is used to distinguish the group D enterococcus species (*S. faecalis* and *S. faecium*) from the group D nonenterococcus species (*S. bovis* and *S. equinus*). The enterococci will grow and produce acid in broth medium containing 6.5 percent NaCl, whereas the nonenterococci are inhibited from growing in this high salt concentration.

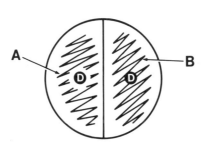

Fig. 119.1. Bacitracin susceptibility tests of a group A *Streptococcus* (*A*), and a non-group A *Streptococcus* (*B*). The growth of the group A *Streptococcus* is inhibited adjacent to the bacitracin disk (*D*), but the growth of the non-group A *Streptococcus* is not inhibited.

3. Identification of selected species
   a. The bovine mastitis streptococci and the equine streptococci are commonly identified to the species level, but most streptococci from other pathogenic processes are evaluated as beta hemolytic, alpha hemolytic, or nonhemolytic.

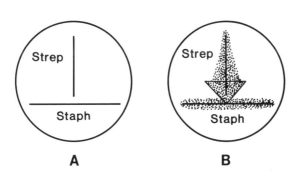

Fig. 119.2. The CAMP test. The test is performed by making a single streak of the *Streptococcus* isolate perpendicular to a strain of *Staphylococcus aureus* that produces beta toxin (*A*). *Streptococcus agalactiae* produces CAMP factor, which causes a zone of increased hemolysis with the shape of an arrowhead at the junction of the two streak lines (*B*).

b.   Bovine mastitis streptococci
   (1) *S. agalactiae*, an obligate pathogen of the bovine
        mammary gland, must be distinguished from the other
        mastitis streptococci (Table 119.2).
c.   Equine streptococci
   (1) *S. equi*, the etiologic agent of strangles, must be
        distinguished from the other *Streptococcus* species
        that commonly infect the horse (Table 119.3).

Table 119.2. Identifying characteristics of mastitis streptococci

Species	Group B	CAMP Test	Esculin Hydrolysis
S. agalactiae	+	+	−
S. dysgalactiae	−	−	−
S. uberis	−	−,+	+
Other streptococci	−	−	−

Table 119.3. Identifying characteristics of equine streptococci

| Species | Group C | Fermentation | | |
		Glucose	Sorbitol	Trehalose
S. equi	+	+	−	−
S. equisimilis	+	+	−	+
S. zooepidemicus	+	+	+	−

II. GENERA OF AEROBIC GRAM-POSITIVE RODS

A.   *Actinomyces pyogenes* and the genera *Bacillus, Corynebacterium,
     Dermatophilus, Erysipelothrix, Listeria, Nocardia,* and *Rhodococcus*
     contain pathogenic species that have marked differences in their
     colony morphologies and ability to produce hemolysis on blood agar.
     Their growth on MacConkey agar is either very sparse or absent.
     Criteria commonly used to presumptively identify these genera and
     selected pathogenic species include oxygen requirements for growth,
     cellular morphology, acid-fastness, ability to form endospores, and
     motility (Table 119.4).

Table 119.4. Hemolytic and cellular characteristics of selected pathogenic aerobic gram-positive rods

Species	Hemolysis	Cellular Morphology	Endospores	Acid-fast	Motil
Actinomyces pyogenes	+	Small coccobacilli	−	−	−
Bacillus anthracis	−	Large bacilli, square ends	+	−	−
Corynebacterium pseudotuberculosis	V	Bacilli	−	−	−
C. renale	−	Bacilli	−	−	−
C. ulcerans	V	Bacilli	−	−	−
Dermatophilus congolensis	+	Filamentous bacilli	−	−	Zoosp
Erysipelothrix rhusiopathiae	+	Pleomorphic bacilli	−	−	−
Listeria monocytogenes	+	Small bacilli, round ends	−	−	+ (20
Nocardia species	−	Pleomorphic bacilli	−	Partial	−
Rhodococcus equi	−	Bacilli	−	−	−

Note: V = variable reactions.

1. Oxygen growth requirements and hemolytic reactions on blood agar
   a. *Nocardia* species and *R. equi* are obligate aerobes, whereas *A. pyogenes*, *B. anthracis*, the pathogenic *Corynebacterium* species, *D. congolensis*, *E. rhusiopathiae*, and *L. monocytogenes* are facultative anaerobes.
   b. *B. anthracis*, *C. renale*, the *Nocardia* species, and *R. equi* are nonhemolytic on blood agar, whereas *A. pyogenes*, *D. congolensis*, *E. rhusiopathiae*, and *L. monocytogenes* are hemolytic. Hemolysis is variable for *C. pseudotuberculosis* and *C. ulcerans*.
2. Characteristics used to distinguish *B. anthracis* from nonpathogenic *Bacillus* species
   a. Cellular characteristics
      (1) Gram-stained smears from tissues or blood with large gram-positive rods with square ends and capsules are highly suggestive of *B. anthracis*.
      (2) Cultures of *B. anthracis* contain both large gram-positive vegetative cells and spores. The endospores have a subterminal location.
      (3) *B. anthracis* is nonmotile, whereas the nonpathogenic *Bacillus* species are motile by peritrichous flagella.
   b. Culture characteristics
      (1) *B. anthracis* is nonhemolytic, whereas the other *Bacillus* species are usually hemolytic. Virulent *B. anthracis* colonies have a characteristic "Medusa head" appearance.
   c. Biochemical characteristics
      (1) *B. anthracis* ferments salicin and reduces nitrate but does not liquefy gelatin or produce urease. The ability to utilize these substrates by nonpathogenic *Bacillus* species is either species-dependent or variable within a species.
3. Biochemical characteristics are used to distinguish the pathogenic genera and species of aerobic, nonsporeforming, gram-positive rods.
   a. These microorganisms can be presumptively identified based on their catalase reactivity, ability to reduce nitrate, TSI agar reactions, and urease activity (Table 119.5).

AEROBIC GRAM-NEGATIVE BACTERIA

I. GROUPS OF GENERA OF AEROBIC GRAM-NEGATIVE RODS
   A. The aerobic gram-negative rods are placed in four groups, based on their ability to grow on blood agar and/or MacConkey agar when incubated aerobically at 37°C, their oxidase reactivity, and their glucose metabolism (Table 119.6).
      1. The genera that have pathogenic species for domestic animals are listed in Table 119.7.

Table 119.5. Biochemical characteristics of selected pathogenic aerobic gram-positive rods

Species	Catalase	Nitrate Reduction	Glucose	Lactose/Sucrose	H_2S	Urea
Actinomyces pyogenes	-	-	+	+	-	-
Corynebacterium pseudotuberculosis	+	V	+	+	-	V
C. renale	+	V	+	+	-	+
C. ulcerans	+	-	+	V	-	+
Dermatophilus congolensis	+	+	+	+	-	+
Erysipelothrix rhusiopathiae	-	-	+	+	+	-
Listeria monocytogenes	+	-	+	+	-	-
Nocardia species	+	+	-	-	-	+
Rhodococcus equi	+	+	-	-	-	V

Note: + = 90% or more of isolates are positive; - = 90% or more of the isolates are negative,
V = 11 to 89% of the isolates are positive.

Table 119.6. Characteristics of four groups of aerobic gram-negative rods

Group No.	Growth		Oxidase	Glucose Fermentation
	Blood Agar	MacConkey Agar		
I	+	+	-	+
II	+	+	-	-[a]
III	+	-,+	+	+[b]
IV	+	-,+	+	-

[a] Glucose is utilized oxidatively.
[b] Includes genera and selected pathogenic species that are either asaccharolytic or utilize glucose oxidatively.

Table 119.7. Genera in each group of aerobic gram-negative rods

Group I[a]	Group II	Group III	Group IV
Citrobacter	*Acinetobacter*	*Actinobacillus*	*Alcaligenes*
Edwardsiella		*Aeromonas*	*Bordetella*
Enterobacter		*Pasteurella*	*Moraxella*
Escherichia			*Pseudomonas*
Klebsiella			
Morganella			
Proteus			
Providencia			
Salmonella			
Serratia			
Yersinia			

[a] All genera are in the family Enterobacteriaceae.

II.   GROUP I, FAMILY ENTEROBACTERIACEAE

A.   Eleven genera in the family Enterobacteriaceae have species that are pathogens of domestic animals: *Citrobacter*, *Edwardsiella*, *Enterobacter*, *Escherichia*, *Klebsiella*, *Morganella*, *Proteus*, *Providencia*, *Salmonella*, *Serratia*, and *Yersinia*.

1.   All members of the family Enterobacteriaceae are gram-negative bacilli approximately 1 um in width and 2 to 6 um in length.

2.   All are facultative anaerobic and will grow on both blood agar and MacConkey agar when incubated either aerobically or anaerobically at 37°C.

3. All have both a respiratory and a fermentative metabolism and utilize glucose oxidatively when incubated aerobically and glucose fermentatively when incubated anaerobically.

B. Characteristics commonly used to distinguish the genera.
 1. Colony characteristics and hemolytic patterns on blood agar
  a. Colonies of most enterobacteria are large, gray, and mucoid, but a few species have characteristic colonies.
  b. Most pathogenic strains of *Escherichia coli* are beta hemolytic, but almost all the other members of the family Enterobacteriaceae are nonhemolytic.
 2. Colony characteristics and lactose utilization on MacConkey agar
  a. Colonies of the lactose-positive genera (*Citrobacter, Enterobacter, Escherichia, Klebsiella*, and *Serratia*) can be distinguished from the lactose-negative genera (*Edwardsiella, Morganella, Proteus, Providencia, Salmonella*, and *Yersinia*) on MacConkey agar. The colonies of lactose-positive bacteria are red, and the colonies of the lactose-negative bacteria are colorless. Slow or weak lactose fermenters (*Citrobacter, Klebsiella*, and *Serratia*) may appear colorless after 24 hours or slightly pink in 24 to 48 hours.
   (1) The red pigmentation within the colony and the red precipitate in the medium adjacent to the colony indicates acid production from the utilization of lactose, the only carbohydrate in the medium.
  b. Colony characteristics of selected genera and species
   (1) Colonies of *Enterobacter agglomerans* are large and mucoid with red centers and colorless peripheries.
   (2) Colonies of *E. coli* are large, regular, and brick-red.
   (3) Colonies of *Klebsiella* species are large and mucoid with red centers and dark pink peripheries.
   (4) Colonies of *Proteus* species and *Salmonella* species are small and colorless and transparent or slightly opaque.
 3. Characteristics on various selective and differential agar media
  a. Brilliant green agar is a selective and differential medium used primarily for the isolation of salmonellae from feces and other clinical specimens.
   (1) Brilliant green dye, lactose, and sucrose are incorporated into the medium. The brilliant green dye is selective and inhibits gram-positive and most gram-negative bacteria, particularly those that ferment lactose and/or sucrose. If acid is produced, lactose has been presumed to be fermented. Lactose-negative bacteria such as the salmonellae have red or pink colonies surrounded by brilliant red zones in the medium, whereas lactose-positive bacteria have yellow to greenish yellow colonies surrounded by intense yellow-green zones in the medium.

b. Eosin methylene blue (EMB) agar is a selective and differential medium for the isolation and differentiation of the lactose-positive and lactose-negative bacteria in the family Enterobacteriaceae.

(1) Lactose and two analine dyes, eosin Y and methylene blue, are incorporated into the medium. The dyes markedly inhibit gram-positive and fastidious gram-negative bacteria. Strong lactose fermenters (*E. coli*) produce colonies that are greenish black with a metallic sheen. Slow or weaker lactose fermenters (*Klebsiella* and *Enterobacter*) produce purple colonies, and the lactose-negative genera (*Morganella, Proteus, Providencia,* and *Salmonella*) produce colorless colonies.

c. *Salmonella-Shigella* agar is a selective and differential medium for the isolation and identification of pathogenic enteric bacilli, especially *Salmonella* and *Shigella*, from feces.

(1) The medium contains brilliant green dye and a mixture of bile salts. This medium inhibits the growth of all gram-positive bacteria and most lactose-positive coliforms and prevents the swarming of *Proteus* species. Lactose, ferric citrate, sodium thiosulfate, and neutral red are also incorporated into the medium. Ferric citrate is the H_2S indicator. Sodium thiosulfate is used as a sulfur source for H_2S production, and neutral red is the pH indicator. Lactose-negative bacteria form colorless colonies and lactose-positive bacteria pink to red colonies. The H_2S-positive salmonellae have black-centered colonies.

d. Tergitol 7 agar is a selective and differential medium for the isolation of coliforms, particularly *E. coli*, from the feces.

(1) The medium contains tergitol 7 (sodium heptadecyl sulfate). Lactose is the only carbohydrate, and bromothymol blue serves as a pH indicator. Tergitol 7 inhibits gram-positive bacteria. The lactose-positive enterics (*E. coli* and *Enterobacter*) form yellow colonies with a yellow halo. The enteric pathogenic strains of *E. coli* may be smooth, mucoid, or rough. The *Enterobacter* colonies often are yellowish green. The lactose-negative enterics (*Salmonella* and *Proteus*) form blue colonies.

4. Selective and enrichment broth media

a. Selenite broth is a selective and differential enrichment media used for the primary cultivation of salmonellae from the mixed fecal microflora.

(1) Sodium selenite inhibits gram-positive bacteria and enterics except *Salmonella*. Two common pathogens of swine, *S. choleraesuis* and *S. typhisuis*, also are often inhibited. In this procedure, approximately 2 g feces are added to 30 ml selenite broth and incubated 6 to 8 hours at 37°C. During this period, the salmonellae are allowed to proliferate, but the growth of other enteric bacteria is inhibited or greatly reduced. After the incubation period, the broth culture is then streaked on selective agar media for colony isolation. The agar plates are then incubated for 18 to 24 hours aerobically at 37°C and the colonies identified as previously described.

b. Tetrathionate broth is a selective and differential enrichment media used for the primary cultivation of salmonellae from the mixed fecal microflora.

(1) Sodium deoxycholate, brilliant green dye, and sodium thiosulfate are incorporated into the medium. Tetrathionate is formed from sodium thiosulfate when the potassium iodine solution is added to the broth just prior to fecal inoculation. The medium inhibits gram-positive bacteria and the majority of the normal intestinal flora. The fecal inoculation of the tetrathionate broth, incubation, and subculturing procedures on selective agar media are similar to those used for selenite broth.

C. Biochemical and motility characteristics (Table 119.8)

1. All members of the family Enterobacteriaceae are oxidase-negative, and all species will reduce nitrate except *E. agglomerans*.

2. Biochemical reactions in TSI agar

   a. Glucose fermentation

   (1) All the Enterobacteriaceae ferment glucose.

   b. Lactose fermentation

   (1) Five genera (*Citrobacter*, *Enterobacter*, *Escherichia*, *Klebsiella*, and *Serratia*) ferment lactose. Two of these genera (*Enterobacter* and *Escherichia*) are strong lactose fermenters and three (*Citrobacter*, *Klebsiella*, and *Serratia*) tend to be weak or slow lactose fermenters. The other six genera (*Edwardsiella*, *Morganella*, *Proteus*, *Providencia*, *Salmonella*, and *Yersinia*) are lactose-negative.

   (2) The lactose reactions of these genera in TSI agar should correlate with their utilization of lactose and uptake of the neutral red dye on MacConkey agar. The ONPG test may be utilized to confirm a lactose reaction.

Table 19.8. Biochemical characteristics and motility of selected species in family Enterobacteriaceae

Characteristic	Citrobacter freundii	Edwardsiella tarda	Enterobacter agglomerans	Enterobacter cloacae	Escherichia coli	Klebsiella oxytoca	Klebsiella pneumoniae	Morganella morganii	Proteus mirabilis	Proteus vulgaris	Providencia rettgeri	Providencia stuartii	Salmonella serovars [a]	Serratia liquefaciens	Serratia marcescens	Yersinia enterocolitica [b]	Yersinia pseudotuberculosis
Oxidase	-	-	-	-	-	-	-	-	-	-	-	-	-	-	-	-	-
Nitrate reduction	+	+	-	+	+	+	+	+	+	+	+	+	+	+	+	+	+
TSI agar reactions																	
D-glucose, acid/gas production	+/+	+/+	+/V	+/+	+/+	+/+	+/V	+/V	+/+	+/+	+/-	+/-	+/+	+/V	+/V	+/-	+/-
Lactose	V	-	+	+	+	+	+	-	-	-	-	-	-	-	-	-	-
Sucrose	V	-	V	+	V	+	V	-	V	+	V	V	-	+	+	V	-
H2S production	+	+	-	-	-	-	-	-	+	+	-	-	+	-	-	-	-
ONPG	+	-	+	+	+	+	+	-	-	-	-	-	-	+	+	+	-
Citrate	+	-	V	+	-	+	+	-	V	-	+	+	+	+	+	-	-
Methyl red	+	+	V	-	+	V	V	+	+	+	+	+	+	V	V	+	+
Voges-Proskauer	-	-	V	+	-	+	+	-	V	-	-	-	-	+	+	TD	TD
Arginine dihydrolase	-	-	-	+	V	-	-	-	-	-	-	-	+	-	-	-	-
Lysine decarboxylase	-	+	-	-	V	+	+	-	-	-	-	-	+	+	+	-	-
Ornithine decarboxylase	+	+	V	+	V	-	-	+	+	-	-	-	+	+	+	+	-
Phenylalanine deaminase	-	-	-	-	-	-	-	+	+	+	+	+	-	-	-	-	-
Indole production	-	+	V	-	+	+	-	+	-	+	+	+	-	-	-	V	-
Urease	V	-	V	V	-	+	+	+	+	+	+	V	-	-	V	+	+
Motility	+	+	V	+	V	-	-	+	+	+	+	V	+	+	+	+	+

Note: + = 90% or more of isolates are positive; - = 90% or more of the isolates are negative; V = 11 to 89% of isolates are positive; TD = temperature dependent.

[a] All Salmonella serovars are motile except the avian host-adapted serovars S. gallinarum and S. pullorum.

[b] Motile at 22°C but not at 37°C.

c. Sucrose fermentation
   (1) Sucrose is fermented by *Y. enterocolitica*, some *Proteus* strains, and a few other members of the family Enterobacteriaceae.
   (2) Since sucrose fermentation will turn the slant of the TSI tube acid, as will lactose fermentation, it may be necessary to inoculate both a sucrose broth and a lactose broth to confirm if an isolate is either lactose-positive or lactose-negative.

d. H_2S production
   (1) Of the lactose-negative organisms, the *Proteus* species and most of the *Salmonella* serovars produce H_2S in TSI agar. *Edwardsiella tarda* also will produce H_2S, but the other species in the genus are negative.
   (2) *C. freundii* is the only lactose-positive species that produces H_2S in TSI agar. The other *Citrobacter* species do not produce H_2S.

III. GROUP II, GENUS *ACINETOBACTER*

A. *A. calcoaceticus* is the only species in the genus.
   1. Common characteristics of the species
      a. The bacterium is an obligate aerobe and will grow on both blood agar and MacConkey agar when incubated aerobically at $37^{\circ}C$. Some strains of *A. calcoaceticus* produce hemolysis on blood agar.
      b. This nonmotile gram-negative bacilli is approximately 1 um in diameter and 2 um in length.
      c. *A. calcoaceticus* is oxidase-negative.
   2. Comparison of genus *Acinetobacter* and family Enterobacteriaceae is shown in Table 119.9.
   3. Biochemical criteria are used to identify *A. calcoaceticus* to the species level. The different strains of the bacterium have highly variable reactions on various substrates, particularly carbohydrates.

Table 119.9. Characteristics of genus *Acinetobacter* and family Enterobacteriaceae

Characteristic	Genus *Acinetobacter*	Family Enterobacteriaceae
Oxygen requirements	Obligate aerobic	Facultative anaerobic
Growth on blood agar	Only aerobically	Aerobically and anaerobically
Hemolysis	+ or -[a]	+ or -[a]
Oxidase reaction	-	-
Glucose fermentation	-	+
Motility	-	+ or -[a]
Nitrate reduction	-	+[b]

[a] Species- or strain-dependent.
[b] All species reduce nitrate except *E. agglomerans*.

IV. GROUP III, GENERA *ACTINOBACILLUS, AEROMONAS,*
AND *PASTEURELLA*

    A. These genera are oxidase-positive and facultative anaerobic with a
fermentative metabolism.

       1. Characteristics of selected species are listed in Tables 119.10
and 119.11.

V. GROUP IV, GENERA *ALCALIGENES, BORDETELLA, MORAXELLA,*
AND *PSEUDOMONAS*

    A. The genera are oxidase-positive and obligate aerobic with a
respiratory metabolism. Some *Pseudomonas* species are oxidase-
negative.

       1. Characteristics of selected species are listed in Tables 119.12
and 119.13.

Table 119.10. Culture characteristics of selected species of
Actinobacillus, Aeromonas, and *Pasteurella*

Species	Blood Agar Growth	Hemolysis	MacConkey Agar Growth
Actinobacillus equuli	+	+ or −[a]	+
A. lignieresii	+	−	+
A. seminis	+	−	−
A. suis	+	+	+
Aeromonas hydrophilia	+	+	+
Pasteurella haemolytica	+	+	+
P. multocida	+	−	−

[a]Strain-dependent.

Table 119.11. Biochemical characteristics of selected species of *Actinobacillus,*
Aeromonas, and *Pasteurella*

Species	Oxidase	TSI Agar Reactions Glucose	Lactose	Sucrose	H₂S	Indole	Urease
Actinobacillus equuli	+	+	+	+	SD	−	+
A. lignieresii	+	+	V	+	+	−	+
A. suis	+	+	+	+	−	−	+
Aeromonas hydrophilia	+	+	+	+	+	+	−
Pasteurella haemolytica	+	+	+	+	−	−	−
P. multocida	+	+	−	+	−	+	−

Note: + = 90% or more of the isolates are positive; − = 90% or more of the
isolates are negative; V = variable reactions from 11 to 89% positive; SD =
strain-dependent.

Table 119.12. Culture characteristics of selected species of
Alcaligenes, Bordetella, Moraxella, and *Pseudomonas*

Species	Blood Agar Growth	Hemolysis	MacConkey Agar Growth
Alcaligenes faecalis	+	−	+
Bordetella bronchiseptica	+	+	+[a]
Moraxella bovis	+	+	−
Pseudomonas aeruginosa	+	V	+
P. mallei	+		+
P. pseudomallei	+	V	+

Note: + = 90% or more of the isolates are positive; − = 90%
or more of the isolates are negative; V = variable reactions from
11 to 89% positive.
[a]Glucose is often added to media to facilitate growth.

Table 119.13. Biochemical and motility characteristics of selected species of *Alcaligenes, Bordetella, Moraxella,* and *Pseudomonas*

Species	Oxidase	Glucose Oxidation	Indole	Urease	Motility
Alcaligenes faecalis	+	+	–	–	+
Bordetella bronchiseptica	+	–	–	+	+
Moraxella bovis	+	–	–	–	–
Pseudomonas aeruginosa	+	+	–	V	+
P. mallei	+	+	–	V	–
P. pseudomallei	+	+	–	V	+

Note: + = 90% or more of the isolates are positive; – = 90% or more of the isolates are negative; V = variable reactions from 11 to 89% positive.

---

120 | Antimicrobial Susceptibility Testing Procedures for Aerobic Bacteria

I. ANTIMICROBIAL THERAPY AND DRUG RESISTANCE

A. Drug therapy
1. Bacterial infections are among the few diseases in veterinary medicine for which specific therapy is available.
2. Antimicrobial therapy aims to treat infection with a drug to which the causal bacterium is sensitive. The determination of which drug to use is based either on the culture and in vitro antimicrobial sensitivity testing of the bacterial pathogen or on a clinical diagnosis that indicates the most likely pathogen in a given condition and its usual antibiotic sensitivity.

B. Bactericidal and bacteriostatic drugs
1. Antimicrobial drugs are classified as bactericidal when they kill the infecting bacteria and as bacteriostatic when they prevent multiplication but do not kill the bacteria.
   a. Depending on the antibiotic, the local concentration of the drug will often determine if its action is bactericidal or bacteriostatic.
   b. An essential requirement for an antibiotic is selective toxicity, meaning that the antibiotic has the ability to kill or inhibit the growth of procaryotic cells without harming the eucaryotic cells of the host.

C. Sources of antibiotics
1. Most antibiotics are products of soil streptomycetes and bacteria of the genus *Bacillus*.

        a.   Penicillin, a product of *Penicillin notatum*, was discovered in 1929 and was first available for clinical use in domestic animals and man in the 1940s. The success of this drug introduced the antibiotic era.

        b.   Antibiotics and other antimicrobial agents in current use include the penicillins, cephalosporins, aminoglycosides, macrolides, chloramphenicol, tetracyclines, polymyxins, isoniazid, and rifampin.

        c.   Many recently introduced antibiotics have been prepared by the chemical manipulation of existing drugs. These drugs include the semisynthetic penicillins and cephalosporins.

  D. Drug resistance

      1. A major problem in antibiotic therapy is the emergence of drug-resistant bacteria.

      2. The frequency of antimicrobial resistance depends on the bacterium and the antibiotic concerned.

        a.   Members of the family Enterobacteriaceae and *Staphylococcus* species are frequently resistant to various antibiotics and rapidly acquire plasmid-mediated antimicrobial resistance, whereas the obligate anaerobic bacteria and *Streptococcus* species rarely develop antimicrobial resistance.

        b.   Resistance to the aminoglycosides, penicillins, and tetracyclines commonly occurs in many aerobic bacteria. Resistance rarely develops to metronidazole, which is only active against anaerobic bacteria.

      3. Drug resistance is commonly associated with antibiotic use.

        a.   Resistant bacterial strains have a selective advantage in the presence of the antibiotic and will multiply at the expense of sensitive bacteria.

        b.   The widespread and indiscriminate use of antibiotics in domestic animals has favored the survival and increase of drug-resistant bacteria. Therefore, the veterinary clinician should be familiar with the concepts and procedures for antimicrobial susceptibility testing, particularly for the aerobic bacteria.

II. ANTIMICROBIAL SUSCEPTIBILITY TESTING METHODS

  A. Minimum inhibitory concentration (MIC) tests

      1. Broth dilution method

        a.   This is the standard reference method for determining the MIC of an antimicrobial agent.

           (1) The MIC is the lowest concentration of antibiotic (ug/ml) that prevents the in vitro growth of bacteria.

        b.   Procedures

           (1) Nutrient broth is used to support the growth of the aerobic bacterial species.

           (2) Quantities of antibiotics, which are serially diluted, are added to each tube except for the control tube, which does not contain antibiotics.

(3) The control broth and broth antimicrobial tubes are inoculated with the test organism and incubated aerobically at 37°C for 18 hours.

  c. Interpretation of results

    (1) At the end of the incubation period, the tubes are visually examined for growth (turbidity). The MIC is the lowest concentration of antibiotic that prevents the growth (no turbidity) of bacteria (Fig. 120.1).

  d. MICs are the basis for the zone diameters used in the agar disk diffusion method. The Kirby-Bauer method (below) is standardized and used in most veterinary clinical laboratories to test aerobic bacteria.

  2. Microtube broth dilution method

    a. This method is similar in principle to the broth dilution method except that a series of microtubes are used.

      (1) It is becoming increasingly popular in many veterinary diagnostic laboratories and is often used instead of the Kirby-Bauer method.

B. Kirby-Bauer agar disk diffusion method

  1. This method is a standard antimicrobial susceptibility for most aerobic bacteria.

    a. Standardized medium

      (1) Mueller-Hinton agar, the culture medium, will support the growth of most significant aerobic bacteria.

    b. Standardized inoculum

      (1) The test organism is inoculated into trypticase soy broth, which is incubated aerobically at 37°C until

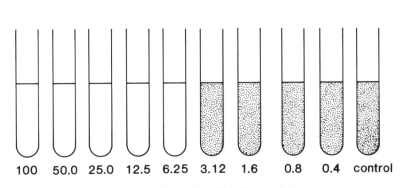

100   50.0   25.0   12.5   6.25   3.12   1.6   0.8   0.4   control

Concentration of antibiotic µg/ml

Fig. 120.1. Broth dilution antimicrobial susceptibility of an antibiotic with a minimum inhibitory concentration of 6.25 ug/ml.

the growth attains a turbidity equivalent to a
MacFarland number 1 standard. This is equivalent to a
concentration of about 10^8 bacteria.
(2) The agar surface is swabbed completely with a
suspension of organisms and then allowed to dry.
c. Standardized antibiotic disks
(1) Paper disks impregnated with standardized
concentrations of various antibacterial drugs are
placed on the agar surface.
d. Standardized incubation
(1) The antibiotic susceptibility plates are incubated
aerobically at $37^{\circ}C$ for 18 hours and then the zones of
inhibition adjacent to the disks are measured in
millimeters. For each antibiotic tested, different
zone diameters are designated susceptible, resistant,
or intermediate.
2. This test has not been standardized for slow growing aerobic
bacteria, aerobic bacteria with fastidious growth requirements,
or obligate anaerobic bacteria.

<table>
<tr><td>PART 2</td><td>Anaerobic Extracellular Bacteria</td></tr>
</table>

<table>
<tr><td>121</td><td>Culture and Identification Procedures for Obligate Anaerobic Bacteria</td></tr>
</table>

I. CLINICAL SIGNIFICANCE OF ANAEROBIC BACTERIA
  A. During the last 20 to 30 years, there has become an increased awareness of the importance of obligate anaerobic bacteria as significant pathogens of domestic animals and man.
    1. Anaerobic bacteria constitute a major component of the normal microbial flora.
    2. The majority of anaerobic infections are caused by bacteria from endogenous sources.
    3. Predisposing factors involved in the pathogenesis of anaerobic infections include poor blood supply, surgery or other trauma, tissue necrosis, malignancy, various diseases, and growth of facultative anaerobes in tissue. All these factors tend to lower the oxidation-reduction potential (Eh) and oxygen tension and help provide a favorable environment for anaerobic growth.

II. BASIC CULTIVATION REQUIREMENTS
  A. The inability of anaerobic bacteria to utilize oxygen as a terminal electron acceptor or even to survive in its presence has necessitated the development of special techniques for the cultivation of anaerobic bacteria.
    1. Anaerobic bacteria are those bacteria that do not require oxygen as a terminal electron acceptor for growth or metabolic activities.
      a. Although anaerobic bacteria may possess certain cytochromes, the anaerobes lack those cytochromes required to transfer electrons to molecular oxygen. Thus their energy comes from fermentation reactions.
      b. The growth of anaerobes in culture is favored by the exclusion of oxygen from the system and by a low Eh within the medium.

2.   There are two basic requirements for the cultivation of anaerobic bacteria: the elimination of oxygen from all environments to which the anaerobes are exposed and the maintenance of low oxidation-reduction potentials in all culture media.

    a.   The level of anaerobiosis required for different species of anaerobes varies widely; however, most anaerobes that are pathogens of domestic animals and man are relatively resistant to brief exposure to oxygen.

III. CULTIVATION METHODS

A.   Several traditional laboratory techniques are used to achieve anaerobic culture conditions.

    1.   The addition of reducing agents to culture media results in both a removal of oxygen and a lowering of the oxidation-reduction potential.

        a.   Cooked meat particles, cysteine, dithiothreitol, glutathione, metallic iron, and thioglycollate are commonly added to liquid and agar media.

    2.   Low concentrations of agar are added to fluid media to restrict the convection of air from the atmosphere.

    3.   Liquid media are boiled before use to drive off dissolved oxygen.

    4.   An impermeable liquid such as paraffin is frequently used to overlay liquid or semiliquid culture media.

    5.   Anaerobes are inoculated into the butt of agar tubes, where they grow preferentially toward the bottom of the culture.

B.   Three specialized methods are commonly used for the cultivation of anaerobes.

    1.   Anaerobic roll tube method

    2.   Anaerobic jar technique

    3.   Anaerobic chamber technique

IV. CULTURE MEDIA

A.   Various culture media are utilized for the recovery of anaerobes from clinical specimens. A few of the more common ones are described.

    1.   Enriched blood agar

        a.   Brain heart infusion agar with 5 percent sheep blood supplemented with hemin, menadione, and yeast extract will support the growth of most anaerobes.

    2.   Phenylethyl alcohol blood agar

        a.   Enriched blood agar supplemented with phenylethyl alcohol is a selective medium that will inhibit the growth of facultative anaerobic gram-negative bacteria and support the growth of both gram-positive and gram-negative obligate anaerobes as well as facultative anaerobic gram-positive cocci.

3. Kanamycin-vancomycin blood agar
   a. Enriched blood agar supplemented with the antibiotics kanamycin and vancomycin is a selective medium used for the recovery of anaerobic gram-negative bacilli.
4. Thioglycollate media
   a. Thioglycollate medium contains thioglycollate and cysteine that keep the medium reduced by absorbing oxygen. It is used primarily as a backup culture in case the anaerobes fail to grow on agar plates, which are usually used for primary isolation.
   b. Thioglycollate broth supplemented with hemin and menadione is often used to cultivate anaerobes with fastidious growth requirements.

V. ANAEROBIC CULTIVATION SYSTEMS
   A. Three types of anaerobic systems for the cultivation of anaerobic bacteria are used.
   1. Roll tube method
      a. The roll tube method utilizes prereduced anaerobically sterilized (PRAS) media. The inoculation and subculturing of the PRAS agar and broth media are performed under a stream of oxygen-free carbon dioxide, which minimizes exposure to air and helps to maintain a reduced oxidation-reduction potential in the medium.
      b. This system is seldom used in the veterinary clinical bacteriology laboratory.
   2. Anaerobic glove box method
      a. Anaerobic glove boxes, which can be constructed of various materials, have an entry lock where specimens and media are passed into the anaerobic chamber. The bacteriologist uses the gloves to perform the isolation and identification of anaerobic bacteria without exposure to air.
         (1) A gas mixture of 80 percent nitrogen, 10 percent hydrogen, and 10 percent carbon dioxide is commonly used to maintain anaerobiosis within the glove box.
   3. Anaerobic jar methods
      a. Two anaerobic jar systems are commonly used: the evacuation replacement method and the GasPak method.
         (1) In the evacuation replacement method, the air in the jar is flushed with a mixture of nitrogen, hydrogen, and carbon dioxide to produce an anaerobic environment.
         (2) In the commercial GasPak method, a Brewer jar with a hydrogen-carbon dioxide generator is used to provide oxygen-free conditions. Briefly, the inoculated agar plates are placed in the jar. The disposable hydrogen-carbon dioxide generator is activated by

adding water to the envelope. Sodium borohydride generates hydrogen gas, which reacts with the atmospheric oxygen in the jar in the presence of the palladium catalyst in the lid of the jar to form water. Five to 10 percent carbon dioxide, which stimulates the growth of many anaerobic bacteria, is generated from a tablet of citric acid and sodium bicarbonate. A methylene blue dye indicator strip is used to monitor anaerobiosis (Fig. 121.1).

(3) The Brewer jar method is commonly used by both clinical microbiology laboratories and practicing veteriarians. However, the Brewer jar is inferior to the anaerobic glove box, since the bacteria in the Brewer jar are exposed to relatively high concentration of oxygen before anaerobiosis is attained.

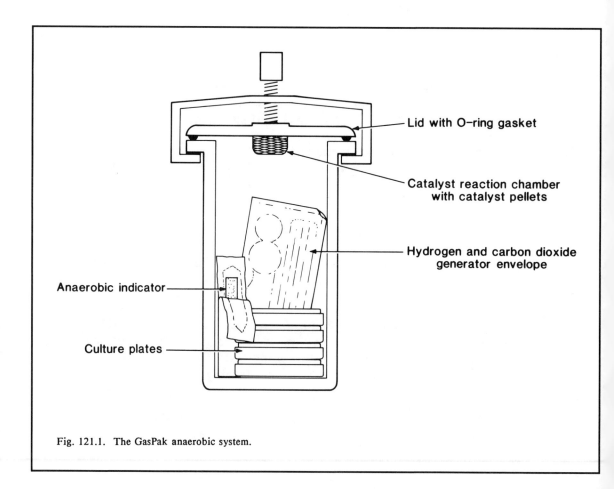

Fig. 121.1. The GasPak anaerobic system.

VI. OXYGEN SENSITIVITY OF ANAEROBIC BACTERIA

A. The various species within the genera classified as obligate anaerobes are designated by their sensitivity to oxygen: strict, moderate, and aerotolerant.

1. Strict anaerobes will not form colonies on agar surfaces exposed to 0.5 percent or more oxygen.

  a. Very few veterinary pathogens are strict obligate anaerobes, with the exception of *Clostridium novyi* type B.

2. Moderate anaerobes are capable of growth at oxygen levels of less than 2 or 3 percent.

  a. Most of the veterinary pathogens are moderate anaerobes, such as *Bacteroides melaninogenicus* and *Fusobacterium necrophorum*.

3. Aerotolerant anaerobes do not use molecular oxygen and are inhibited by it to some extent. These bacteria grow best under anaerobic conditions and grow scantily in an aerobic incubator. An example is *Clostridium tertium*.

  a. Microaerophilic bacteria require oxygen as a terminal electron acceptor for growth but grow minimally, if at all, in aerobic conditions (20 to 21 percent oxygen) or under anaerobic conditions.

B. Some microaerophiles (e.g., *Actinomyces viscosus*) and facultative anaerobes (e.g., *A. pyogenes*) are classified in the genera with obligate anaerobes (e.g., *A. bovis* and *A. israelii*).

C. The oxygen sensitivity of bacteria has been correlated with their levels of superoxide dismutase, catalase, and peroxidases.

1. Superoxide dismutase catalyzes the reaction to produce hydrogen peroxide (H_2O_2) from its substrate, the superoxide radical (O_2^-) formed by the monovalent reduction of molecular oxygen. The free superoxide radical is toxic to bacteria.

2. Catalase degrades hydrogen peroxide to water and molecular oxygen, whereas peroxidases eliminate peroxides other than hydrogen peroxide. Peroxides can be highly toxic to bacteria.

3. Comparison of some properties of aerobic and anaerobic bacteria

  a. Many obligate aerobes and facultative anaerobes produce superoxide dismutase, catalase, and/or peroxides; hence superoxide radicals, hydrogen peroxide, and other peroxides do not accumulate to toxic levels.

  b. Many aerotolerate anaerobes contain superoxide dismutase at levels about 30 percent of the concentration found in aerobic bacteria. Aerotolerant anaerobes survive in air because they produce hydrogen peroxide at a very low rate.

  c. Some moderate anaerobes produce catalase and possibly very low levels of superoxide dismutase.

  d. Strict anaerobes are considered not to produce either catalase or superoxide dismutase. Therefore aeration is almost always lethal.

D. Aerotolerance tests are used to determine the oxygen requirements of freshly isolated bacteria from anaerobic culture systems.
   1. Briefly, each colony type from the anaerobic isolation plate is subcultured onto one anaerobic and one aerobic blood agar plate (Table 121.1). The anaerobic plate is incubated in an anaerobic atmosphere for 18 to 24 hours at $37^{o}C$, and the aerobic plate is incubated either in a candlejar or in an atmosphere of air and 5 percent carbon dioxide for 18 to 24 hours at $37^{o}C$.

Table 121.1. Aerotolerance tests

	Growth on Agar Media	
Oxygen Classification of Isolate	Aerobic plate	Anaerobic plate
Obligate aerobe or microaerophile	+	-
Facultative anaerobe	+	+
Obligate anaerobe	-	+

Note: + = growth; - = no growth.

E. Indicators of anaerobiosis
   1. Oxidation-reduction indicators, which measure the redox potential in millivolts (mv) at pH 7.0, are often used to measure various levels of anaerobiosis.
      a. Methylene blue with a redox potential of +11 mv is blue when oxidized and colorless when reduced. This indicator is commonly used to monitor the atmospheric conditions in anaerobic jars and anaerobic chambers.
      b. Resazurin with a redox potential of -41 mv is red when oxidized and colorless when reduced. This indicator is commonly incorporated into liquid and semisolid media.
         (1) Most anaerobic bacterial pathogens will survive and grow if the redox potential is -41 mv or lower.
      c. Phenosafranine with a redox potential of -252 mv is red when oxidized and colorless when reduced. This indicator is used when strict obligate anaerobes are cultured, such as *C. novyi* type B.

VII. CLASSIFICATION AND IDENTIFICATION OF ANAEROBIC BACTERIA
   A. Genera of obligate anaerobes
      1. The major groups of anerobic bacteria are based on their Gram reaction, spore formation, and cellular morphology (Table 121.2).
      2. Modern taxonomic criteria for identifying the anaerobic genera have been based on the production patterns of volatile and nonvolatile fatty acids produced from fermentation reactions (Table 121.3).
         a. Gas liquid chromatography is used to identify the types and amounts of fatty acids, which are metabolic products produced in peptone-yeast extract-glucose (PYG) broth

Table 121.2. Characteristics of genera with obligate anaerobic species

Characteristics	Genera[a]
Gram-positive cocci	*Peptococcus*
	Peptostreptococcus
Gram-positive sporeforming rods	*Clostridium*
Gram-positive nonsporeforming rods	*Actinomyces*[b]
	Bifidobacterium
	Eubacterium
	Propionibacterium
Gram-negative cocci	*Veillonella*
Gram-negative rods	*Bacteroides*
	Fusobacterium
Gram-negative helical rods	*Treponema*

[a]Some pathogenic species within these genera are microaerophiles.
[b]The genus *Actinomyces* is now classified as facultative anaerobic. Anaerobic culture and identification procedures are used to isolate and identify some microaerophilic and anaerobic members.

Table 121.3. Fatty acids from glucose metabolism

Volatile	Nonvolatile
Formic	Lactic
Acetic	Pyruvic
Propionic	Succinic
Butyric	
Isobutyric	
Valeric	
Isovaleric	
Caproic	
Isocaproic	

cultures. Ether is used to extract the volatile fatty acids from the cultures. The nonvolatile fatty acids are first methylated and then extracted with chloroform.

b. The ratio of protein to fermentable carbohydrate in a culture medium can have a profound influence on the acid metabolic products elaborated in it by various anaerobic bacteria.

B. Species of obligate anaerobes
1. The species in the anaerobic genera are identified primarily on the basis of biochemical criteria.
   a. Bacteria in the genera *Actinomyces*, *Clostridium*, *Bacteroides*, and *Fusobacterium* are frequently identified to the species level, while bacteria in the other anaerobic genera are often identified only to the genus level.

C. Differential media and biochemical tests
1. Egg yolk agar is used to detect proteolysis, lipase production, and lecithinase production.
   a. Proteolysis is indicated by a clearing of the medium in the vicinity of the bacterial growth.
   b. Lipase production is detected by the presence of an iridescent sheen on the surface of colonies and on the medium immediately surrounding the growth.

      c. Lecithinase production is detected by the formation of a zone of insoluble precipitate in the medium surrounding the bacterial growth.

  2. Biochemical tests commonly used to identify anaerobes.
      a. Catalase
      b. Esculin hydrolysis
      c. Gelatin hydrolysis
      d. H_2S production
      e. Indole
      f. Nitrate reduction
      g. Urease
      h. Carbohydrate fermentation of a variety of sugars

  3. Antibiotic inhibition tests are commonly used in identifying the gram-negative species in the genera *Bacteroides* and *Fusobacterium*.
      a. Kanamycin, penicillin, and rifampin are commonly employed in these test. Paper disks impregnated with these antibiotics are placed on agar plates, and the zones of growth inhibition around the disks are measured. Zones are recorded as either sensitive or resistant.

---

122 | Antimicrobial Susceptibility Testing Procedures for Anaerobic Bacteria

---

I. INDICATIONS FOR ANTIMICROBIAL SUSCEPTIBILITY TESTING
  A. Antimicrobial resistance in anaerobic bacteria
    1. At present, most veterinary clinicians and clinical microbiologists assume that obligate anaerobic bacterial pathogens of domestic animals are uniformly susceptible to the antimicrobials commonly used to treat anaerobic bacterial infections.
      a. Antimicrobials with moderate to excellent antibacterial activity include penicillin G, ampicillin, carbenicillin, cephaloridine, tetracycline, and clindamycin.
      b. Antimicrobials that are inactive against anaerobes include the aminoglycosides (amikacin, gentamicin, kanamycin, neomycin, and streptomycin) and polymyxin B and E (colistin).

2. Human isolates of *Bacteroides* species and *Fusobacterium* species within the last 15 years have shown a marked increase of antimicrobial resistance. Experimentally antimicrobial resistance that is plasmid-mediated has been transferred within various species of gram-negative obligate anaerobes and to *Escherichia coli.*
   a. This form of antimicrobial resistance also has been recorded in gram-negative bacteria isolated from domestic animals.
   b. Chromosome-mediated antimicrobial resistance also has been demonstrated in some *Bacteroides* species.
3. In vitro experiments have demonstrated that aerobic bacteria that excrete enzymes that inactivate antibiotics will protect anaerobic bacteria in mixed cultures from the antimicrobial activity of the drug. Therefore it is prudent to test the aerobic bacteria, particularly bacteria in the family Enterobacteriaceae and the genus *Staphylococcus* when found in mixed culture with anaerobes, even if the aerobic bacteria is not considered to be a significant pathogen in the lesion.

II. THREE ANTIMICROBIAL SUSCEPTIBILITY TESTING METHODS
   A. Agar dilution method
      1. The agar dilution procedure was developed as a standardized method for the antimicrobial susceptibility testing of anaerobes. This is used as a reference method by the National Committee for Clinical Laboratory Standards (NCCLS) for evaluating other methods but is rarely used by clinical veterinary bacteriology laboratories.
   B. Conventional broth disk method
      1. The antimicrobials are added to broth tubes, using commercially available paper disks impregnated with various antimicrobial agents.
      2. Procedures
         a. The medium is prereduced anaerobically sterilized (PRAS) brain-heart infusion broth supplemented with hemin, menadione, and yeast extract. PRAS will support the growth of most anaerobic bacterial species.
         b. Antimicrobial impregnated paper disks are added to the broth medium until the proper concentration (ug/ml) is achieved. Serial dilutions of each antimicrobial tested are made.
         c. The broth antimicrobial and control tubes are inoculated with the test organism and incubated anaerobically for 18 to 24 hours at 37°C.
      3. Intrepretation of results
         a. The growth (turbidity) in each tube containing an antimicrobial is compared with the growth in the control tube. Each anaerobic bacterium is either susceptible or

resistant to each concentration of the various
antimicrobials tested.
(1) Susceptible organisms show no turbidity.
(2) Resistant organisms have a turbidity equivalent to the
control tube.
C.   Category broth disk method
1.   This method is a modification of the conventional broth dilution
procedure, in which the test anaerobes are evaluated against
only two or three concentrations of each antimicrobial.
2.   Procedures
a.   The methods used are very similar to the conventional broth
dilution method.
3.   Intrepretation of results (Table 122.1)

Table 122.1. Reporting of results of the category broth disk method

Category of Susceptibility	Control Tube	Concentration of Antimicrobial		
		Low	Medium	High
Very susceptible	+	–	–	–
Moderately susceptible	+	+	–	–
Moderately resistant	+	+	+	–
Very resistant	+	+	+	+

a.   The results are reported as categories of susceptibility or
minimum inhibitory concentrations. The end point is the
lowest concentration where no growth (turbidity) occurred.

PART 3	Obligate Intracellular Bacteria

123	Diagnostic Procedures for Obligate Intracellular Bacteria

FAMILY CHLAMYDIACEAE

I. GENUS *CHLAMYDIA*
  A. *C. psittaci*
    1. Egg inoculation
      a. Chlamydiae can be grown in the yolk sacs of 6- to 8-day-old chicken embryos.
      b. Clinical specimens harboring *C. psittaci* are inoculated into the yolk sacs of embryonated eggs, where the bacteria propagate and form characteristic intracytoplasmic chlamydial inclusions in infected epithelial cells.
        (1) The chlamydiae in the yolk sac membranes can be demonstrated by staining with Giemsa, Gimenez, or Macchiavello methods. With the Giemsa method, the intracytoplasmic bacteria stain bluish purple; with the Gimenez and Macchiavello methods the bacteria stain bright red.
        (2) The organisms also can be demonstrated by specific fluorescence, using a fluorescent antibody conjugate.
      c. Infected egg embryos usually die in 3 to 8 days after inoculation.
    2. Cell cultures
      a. Monolayers of McCoy cells are commonly used to recover *C. psittaci* from clinical specimens. Several other established cell lines also have been used successfully.
        (1) It is often necessary to reduce the metabolic activity of the cells to be used for the isolation of chlamydiae. Such a reduction can be achieved by irradiation or treatment with cytostatic compounds such as cycloheximide.

          (a) The cycloheximide treatment of cell monolayers can be performed in association with the inoculation of the sample onto the cell culture.

    (2) Centrifugation of the chlamydiae and cell culture monolayers is often used to facilitate the contact between the bacteria and eucaryotic cells and to increase the endocytotic activity of the host cells.

    (3) The inoculated cell cultures are observed for 72 hours after incubation at $37^{\circ}C$ to detect chlamydial inclusions.

          (a) Chlamydial inclusions in the monolayers are detected by the Giemsa stain or by immunologic techniques, including immunofluorescence and immunoperoxidase.

3. Laboratory animal inoculation
   a. Mice, which are very susceptible to *C. psittaci*, are inoculated either intraperitoneally or intracranially with suspected material. Impression smears of various tissues are stained and examined for chlamydiae, or the serum is examined for antibodies to the infective agent.

4. Cytology
   a. Direct impression smears from affected tissues are stained with Giemsa, Gimenez, or Macchiavello methods to detect the chlamydiae in infected epithelial cells and the vascular endothelium.

5. Serology
   a. The complement-fixation (CF) test is a reliable method of diagnosing infections in domestic animals.
   b. The CF test detects antibodies to group-specific antigens found in both *C. psittaci* and *C. trachomatis*.
      (1) Titers equal to or greater than 1:16 are considered presumptive evidence of chlamydial infection.
      (2) Paired sera obtained during the acute and convalescent stages of infection will often have a 4-fold or greater increase in titer.

6. Methods to distinguish *C. psittaci* from *C. trachomatis*
   a. *C. trachomatis* can be distinguished from *C. psittaci* by the formation of cell inclusions stained by iodine.
   b. The growth of *C. trachomatis* is inhibited by sulfonamides, whereas *C. psittaci* is resistant.

FAMILY RICKETTSIACEAE

I. GENUS *COWDRIA*
  A. *C. ruminantium*
    1. Clinical diagnosis
      a. In endemic areas, a clinical diagnosis of heartwater can

usually be made on the basis of clinical symptoms and
necropsy lesions.
2. Embryonated eggs and cell cultures
   a. *C. ruminantium* has not been cultivated in embryonated eggs
      or in cell cultures.
3. Laboratory animal inoculation
   a. Mice are inoculated intraperitoneally with suspected
      material, and after a 14- to 21-day period, infected
      tissues from the mice are inoculated into susceptible
      ruminants.
      (1) Cattle, goats, and sheep can be readily infected by
          this method and demonstrate clinical signs of
          heartwater after a 10- to 21-day incubation period.
4. Cytology
   a. Impression smears made from the cerebral cortex and
      hippocampus of infected ruminants are stained by the
      Giemsa method to demonstrate rickettsialike bacteria.
   b. Colonies of *C. ruminantium* can be demonstrated within the
      cytoplasm of the vascular endothelial cells when stained by
      the Giemsa method.

II. GENUS *COXIELLA*
   A. *C. burnetii*
      1. Egg inoculation
         a. Placenta material, uterine discharges, or other excretions
            and secretions from infected animals are inoculated into
            the yolk sacs of embryonated eggs. Large masses of red-
            colored coccobacilli can be demonstrated in yolk sac
            preparation stained by Macchiavello's method.
            (1) The organisms in the eggs undergo a phase shift in
                which the virulent phase I cells lose part of their
                cell wall lipopolysaccharide when they convert to the
                avirulent phase II cells. This process is analogous
                to a smooth to rough transformation of gram-negative
                enterics.
      2. Laboratory animal inoculation
         a. Guinea pigs, hamsters, mice, and rabbits are susceptible to
            C. burnetii infections. These laboratory animals are
            inoculated intraperitoneally with material from Q fever-
            infected animals.
         b. Guinea pigs are very susceptible to *C. burnetii* and are the
            most commonly used laboratory animal. The finding of Q
            fever antibodies in guinea pig serum is sufficient evidence
            to make a diagnosis of *C. burnetii*.
      3. Cytology
         a. A tentative diagnosis can be made by demonstrating bacteria
            in stained impression smears from placental and uterine
            discharges of cattle and sheep infected with Q fever.

(1) The bacteria stain readily with Giemsa stain, appearing reddish blue or purple, and bright red with the Macchiavello method.
4. Serology
   a. The CF test is the most widely used serologic test. Titers are usually detectable 2 to 3 weeks after infection, attain maximum levels after 1 to 2 months, and then slowly decline over a period of several months.
      (1) Antibodies against *C. burnetii* are highly specific regardless of the diagnostic techniques employed. A 4-fold or greater rise in titers has diagnostic significance.

III. GENUS *EHRLICHIA*
A. *E. canis*
   1. Clinical diagnosis
      a. In endemic areas, a clinical diagnosis of canine ehrlichiosis can be based on clinical signs and the presence of the brown dog tick.
   2. Embryonated eggs and cell cultures
      a. *E. canis* has not been cultivated in embryonated eggs or in cell cultures.
   3. Cytology
      a. Colonies of the bacteria can be demonstrated in the cytoplasm of monocytes in blood smears stained by the Giemsa method. The organisms stain deep blue or purple.
B. *E. equi*, *E. phagocytophila*, and *E. risticii*
   1. Embryonated eggs and cell cultures
      a. These organisms have not been cultivated in embryonated eggs or in cell cultures.
   2. Cytology
      a. Demonstration of rickettsialike bacteria in leukocytes in blood smears stained by the Giemsa method is used to confirm a clinical diagnosis of ehrlichiosis.

IV. GENUS *NEORICKETTSIA*
A. *N. helminthoeca*
   1. Clinical diagnosis
      a. In endemic areas, a clinical diagnosis of salmon poisoning can usually be made on the basis of clinical symptoms and the presence of fluke eggs in the dog's feces.
   2. Cell cultures
      a. Primary canine monocyte cultures will propagate the bacterium.
   3. Cytology
      a. *N. helminthoeca* are found diffusely arranged or in tight clusters within the cytoplasm of macrophages and reticuloendothelial cells of lymph nodes, spleen, and

tonsils. The bacteria can often be demonstrated in stained smears of fluid aspirated from the mandibular lymph nodes. The organisms stain red with Macchiavello's stain and purple with Giemsa's stain.

V. GENUS *RICKETTSIA*
  A. *R. rickettsii*
    1. Clinical diagnosis
      a. In endemic areas, a clinical diagnosis of canine Rocky Mountain spotted fever can usually be made on the basis of clinical symptoms and the presence of the tick vectors.
    2. Egg inoculation
      a. Rickettsiae are inoculated into the yolk sac of embryonated eggs that have been incubated 7 to 10 days when the development of the chick embryo is well advanced. After the inoculated egg is incubated an additional 4 to 5 days, the egg is opened and the yolk sac membrane removed and examined for rickettsiae. The bacteria can be demonstrated in the yolk sac by staining with Giemsa, Gimenez, or Macchiavello methods.
    3. Cell cultures
      a. Various primary or established cell cultures, including chick embryo fibroblasts and Golden hampster BHK-21 cells, are used to propogate the bacterium. After 5 to 8 days incubation, plaque formation occurs in the monolayers.
    4. Laboratory animal inoculation
      a. Guinea pigs are very susceptible to *R. rickettsii*. Specific antibody appears by the end of the first week of infection and can be detected by serologic tests.
    5. Cytology
      a. Direct impression smears from affected tissues are stained purple by the Giemsa stain and red by the Gimenez and Macchiavello techniques to detect the intracellular rickettsiae.
    6. Serology
      a. Weil-Felix test
        (1) The Weil-Felix test is the oldest and simplest serologic test for detecting rickettsial infections, but unfortunately it is not the most accurate serologic test. The agglutination reactions are based on serum antibody from primary rickettsial infection with the somatic antigens of three *Proteus vulgaris* strains: OX-2, OX-19, and OX-K.
        (a) *R. rickettsii*, a member of the spotted fever group, has the greatest cross reaction to the OX-19 antigen, a weaker reaction to the OX-2 antigen, and no cross reaction with the OX-K antigen.

b.   CF test
   (1)   The CF test is one of the most useful and widely used
        serologic tests for rickettsiae. It detects both
        group-specific antigens, which are found in the
        soluble portion of the rickettsial cell, and the
        species-specific antigens associated with the
        bacterial cell wall.
        (a)   Unfortunately the antigens of *R. rickettsii* tend
              to be anticomplementary, thus making it difficult
              to obtain accurate results with the complement-
              fixing antibodies in the sera.

FAMILY ANAPLASMATACEAE

I.   GENUS *ANAPLASMA*
   A.   *Anaplasma* species
       1.   Cytology
           a.   Demonstration of *Anaplasma* bodies in erythrocytes in blood
                smears stained with the Giemsa method.
       2.   Serology
           a.   For cattle infected with *A. marginale*, the card
                agglutination and CF tests are used to detect cattle that
                have been exposed to infection or are carriers of the
                disease.

II.   GENUS *EPERYTHROZOON*
   A.   *Eperythrozoon* species
       1.   Cytology
           a.   Demonstration of organisms both adhered to the surface of
                erythrocytes and free in the plasma in blood smears stained
                with the Giemsa method.

III.   GENUS *HAEMOBARTONELLA*
   A.   *H. felis*
       1.   Cytology
           a.   Demonstration of *H. felis* on the surfaces of erythrocytes
                in blood smears or impression smears of bone marrow stained
                by the Giemsa method.

SECTION VII

Zoonotic Bacterial Diseases

124 | Zoonotic Bacterial Diseases

I. ZOONOTIC DISEASES

A. Zoonoses are those diseases and infections naturally transmitted between man and other vertebrate animals.

1. Zoonotic diseases may be classified according to the major reservoir of the bacterial agent, the mode of transmission of the bacterium among natural host species, or the major human population at risk.

II. CLASSIFICATION SCHEMA (Tables 124.1 and 124.2)

Table 124.1. Characteristics of selected extracellular and facultative intracellular bacteria

Bacterial Species	Reservoir Classification			Mechanism of Transmission			
	Anthropozoonosis	Zooanthroposis	Amphixenosis	Direct	Cyclo	Meta	Sapro
Gram-positive cocci							
Staphylococcus species	+	+	+	+			+
Streptococcus species	+	+	+	+			+
Gram-positive rods							
Erysipelothrix rhusiopathiae	+			+			+
Listeria monocytogenes	+			+			+
Mycobacterium avium	+			+			
M. bovis	+	+		+			
M. tuberculosis	+	+		+			
Gram-positive sporeforming rods							
Bacillus anthracis	+			+			+
Clostridium tetani	+						+
Gram-negative rods							
Brucella species	+			+			
Escherichia coli	+	+	+	+			
Francisella tularensis	+			+	+	+	
Pasteurella species	+			+			
Pseudomonas mallei	+			+			
P. pseudomallei	+			+		+	+
Salmonella serovars	+	+	+	+			+
Yersinia pestis	+			+		+	
Gram-negative spirochetes							
Leptospira serovars	+			+			+

Table 124.2. Characteristics of selected obligate intracellular bacteria

Bacterial Species	Reservoir Classification			Mechanism of Transmission			
	Anthropozoonosis	Zooanthroposis	Amphixenosis	Direct	Cyclo	Meta	Sapro
Gram-negative rods							
Chlamydia psittaci		+		+			+
Coxiella burnetii		+		+			
Rickettsia rickettsii		+				+	

A.   Major reservoir of agent
   1.   Anthropozoonoses are those infections with their reservoir in nonhuman vertebrates such as domestic animals. Man is then infected by contact with diseased animals. Most zoonoses that affect veterinarians belong to this group.
   2.   Zooanthroposes have their reservoir in man. Man is the natural host of the bacterial agent, and domestic animals may acquire the infection by contact with infected humans.
   3.   Amphixenoses are those infections that include both man and other animals as part of the reservoir. Domestic animals and man serve equally well as natural hosts. It is often difficult to determine if human infections are acquired from domestic animals or from other humans.
B.   Primary mode of transmission
   1.   Direct zoonoses require only one vertebrate host to maintain the bacterial agent.
   2.   Cyclozoonoses require two or more vertebrate hosts for maintenance of the bacterial agent.
   3.   Metazoonoses require both a vertebrate and invertebrate host for the maintenance of the bacterial agent.
   4.   Saprozoonoses require both a vertebrate and a nonanimal reservoir. The bacterial agent is maintained in the soil, water, or another type of inanimate object.
C.   Human populations at risk
   1.   Zoonoses are occupational hazards for veterinarians who care for diseased animals. The risks for specific diseases vary with the particular type of animal production and geographic location of veterinarians.

Glossary

Abscess. A localized accumulation of pus.

Acid-fast. Not decolorized by acid alcohol solutions. Acid-fastness is a unique characteristic of mycobacteria.

Active immunity. Immunity acquired by an animal as a result of its own response to pathogenic bacteria or their products, either through infection or immunization.

Active transport. The passage of a substance into a bacterial cell with the expenditure of energy.

Adenosine triphosphate (ATP). A major carrier of phosphate energy in a biologic system. ATP is composed of adenine, D-ribose, and three phosphoric acid groups.

Adhesin. Component on the bacterial surface that mediates attachment to host cells. See **Fimbria.**

Adjuvant. Any substance that enhances the immune response to an antigen or antigens. Adjuvants are commonly incorporated into bacterial vaccines.

Aerobe. A bacterium that can grow in the presence of atmospheric oxygen. Aerobes include both obligate aerobic bacteria and facultative anaerobic bacteria.

Aerogenic. Producing free gaseous products in the metabolism.

Agalactia. The absence of the secretion of milk.

Agar. A polysaccharide derivative of seaweed that is used as a solidifying agent in bacteriologic media.

Agglutination. The clumping of bacteria as they combine with specific antibody. Particulate antigens such as bacteria are used in agglutination tests.

Agglutinin. An antibody that causes agglutination.

Alternate complement pathway. A pathway activated at C3, bypassing complement components C1, C2, and C4.

Amino acid. The monomeric unit of polypeptides and proteins. Amino acids contain amino ($-NH_2$) and carboxyl ($-COOH$) groups.

Amphitrichous. Having one flagellum at each pole of the cell.

Anaerobe. A bacterium that can grow in the absence of atmospheric oxygen. The term generally applies only to obligate anaerobic bacteria.

Anaerobiosis. Life in the absence of oxygen.

Anamnestic response. The secondary immune response of a host to an antigen.

Anergy. A condition in which an animal previously sensitized to an antigen has a markedly diminished or absent cell-mediated reactivity to that antigen.

Angstrom unit. A unit of length that equals 10^{-10} meter.

Antibiogram. The antimicrobial susceptibility pattern of a specific bacterial strain.

Antibiotic. A biologic substance developed from a microbe that is either bacteriostatic or bacteriocidal.

Antibody. Immunoglobulin formed in response to antigens that are recognized by the body as foreign. Once antibodies are formed, they react with the particular inducing antigen.

Antigen. Any component of the bacterium or bacterial product that when introduced into an animal's body causes the production of specific antibodies.

Antigen binding site. See **Fab fragment.**

Antigenic determinant. The site on the antigen molecule to which specific antibody combines.

Antimicrobial. Any antibiotic or chemotherapeutic substance used to treat microbial infections.

Antiserum. Serum containing specific antibodies to a specific antigen. A hyperimmune antiserum contains a high titer of antibodies and is used to confer passive immunity on a recipient.

Antitoxin. A specific antibody capable of neutralizing a specific bacterial toxin.

Asaccharolytic. Incapable of degrading carbohydrates.

Asepsis. The absence of infectious bacteria in living tissue.

Aseptic. Free from bacteria capable of causing infection or contamination.

Attenuated. Having a reduced virulence.

Autogenous bacterin (or **vaccine**). A bacterin or vaccine prepared from bacteria causing disease in a herd or individual and subsequently used to immunize the herd or individual. See **Bacterin** and **Vaccine.**

Autolysis. The lysis of bacterial cells resulting from the action of their own enzymes.

Autotroph. A bacterium that obtains energy by the oxidation of inorganic compounds. Some autotrophs can utilize carbon dioxide as a sole carbon source.

Axenic. A pure culture of a bacterial strain.

Axial filament. See **Periplasmic flagellum.**

Bacillus (pl. **bacilli**). A rod-shaped bacterium.

Bacillus Calmette-Guerin vaccine. See **BCG vaccine.**

Bacteremia. A disease condition in which bacteria are present in the blood. The affected animal may or may not be symptomatic.

Bacterin. A killed suspension of bacteria used for the immunization of domestic animals.

Bacteriocidal. Able to kill bacteria. The term applies to any compound or mechanism capable of killing bacteria.

Bacteriocin. A bacteriocidal substance produced by some strains of bacteria that inhibits the growth of other bacteria.

Bacteriology. The science that deals with bacteria.

Bacteriophage (or **phage**). A virus that infects bacteria and is released as a result of lysis of the bacterial cells.

Bacteriostatic. Able to cause the inhibition of a bacterium's growth and multiplication. The term applies to any compound or mechanism capable of inhibiting a bacterium's growth.

Bacterium. A procaryotic cell. See **Procaryote.**

B-cell. A lymphocyte that can differentiate into an antibody-producing plasma cell. B-cells also are called B-lymphocytes.

BCG vaccine. An attenuated strain of *Mycobacterium bovis* used to immunize against tuberculosis. BCG is the abbreviation for Bacillus Calmette-Guerin.

Beta-lactamase. An enzyme produced by some bacteria that can break the beta-lactam ring of a penicillin molecule.

Binary fission. An asexual single nuclear division, followed by division of the cytoplasm to form two daughter cells of approximately equal size. Bacteria proliferate by binary fission.

Buffer. Any substance in solution that tends to maintain a constant pH even though small amounts of acid or alkali are added.

Capnophilic. Growing best in the presence of carbon dioxide.

Capsule (or slime layer). A chemical structure located external to the bacterial cell wall. Capsular antigens are classified as K antigens.

Carrier. An individual that harbors and disseminates an infectious bacterial agent but does not exhibit clinical symptoms of the disease.

Catalase. An enzyme that catalyzes the decomposition of hydrogen peroxide into water and oxygen.

Cell-mediated immunity. A specific acquired immunity mediated by T-lymphocytes. Cell-mediated immunity is a protective mechanism for some bacterial infections, particularly those caused by facultative intracellular and obligate intracellular pathogens.

Chemotaxis. Movement of an organism or cell toward a substance (positive chemotaxis) or away from a substance (negative chemotaxis), which establishes a chemical concentration gradient. Phagocytic cells and bacteria can exhibit chemotaxis.

Chromosome. It contains the genes. Procaryotic cells have a single circular chromosome composed of double-stranded DNA. Eucaryotic cells have numerous linear chromosomes.

Clone. The asexual progeny of a single bacterium.

Coagulase. An enzyme produced by some bacteria that is capable of clotting citrated blood or plasma.

Coccobacillus (pl. coccobacilli). An oval bacterium. The term is often used to describe bacteria in the genera *Brucella* and *Haemophilus*.

Coccus (pl. cocci). A spherical bacterium.

Coliform. Any facultative anaerobic, gram-negative bacillus that is an inhabitant of the intestinal tract of animals and produces acid from the fermentation of lactose. The term is often used to denote the lactose-positive members of the family Enterobacteriaceae.

Collagenase. An enzyme that causes the breakdown of collagen.

Colony. A mass of bacteria on a culture medium, such as an agar plate, that is visible to the naked eye. A colony develops from a single cell or a group of cells.

Communicable disease. A bacterial disease capable of being transmitted from one individual to another.

Complement. A complex of at least eleven serum proteins that react with a variety of antigen-antibody complexes and often exert a lytic effect on certain bacteria.

Conjugation. The transfer of genetic material from one bacterial cell to another cell via a conjugation bridge.

Contagious. Capable of being transmitted from one individual to another, such as a bacterial agent.

Coryneform. Referring to the unique cellular morphologic characteristics of selected species in the genus *Corynebacterium*, particularly *C. diphtheriae*. These cells are pleomorphic straight or curved rods, frequently with club-shaped swellings and a palisade arrangement. See **Diphtheroid.**

Culture. The cultivation and growth of bacterial populations, usually in an artificial medium. A few bacteria are grown and propagated in tissue culture or embryonated eggs.

Culture filtrate. A bacteria-free filtrate from a broth culture that has been passed through a filter.

Cytochromes. Iron-containing proteins found in aerobic bacteria that transfer electrons or hydrogen ions along an oxidative pathway.

Cytoplasm. The protoplasm of a eucaryotic or procaryotic cell exclusive of the nucleus.

Cytotoxic. Having a toxin-caused damaging effect on a cell.

Dalton. A unit of molecular weight equal to the weight of one hydrogen atom.

Deaminase. An enzyme that removes an amino group from a molecule, particularly of an amino acid.

Deamination. The chemical process of removing an amino group from an amino acid.

Decarboxylase. An enzyme that removes the carboxyl group from a molecule, particularly of an amino acid.

Decarboxylation. The chemical process of removing a carboxyl group from a molecule, particularly of an amino acid.

Dehydrogenase. An enzyme that catalyzes the transfer of electrons or hydrogen ions from a substrate to a recipient molecule.

Dehydrogenation. The removal of hydrogen from a molecule.

Deoxyribonucleic acid (DNA). The carrier of genetic information in most organisms. The DNA in the bacterial chromosome, eucaryotic chromosomes, and plasmids is composed of a double-stranded chain of deoxyribonucleotides. The purine and pyrimidine bases in DNA are adenine, cytosine, guanine, and thymine.

Deoxyribose. A pentose found in DNA.

Diaminopimelic acid. An amino acid found in the cell walls of most species of bacteria.

Diapedesis. The transudation of cells through the intact walls of blood vessels.

Differential medium. A bacteriologic medium that can detect different enzymatic activity in different kinds of bacteria (e.g., MacConkey agar can differentiate lactose fermentors from nonlactose fermentors).

Dimorphic. Referring to a bacterium with the ability to grow in two forms.

Diphtheroid. Referring to cells with an irregular morphology, and often specifically to the cellular morphology of *Corynebacterium diphtheriae*. See **Coryneform.**

Dipicolinic acid. A compound found in high concentration in bacterial spores but not in vegetative cells.

Diplococcus. A bacterium always found in pairs.

Disaccharide. A carbohydrate composed of two monosaccharides.

Dysentery. An intestinal bacterial infection characterized by diarrhea containing blood and mucus.

Ecology. The study of the interrelationship of organisms (e.g., bacteria) and their environment.

Edema. An excessive fluid accumulation in tissues.

Endemic. Referring to a bacterial disease present in a population of animals at all times but not always recognizable clinically. In endemic areas, the incidence of the disease is low.

Endogenous bacterium. A bacterium that originates within the host. Endogenous microorganisms are often part of the animal's normal flora.

Endospore. A specialized nonproductive structure formed within a vegetative cell. Only one spore is formed in each bacterial cell.

Endotoxin. The lipopolysaccharide component of gram-negative bacterial cell walls, which possesses endotoxic activity. Lipid A is responsible for the nonspecific endotoxic activity of the lipopolysaccharide.

Enteric bacterium. A bacterium that inhabits the gastrointestinal tracts of animals (e.g., coliforms are enteric bacteria).

Enteritis. An inflammation of the intestine.

Enterotoxin. A bacterial exotoxin specific for cells in the intestine.

Epidemic. Having an incidence greater than the expected endemic level.

Episome. A segment of DNA capable of integrating into the bacterial chromosome. The episome replicates as part of the bacterial chromosome.

Epitope. See **Antigenic determinant.**

Esterase. An enzyme that catalyzes the hydrolysis of esters, particularly in fats.

Etiology. The cause(s) or origin of a disease.

Eucaryote. An organism whose cells have a true nucleus with a nuclear membrane, such as animals, plants, fungi, and yeasts.

Exogenous bacterium. A bacterium that originates outside the host.

Exotoxin. A toxic substance formed by bacteria that is found outside the bacterial cell. Most bacterial exotoxins are proteins and have a specific toxic effect.

Extracellular bacterium. A bacterium that grows and proliferates only outside of cells.

Exudate. The material formed at the site of inflammation or a bacteria-induced lesion. Common components found in the exudate include bacteria, phagocytic cells, and various types of tissue debris.

Fab fragment. The antigen-binding portion of the immunoglobulin molecule.

Facultative anaerobe. A bacterium that can grow under either aerobic or anaerobic conditions.

Facultative intracellular bacterium. A bacterium that can grow and proliferate either extracellularly or intracellularly within living cells.

F antigens. See **Fimbria.**

Fastidious bacterium. A bacterium that is difficult to cultivate using ordinary culture procedures. Fastidious bacteria often have complex nutritional requirements.

Fc fragment. The crystallizable portion of the immunoglobulin molecule. The Fc fragment can bind complement and provides an attachment site for phagocytic cells, that possess Fc receptors.

Fermentation. The anaerobic utilization of carbohydrates and related compounds in which an organic compound serves as the final electron (hydrogen) acceptor.

Filamentous bacterium. A bacterium whose cells are long filaments. The majority of the filamentous bacteria have a highly pleomorphic cellular morphology.

Fimbria (or **pilus;** pl. **fimbriae**). A short, hairlike projection on the surface of certain bacteria. These proteins act as adhesins in the colonization of selected body surface structures, and some specialized fimbriae may serve as conduits for the transfer of genetic material between bacterial cells during conjugation. Some fimbriae are classified as F antigens.

Flagellar antigen. An antigenic protein derived from the flagellum, often called H antigens. See **Flagellum** and **H antigen.**

Flagellum (pl. **flagella**). A protein appendage on bacterium that is used as an organ of locomotion.

Flora. Microorganisms typically found in a given environment.

Fomite. Any inanimate object or substance that can serve as a mode of transmission for infectious bacteria from one host to another.

Forespore. The structure in sporeforming vegetative bacterial cells that becomes the endospore.

Fusiform. Spindle-shaped and tapered at the ends.

Gamma globulin. Antibodies associated with the gamma globulin fraction of blood proteins. See **Immunoglobulin.**

G+C content. The molar percentage of the total base content in the DNA. It can also be expressed as a molar ratio of A+T:G+C.

Gelatin. A substance used in culture media for the determination of a specific proteolytic activity of bacteria.

Gelatinase. An enzyme produced by bacteria that is responsible for the liquefaction of gelatin.

Gene. A functional component of a chromosome or plasmid that codes for a specific polypeptide.

Genome. Composed of chromosome(s) of an organism. The genome of a bacterium is composed of a single circular chromosome; however, the genome of eucaryotic cells such as those found in domestic animals contain a set of chromosomes.

Genotype. The genetic composition of an organism that includes all the genes contained by a cell whether or not they are all expressed.

Germination. The process of vegetative cell formation from a bacterial endospore.

Glycolysis. The anaerobic catabolism of glucose to pyruvic acid (e.g., the Embden-Meyerhof-Parnas pathway is a glycolytic pathway).

Gnotobiotic animal. A germ-free animal.

Gram-negative bacterium. A bacterium readily decolorized with alcohol in Gram's method of staining that will then pick up the color of the counterstain. Safranin is commonly used as the counterstain. Gram-negative bacteria stain pink.

Gram-positive bacterium. A bacterium not readily decolorized with alcohol in Gram's method of staining, thus retaining the crystal violet-iodine complex. Gram-positive bacteria stain purple.

Gram stain. A differential stain for bacteria developed by Hans C. Gram. The stain is based on the inability of gram-positive bacteria to be readily decolorized with alcohol once they have been stained with a combination of crystal violet and iodine.

Granuloma. A mass of granulation tissue often resulting from chronic bacterial infections.

H antigen. See **Flagellar antigen** and **Flagellum**.

Hemagglutination. The agglutination of erythrocytes in the presence of certain types of bacteria or specific antibody.

Hemolysin. A substance that causes the lysis of red blood cells.

Hemolysis. The lysis of erythrocytes.

Heterofermentation. A fermentation process in which a carbohydrate is degraded by a bacterium, resulting in a mixture of organic acids and gases as end products.

Heterotroph. An organism that requires organic compounds for a source of carbon and energy.

Hexose. A monosaccharide with six carbon atoms.

Homofermentation. A fermentation process in which a carbohydrate is degraded by a bacterium, resulting in a single metabolic end product. The streptococci ferment glucose to produce lactic acid as the sole end product.

Horizontal transmission. The tranfer of an infectious bacterium from one animal to another through the environment.

Humoral immunity. Antibody-mediated immunity.

Hyaluronic acid. A mucopolysaccharide that composes the capsule of some bacteria. The intracellular substance in connective tissue also contains hyaluronic acid.

Hyaluronidase. An enzyme capable of degrading hyaluronic acid.

Hydrolysis. The enzymatic cleavage of a compound by the addition of a water (H_2O) molecule. The hydrogen ion (H^+) is incorporated in one fragment and the hydroxyl (OH^-) group in the other.

Immunity. The resistance of the host to the effects of pathogenic bacteria or their toxins.

Immunogen. An antigenic substance that induces immunity.

Immunoglobulin. A class of proteins having antibody activity, evoked as a result of antigenic stimulation. The term is frequently used interchangeably with antibody and immune gamma globulins. See **Antibody** and **Gamma globulin**.

IMViC test. An acronym for four biochemical tests (indole, methyl red, Voges-Proskauer, and citrate). This test is helpful in differentiating some lactose-positive genera in the family Enterobacteriaceae.

Incubation. The maintenance and growth of bacterial cultures under favorable conditions.

Incubation period. The time interval between infection and the appearance of clinical symptoms.

Infection. A disease state due to the invasion of a host by a pathogenic bacterium.

Infectious. Referring to the capability of a pathogenic bacterium to be communicated to susceptible hosts.

Inflammation. The nonspecific response of the host's tissues to bacterial injury, characterized by heat, pain, redness, swelling, and occasionally the loss of function.

Inoculation. The introduction of bacteria into animals, culture media, eggs, or tissue cultures.

Inoculum. The microorganisms being introduced into living tissue or culture media by inoculation.

Invasiveness. The property of a bacterium that enables it to overcome the normal body defenses and cause an overt disease.

In vitro. In the laboratory.

In vivo. Within the body.

Kauffmann-White schema. The classification system used to identify and classify the serovars of *Salmonella* by antigenic analyses of their somatic (O), flagellar (H), and capsular (Vi) antigens.

Krebs cycle. See **Tricarboxylic acid cycle.**

Lactose. A disaccharide composed of glucose and galactose.

Latency. A period in which the host may harbor infectious bacteria and not manifest any clinical symptoms.

Lesion. Any pathogenic change in a tissue caused by a bacterial infection.

Leukocyte. A white blood cell.

Leukotoxin. A substance that is toxic to white blood cells, produced by a pathogenic bacterium.

L-form. A bacterial form devoid of a cell wall. See **Protoplast** and **Spheroplast.**

Lipase. Any enzyme capable of degrading lipid.

Litmus. A pigment extracted from lichen. Litmus is incorporated in some bacteriologic media as a pH indicator or a redox indicator. It turns blue in reaction to alkaline substances and red to acid.

Lophotrichous. Having a tuft of flagella at one or both poles of the cell.

Lymphocyte. A white blood cell. See **B-cell** and **T-cell.**

Lysis. The disruption of a cell by hemolysin, toxin, or the action of specific antibodies plus complement.

Lysogenic. Referring to a bacterium carrying a prophage. See **Bacteriophage.**

Lysogeny. A state in which a bacteriophage genome is integrated with the bacterial chromosome.

Lysozyme. An enzyme with the ability to hydrolyze the peptidoglycan in the bacterial cell wall. Lysozyme can lyse certain types of bacteria, especially gram-positive cells, and is present in many body fluids, including tears.

Macrophage. A large mononuclear cell with phagocytic activity. Macrophages are derived from the reticuloendothelial system.

Maltose. A disaccharide of glucose.

Mesophile. A bacterium whose optimum temperature for growth is in the range of 20°C to 45°C.

Mesosome. A highly convoluted invagination of the bacterial cytoplasmic membrane.

Metachromatic granule. A cytoplasmic granule in the cells of certain bacteria that stains with basic dyes, such as methylene blue.

Microaerophile. A bacterium whose optimum growth occurs in the presence of a small amount of atmospheric oxygen.

Micrometer. A unit of measurement equal to 10^{-6} m.

Monosaccharide. A simple carbohydrate that cannot be decomposed further by hydrolysis (e.g., hexoses and pentoses).

Monotrichous. Having one flagellum at one end of the cell.

Morbidity. The relative incidence of disease expressed as a ratio of clinically ill to healthy animals in a herd or population.

Mortality. The proportion of deaths in a herd or population.

Murein. See **Peptidoglycan.**

Mutant. A daughter cell with an altered genotype.

Mycoplasma. A genus of bacteria that lack cell walls. The term also refers to any bacterium in the genera *Mycoplasma* and *Ureaplasma*.

Nanometer. A unit of measure equal to 10^{-9} m.

Necrosis. The death of cells or tissues.

Nitrate reduction. A process in which nitrate is reduced to nitrite or other degradation products.

Nitroreductase. An enzyme that has the capacity to reduce nitrate.

Normal flora. Any organism living indogenously on or in healthy animals (e.g., bacteria, protozoa, or viruses).

Nucleic acid. A substance composed of nucleotides. DNA and RNA are the two principal types of nucleic acids in bacteria.

Nucleoid. The area in the procaryotic cell containing the chromosomal DNA.

O antigen. See **Somatic antigen.**

Obligate aerobe. A bacterium that can grow only in the presence of free oxygen.

Obligate anaerobe. A bacterium that can grow only in the absence of free oxygen.

Obligate intracellular bacterium. A bacterium that can grow and proliferate only within living cells.

Opportunistic pathogen. A bacterial species that may cause infection under certain circumstances, although not normally regarded as a pathogen.

Opsonin. A substance that binds to bacteria and facilitates phagocytosis by neutrophils and macrophages (e.g., specific antibody and complement).

Organotrophism. A characteristic by which certain bacteria select and localize in specific body tissues.

Oxidation. A chemical reaction in which a substance gains an oxygen atom or loses electrons or a hydrogen atom.

Oxidation-reduction potential. The electron-accepting or electron-yielding potential of a given compound under specified conditions.

Oxidative phosphorylation. The chemical reactions associated with the electron transport system in which inorganic phosphate is converted to high-energy phosphate, adenine triphosphate (ATP).

Passive natural immunity. Immunity acquired by receiving antibody in the colostrum or by placental transfer.

Pasteurization. A heat treatment commonly used to kill pathogenic bacteria in milk, named after Louis Pasteur, the French microbiologist who developed it.

Pathogen. Any bacterium capable of causing disease.

Pathogenesis. The mode of origin and development of a bacterial disease.

Pathognomonic. Referring to a clinical sign or lesion so characteristic of a disease that a diagnosis can be made.

Penicillinase. See **Beta-lactamase.**

Pentose. A monosaccharide with five carbon atoms.

Peptidase. A proteolytic enzyme that hydrolyzes the peptide bonds in polypeptides and proteins.

Peptidoglycan. A substance largely responsible for the rigidity of the bacterial cell wall. It is composed of alternating disaccharides of N-acetyl glucosamine and N-acetylmuramic acid to which short peptide chains are attached.

Peptone. A substance commonly used in bacteriologic media, composed of peptides and proteins formed as an intermediate product in the digestion of protein.

Periplasmic flagellum. A specialized type of appendage on spirochetes in the genera *Borrelia*, *Leptospira*, and *Treponema* used as an organ of locomotion.

Peritrichous. Having flagella around the entire cell.

Permease. An enzyme or enzyme system that transports substances across the cell wall into the bacterial cell.

pH. A measure of acidity or alkalinity, the negative logarithm of the hydrogen ion activity.

Phagocyte. A cell with the capacity to ingest and kill bacteria. Neutrophils and macrophages are the principal phagocytes of domestic animals.

Phagocytosis. The process of ingesting bacteria or other particulate matter by phagocytic cells.

Phenotype. The detectable expression produced by the genotype of a bacterium under a given set of conditions.

Pilus (pl. pili). See **Fimbria.**

Plasma cell. A differentiated B-lymphocyte capable of producing antibodies.

Plasmid. Extrachromosomal DNA that replicates autonomously from the bacterial chromosome.

Pleomorphism. The appearance of bacteria in more than one morphological form.

Pleuropneumonialike organisms (PPLO). An older term to describe some of the mycoplasmas.

Polar flagellation. The presence of flagella at the ends of the bacterial cells. See **Amphitrichous, Lophotrichous,** and **Monotrichous.**

Polypeptide. A polymer of many amino acids bound by the covalent peptide bonds.

Polyribosome. A chain of ribosomes held together by a messenger ribonucleic acid (mRNA) molecule.

Polysaccharide. A polymer of many monosaccharides or disaccharides held together by covalent bonds.

Procaryote. A cell without a nuclear membrane (e.g., bacteria).

Prophage. The stage of a bacteriophage in a lysogenic bacterium in which the bacteriophage DNA is integrated into the bacterial DNA.

Proteases. Proteolytic enzymes capable of hydrolyzing the peptide bonds in proteins.

Protein. A macromolecular polymer of amino acids joined by peptide bonds.

Protoplast. A gram-positive bacterium with little or no residual cell wall.

Psychophile. A bacterium whose optimal growth temperature is below 20°C.

Pyogenic bacterium. A bacterium that produces pus.

Pyremia. A systemic disease characterized by the presence of pyogenic bacteria in the blood.

Pyrogen. An infectious agent or substance that induces fever.

Quelling reaction. The reaction of a specific anticapsular antibody with its specific caspular antigen, allowing the visualization of the capsule.

Reduction. A chemical reaction in which a substance loses an oxygen atom or gains electrons or a hydrogen atom.

Respiration. A type of metabolism in which oxygen serves as the final electron (hydrogen) acceptor in the electron transport system.

Reticuloendothelial system (RES). A body defense system composed of both free and fixed macrophages that reside in various tissues and organs (e.g., bone marrow, lymph nodes, liver, and spleen).

Ribonucleic acid (RNA). Macromolecules that function in the storage and transfer of genetic information and are composed of purine and pyrimidine ribonucleotides. Bacteria have three types of RNA: messenger RNA (mRNA), ribosomal RNA (rRNA), and transfer RNA (tRNA). The four ribonucleotides in RNA are adenine, cytosine, guanine, and uracil.

Ribose. A pentose found in of RNA.

Ribosome. Cytoplasmic RNA-protein complexes that are the site of cellular protein synthesis. Bacteria have 70S ribosomes each composed of a 30S and 50S subunits. Eucaryotic cells have 80S ribosomes composed of 40S and 60S subunits. (S = Svedberg unit, a measurement of sedimentation coefficients.)

Saccharolytic bacterium. A bacterium capable of degrading carbohydrates.

Saprophyte. A bacterium that generally lives on dead and decaying organic matter in the environment.

Selective medium. A bacteriologic medium that allows certain bacteria to grow while inhibiting others (e.g., MacConkey agar contains bile salts and allows the growth of most aerobic gram-negative bacteria but inhibits the growth of most nonenterics).

Sepsis. The presence of infectious bacteria in the tissue of the host.

Septicemia. A disease condition in which bacteria are present in the blood and the affected animal is symptomatic.

Sequela (pl. **sequelae**). A disease condition that results as a consequence of another disease.

Serology. The study of antigen-antibody reactions in vitro.

Somatic antigen. An antigen derived from the bacterial cell wall, often called O antigens (e.g., lipopolysaccharides are somatic antigens in gram-negative bacteria and the teichoic acids are somatic antigens in gram-positive bacteria).

Spheroplast. A gram-negative bacteria with little or no residual cell wall.

Spirochete. A bacterium with a spiral form.

Spore. See **Endospore.**

Sporulation. The process of producing bacterial endospores.

Substrate. A compound acted on by an enzyme.

Superinfection. An infection superimposed on an already existing infection.

Suppuration. The formation of pus.

Synergistic bacterium. A bacterium that, when paired with a bacterium of another certain species, can produce a disease or disease condition that neither bacterium alone could produce.

Taxon (pl. taxa). A scientific classification of living organisms, such as a division, order, class, family, genus, or species.

Taxonomy. The classification of living organisms, such as bacteria, into groups or categories called taxa.

T-cell (or T-lymphocyte). A thymus-dependent lymphocyte that plays a central role in acquired cell-mediated immune responses.

Temperate bacteriophage. A bacteriophage capable of infecting a bacterial cell and integrating its DNA into the bacterium's DNA, rendering that cell lysogenic.

Thermophile. A bacterium that can grow optimally at temperatures of 55°C to 80°C.

Thrombosis. The formation of a clot within a blood vessel.

Titer. The highest dilution of a serum that gives a positive reaction.

Toxemia. The presence of toxins in the blood.

Toxin. A poisonous substance produced by a living organism. Bacteria have two types of toxins, endotoxins and exotoxins. See **Endotoxin** and **Exotoxin.**

Toxoid. An exotoxin that has been treated with various chemical or physical agents to destroy its toxicity without affecting its antigenic properties.

Transcription. The process by which mRNA, using DNA as a template, copies a nucleotide sequence complementary to a segment of the DNA in the chromosome.

Transduction. A bacteriophage-mediated transfer of bacterial DNA from one bacterium to another.

Translation. The process by which tRNA converts the codons on mRNA into polypeptides.

Transovarial transmission. The transmission of bacteria through the female eggs to the offspring.

Transstadial transmission. The survival of a microorganism, such as a bacterium, through one or more stages (e.g., larva, nymph, and adult) of tick development.

Tricarboxylic acid (TCA) cycle. An aerobic metabolic pathway by which pyruvic acid is converted to carbon dioxide and water with the release of energy.

Tubercle. The characteristic lesion induced by *Mycobacterium bovis* and *M. tuberculosis.*

Vaccine. A substance containing antigen from a pathogenic bacterium that on administration to an animal, stimulates a specific active immunity.

Variant. A bacterium having one or more characteristics that differ from the parent bacterial strain.

Vector. Any animate or inanimate agent that carries a pathogenic microorganism from one host to another.

Vehicle. See **Fomite**.

Verticle transmission. The transmission of a bacterium from mother to offspring (e.g., in utero infection of a fetus across the placenta from the dam).

Virulence. The disease-producing potential of a given species or strain of bacterium in quantitative terms.

Zoonosis. An animal disease that may be transmitted to man.

Selected References

Adams, D. O. 1976. The granulomatous inflammatory response: A review. *Am. J. Pathol.* 84:164-91.

Afshar, A., P. Stuart, and R. A. Huck. 1966. Granular vulvovaginitis (nodular venereal disease) of cattle associated with *Mycoplasma bovigenitalium*. *Vet. Rec.* 78:512-19.

Alton, G. G. 1978. Recent developments in vaccination against bovine brucellosis. *Aust. Vet. J.* 54:551-57.

Amatredjo, A., and R. S. F. Campbell. 1975. Bovine leptospirosis. *Vet. Bull.* 43:875-91.

Anderson, M. J., J. S. Whitehead, and Y. S. Kim. 1980. Interaction of *Escherichia coli* K88 antigen with porcine intestinal brush border membranes. *Infect. Immun.* 29:897-901.

Ayers, J. L. 1977. Caseous lymphadenitis in goats and sheep: A review of diagnosis, pathogenesis and immunity. *J. Am. Vet. Med. Assoc.* 171:1251-54.

Bagadi, H. O., and M. M. H. Sewell. 1973. Experimental studies on infectious necrotic hepatitis (black disease) of sheep. *Res. Vet. Sci.* 15:53-61.

Bang, B. 1897. The etiology of epizootic abortion. *J. Comp. Pathol. Ther.* 10:125-49.

Barton, M. D., and K. L. Hughes. 1980. *Corynebacterium equi*: A review. *Vet. Bull.* 50:65-80.

Bauer, A. W., W. M. M. Kirby, J. C. Sherris, and M. Turck. 1966. Antibiotic susceptibility testing by a standardized single disk method. *Am. J. Clin. Pathol.* 45:493-96.

Bellanti, J. A., and D. H. Dayton. 1975. *The Phagocytic Cell in Host Resistance*. New York: Raven.

Bemis, D. A., H. A. Greisen, and M. J. G. Appel. 1977. Pathogenesis of canine bordetellosis. *J. Infect. Dis.* 135:753-62.

Berg, J. N., and R. W. Loan. 1975. *Fusobacterium necrophorum* and *Bacteroides melaninogenicus* as etiologic agents of foot rot in cattle. *Am. J. Vet. Res.* 36:1115-22.

Berg, J. N., W. H. Fales, and C. M. Scanlan. 1979. Occurrence of anaerobic bacteria in diseases of the dog and cat. *Am. J. Vet. Res.* 40:876-81.

Blazevic, D. J., and G. M. Ederer. 1975. *Principles of Biochemical Tests in Diagnostic Microbiology*. New York: John Wiley.

Brewer, J. H., and D. L. Allgeier. 1966. Safe self-contained carbon dioxide-hydrogen anaerobic system. *Appl. Microbiol.* 14:985-88.

Buhles, W. C., Jr., D. L. Huxsoll, and M. Ristic. 1974. Tropical canine pancytopenia: Clinical, hematologic, and serologic response of dogs to *Ehrlichia canis* infection, tetracycline therapy, and challenge inoculation. *J. Infect. Dis.* 130:357-67.

Burgess, G. W. 1982. Ovine contagious epididymitis: A review. *Vet. Microbiol.* 7:551-75.

Bush, B. M. 1976. A review of the aetiology and consequences of urinary tract infections in the dog. *Br. Vet. J.* 132:632-41.

Carman, R. J., and J. C. M. Lewis. 1983. Recurrent diarrhoea in a dog associated with *Clostridium perfringens* type A. *Vet. Rec.* 112:342-43.

Carmichael, L. E., and R. M. Kenney. 1968. Canine abortion caused by *Brucella canis*. *J. Am. Vet. Med. Assoc.* 152:605-16.

Carpenter, C. C. J. 1972. Cholera and other enterotoxin-related diarrheal diseases. *J. Infect. Dis.* 126:551-64.

Carpenter, P. L. 1975. *Immunology and Serology*. Philadelphia: W. B. Saunders.

Carter, G. R., ed. 1984. *Diagnostic Procedures in Veterinary Bacteriology and Mycology*. 4th ed. Springfield: C. C. Thomas.

Christie, R., N. E. Adkins, and E. A. Munch-Peterson. 1944. A note on the lytic phenomenon shown by group B streptococci. *Aust. J. Exp. Biol. Med. Sci.* 23:197-200.

Collins, F. M. 1971. Mechanisms in antimicrobial immunity. *J. Reticuloendothel. Soc.* 10:58-99.

Dannenberg, A. M. J. 1975. Macrophages in inflammation and infection. *N. Engl. J. Med.* 293:489-93.

Dowell, V. R., Jr., and T. M. Hawkins. 1974. *Laboratory Methods in Anaerobic Bacteriology*. DHEW Publication (CDC) 74-8272. Atlanta: Center for Disease Control.

Eiklid, K. and S. Olsnes. 1983. Animal toxicity of *Shigella dysenteriae* cytotoxin: Evidence that the neurotoxic, enterotoxic, and cytotoxic activities are due to one toxin. *J. Immun.* 130:380-84.

Field, M. 1979. Modes of action of *Vibrio cholerae* and *Escherichia coli*. *Rev. Infect. Dis.* 1:918-25.

Francis, J., C. L. Choi, and A. J. Frost. 1973. The diagnosis of tuberculosis in cattle with special reference to bovine PPD tuberculin. *Aust. Vet. J.* 49:246-51.

Friend, S. C., R. G. Thomson, and B. N. Wilkie. 1977. Pulmonary lesions induced by *Pasteurella hemolytica* in cattle. *Can. J. Comp. Med.* 41:219-23.

Gaastra, W., and F. K. deGraaf. 1982. Host-specific fimbrial adhesins of noninvasive enterotoxigenic *Escherichia coli* strains. *Microbiol. Rev.* 46:129-161.

Gibbons, D. F. 1980. Equine salmonellosis: A review. *Vet. Rec.* 106:356-59.

Gribble, D. H. 1969. Equine ehrlichiosis. *J. Am. Vet. Med. Assoc.* 155:462-69.

Hadad, J. J., and C. L. Gyles. 1982. The role of K antigens of enteropathogenic *Escherichia coli* in colonization of the small intestine of calves. *Can. J. Comp. Med.* 46:21-26.

Hanson, L. E. 1973. Immunologic problems in bovine leptospirosis. *J. Am. Vet. Med. Assoc.* 163:919-21.

------. 1982. Leptospirosis in domestic animals: The public health perspective. *J. Am. Vet. Med. Assoc.* 181:1505-9.

Harris, D. L., and R. D. Glock. 1972. Swine dysentery. *J. Am. Vet. Med. Assoc.* 160:561-65.

Henry, S. C. 1979. Clinical observations on eperythrozoonosis. *J. Am. Vet. Med. Assoc.* 174:601-3.

Holdeman, L. V., E. P. Cato, and W. E. C. Moore. 1977. *Anaerobe Laboratory Manual.* 4th ed. Blacksburg: Virginia Polytechnic Institute.

Hood, A. M. 1977. Virulence factors of *Francisella tularensis. J. Hyg.* 79:47-60.

Hoover, E. A., D. E. Kahn, and J. M. Langloss. 1978. Experimentally induced feline chlamydial infection (feline pneumonitis). *Am. J. Vet. Res.* 39:541-47.

Hugh, R., and E. Leifson. 1953. The taxonomic significance of fermentative versus oxidative metabolism of carbohydrates by various gram negative bacteria. *J. Bacteriol.* 66:24-26.

Jensen, R., H. M. Deane, L. J. Cooper, V. A. Miller, and W. R. Graham. 1954. The rumenitis-liver abscess complex in beef cattle. *Am. J. Vet. Res.* 15:202-16.

Johnston, N. E., R. A. Estrella, and W. D. Oxender. 1977. Resistance of neonatal calves given colostrum diet to oral challenge with a septicemia-producing *Escherichia coli. Am. J. Vet. Res.* 38:1323-26.

Kernkamp, H. C. H., M. H. Roepke, and D. E. Jasper. 1946. Orchitis in swine due to *Brucella suis. J. Am. Vet. Med. Assoc.* 108:215-21.

Klipstein, F. A., and R. F. Engert. 1977. Immunological interrelationships between cholera toxin and the heat-labile and heat-stable enterotoxins of coliform bacteria. *Infect. Immun.* 18:110-17.

Krieg, N. R., ed. 1984. *Bergey's Manual of Systematic Bacteriology.* Vol. 1. Baltimore: Williams and Wilkins.

Lancefield, R. C. 1933. A serological differentiation of human and other groups of hemolytic streptococci. *J. Exp. Med.* 57:571-95.

Lawson, G. H. K., and C. Dow. 1965. The pathogenesis of oral *Salmonella cholerae-suis* infection in pigs. *J. Comp. Pathol.* 75:75-81.

Liu, P. V. 1974. Extracellular toxins of *Pseudomonas aeruginosa. J. Infect. Dis.* 130:S94-S99.

Lomax, L. G., and R. D. Glock. 1982. Naturally occurring porcine proliferative enteritis: Pathologic and bacteriologic findings. *Am. J. Vet. Res.* 43:1608-14.

McCandlish, I. A. P., H. Thompson, and N. G. Wright. 1976. Kennel cough: Vaccination against *Bordetella bronchiseptica* infection. *Vet. Rec.* 98:156-57.

MacFaddin, J. F., ed. 1980. *Biochemical Tests for Identification of Medical Bacteria.* 2d ed. Baltimore: Williams and Wilkins.

Mackaness, G. B. 1971. Resistance to intracellular infection. *J. Infect. Dis.* 123:439-45.

Maede, Y., and R. Hata. 1975. Studies on feline haemobartonellosis. II. The mechanism of anemia produced by infection with *Haemobartonella felis. Jpn. J. Vet. Sci.* 37:49-54.

Mare, C. J., and W. P. Switzer. 1965. New species: *Mycoplasma hyopneumoniae*: A causative agent of virus pig pneumonia. *Vet. Med. Small Anim. Clin.* 60:841–46.

Marted, W. R. 1953. The use of bacitracin for identifying group-A haemolytic streptococci. *J. Clin. Pathol.* 6:224–26.

Merkal, R. S., K. E. Kopecky, A. B. Larsen, and R. D. Ness. 1970. Immunologic mechanisms in bovine paratuberculosis. *Am. J. Vet. Res.* 31:475–85.

Miles, A. A., and P. L. Khimji. 1975. Enterobacterial chelators of iron: Their occurrence, detection, and relation to pathogenicity. *J. Med. Microbiol.* 8:477–96.

Moller, V. 1955. Simplified tests for some amino acid decarboxylases and for the arginine dihydrolase system. *Acta Pathol. Microbiol. Scand.* 36:158–72.

Moon, H. W. 1981. Protection against enteric colibacillosis in pigs suckling orally vaccinated dams: Evidence for pili as protective antigens. *Am. J. Vet. Res.* 42:173–77.

Morrison, W. I., and N. G. Wright. 1976. Canine leptospirosis: An immunopathological study of interstitial nephritis due to *Leptospira canicola*. *J. Pathol.* 120:83–89.

Morse, E. V. 1951. Canine brucellosis: A review of the literature. *J. Am. Vet. Med. Assoc.* 119:304–8.

Nayar, P. S. G., and J. R. Saunders. 1975. Infectious bovine keratoconjunctivitis. II. Antibodies in lacrimal secretions of cattle naturally or experimentally infected with *Moraxella bovis*. *Can. J. Comp. Med.* 39:32–40.

Niilo, L. 1980. *Clostridium perfringens* in animal disease: A review of current knowledge. *Can. Vet. J.* 21:141–48.

Oburolo, M. J. 1976. A review of yersiniosis (*Yersinia pseudotuberculosis*) infection. *Vet. Bull.* 46:167–71.

Osebold, J. W., J. W. Kendrick, and A. Njoku-Obi. 1960. Cattle abortion associated with natural *Listeria monocytogenes* infection. *J. Am. Vet. Med. Assoc.* 137:221–26.

Pappenheimer, A. M., Jr., and D. M. Gill. 1973. Diphtheria. *Science* 182:353–58.

Parker, R. H., and P. D. Hoeprich. 1962. Disk method for rapid identification of *Hemophilus* species. *Am. J. Clin. Pathol.* 37:319–27.

Pearson, G. R., and E. F. Logan. 1979. The pathogenesis of enteric colibacillosis in neonatal unsuckled calves. *Vet. Rec.* 105:159–64.

Pienaar, J. G., P. A. Basson, and J. L. deB. Van Der Merwe. 1966. Studies on the pathology of heartwater [*Cowdria* (Rickettsia) *ruminantium*, Cowdry, 1926]. I. Neuropathological changes. *Onderstepoort J. Vet. Res.* 33:115–38.

Plastridge, W. N. 1955. Vibriosis. *Adv. Vet. Sci.* 2:327–79.

Richardson, A. 1975. Salmonellosis in cattle. *Vet. Rec.* 96:329–31.

Roberts, D. S., N. P. H. Graham, J. R. Egerton, and I. M. Parsonson. 1968. Infective bulbar necrosis (heel-abscess) of sheep, a mixed infection with *Fusiformis necrophorus* and *Corynebacterium pyogenes*. *J. Comp. Pathol.* 78:1–8.

Rowland, A. C., and G. H. K. Lawson. 1975. Porcine intestinal adenomatosis: A possible relationship with necrotic enteritis, regional ileitis and proliferative haemorrhagic enteropathy. *Vet. Rec.* 97:178-80.

Runnels, L. J. 1982. Infectious atrophic rhinitis of swine. *Vet. Clin. N. Am.* 4:301-19.

Runyon, E. H. 1970. Identification of mycobacterial pathogens utilizing colony characterisitics. *Am. J. Clin. Pathol.* 54:578-86.

Rutter, J. M. 1975. *Escherichia coli* infections in piglets: Pathogenesis, virulence and vaccination. *Vet. Rec.* 96:171-75.

Scanlan, C. M., and T. L. Hathcock. 1983. Bovine rumenitis-liver abscess complex: A bacteriological review. *Cornell Vet.* 73:288-97.

------. 1983. Bovine campylobacteriosis. *Auburn Vet.* 39:18-23.

Scanlan, C. M., P. D. Garrett, and F. F. Campbell. 1985. Ovine contagious foot rot. *Comp. Contin. Educ. Pract. Vet.* 7:S15-S20.

Scanlan, C. M., P. D. Garrett, and D. B. Geiger. 1984. *Dermatophilus congolensis* infections of cattle and sheep. *Comp. Contin. Educ. Pract. Vet.* 6:S4-S14.

Scanlan, C. M., D. A. Stringfellow, S. S. Hannon, and P. A. Galik. 1983. Laboratory diagnosis of bovine brucellosis. *Auburn Vet.* 39:6-11.

Shaw, W. B. 1971. *Escherichia coli* in newborn lambs. *Br. Vet. J.* 127:214-19.

Shewen, P. E. 1980. Chlamydial infection in animals: A review. *Can. Vet. J.* 21:2-11.

Shope, R. E. 1931. Swine influenza. III. Filtration experiments and etiology. *J. Exp. Med.* 54:373-85.

Smith, H., and H. B. Stoner. 1967. Anthrax toxic complex. *Fed. Proc.* 26:1554-57.

Smith, H. W., and S. Halls. 1968. The experimental infection of calves with bacteremia-producing strains of *Escherichia coli:* The influence of colostrum. *J. Med. Microbiol.* 1:61-78.

Smith, L. D. S., ed. 1975. *The Pathogenic Anaerobic Bacteria.* 2d ed. Springfield: C. C. Thomas.

Sneath, P. H. A., ed. 1984. *Bergey's Manual of Systematic Bacteriology.* Vol. 2. Baltimore: Williams and Wilkins.

Snow, G. A. 1970. Mycobactins: Iron-chelating growth factors from mycobacteria. *Bacteriol. Rev.* 34:99-125.

Splitter, E. J., and R. L. Williamson. 1950. Eperythrozoonosis in swine: A preliminary report. *J. Am. Vet. Med. Assoc.* 116:360-64.

Steel, K. J. 1961. The oxidase reaction as a taxonomic tool. *J. Gen. Microbiol.* 25:297-306.

Sussman, M., ed. 1985. *The Virulence of Escherichia coli: Reviews and Methods.* London: Academic Press.

Thayer, J. D. and J. E. Martin, Jr. 1966. Improved medium selective for cultivation of *N. gonorrhoeae* and *N. meningitidis. Publ. Health Rep.* 81:559-62.

Thomlinson, J. R. 1963. II. Observations on the pathogenesis of gastroenteritis associated with *Escherichia coli. Vet. Rec.* 75:1246-50.

Timoney, J. F. 1976. Erysipelas arthritis in swine: Concentrations of complement and third component of complement in synovia. *Am. J. Vet. Res.* 37:5-8.

Timoney, J. F., H. C. Niebert, and F. W. Scott. 1978. Feline salmonellosis: A nosocomial outbreak and experimental studies. *Cornell Vet.* 68:211-19.

Tizard, I. R., ed. 1987. *An Introduction to Veterinary Immunology.* 3d ed. Philadelphia: W. B. Saunders.

Wilkens, T. D., and T. Thiel. 1973. Modified broth-disk method for testing the antibiotic susceptibility of anaerobic bacteria. *Antimicrob. Agents Chemother.* 3:350-56.

Wilkinson, G. T. 1980. Mycoplasms of the cat. *Vet. Annu.* 20:145-50.

Wilkinson, P. C. 1976. Recognition and response in mononuclear and granular phagocytes: A review. *Clin. Exp. Immun.* 25:355-66.

Winter, A. J. 1979. Mechanisms of immunity in bacterial infections. *Adv. Vet. Sci. Comp. Med.* 23:53-69.

Woolcock, J. B. 1973. Resistance to microbial infection: Vaccines in theory and practice. *Aust. Vet. J.* 49:307-17.

Young, M. F., K. L. Kuttler, and L. G. Adams. 1977. Experimentally induced anaplasmosis in neonatal isohemolytic anemia-recovered calves. *Am. J. Vet. Res.* 38:1745-47.

Index of Scientific Names of Bacteria

Page numbers in italics indicate a chart, figure, or table.

Index of Bacterial Diseases of Domestic Animals and Man

Page numbers in italics indicate a chart or table.

FELINE DISEASES

HUMAN DISEASES

OVINE DISEASES

PORCINE DISEASES